Sulfation of Drugs
and
Related Compounds

Editor

Gerard J. Mulder, Ph.D.

Associate Professor
Department of Pharmacology
University of Groningen
The Netherlands

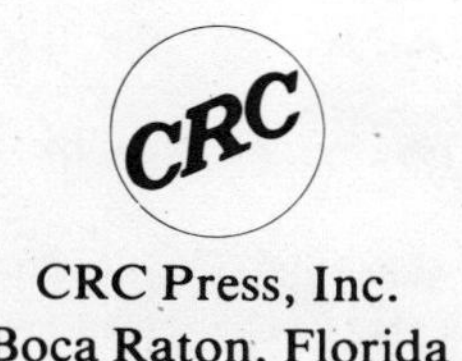

CRC Press, Inc.
Boca Raton, Florida

Library of Congress Cataloging in Publication Data

Main entry under title:

Sulfation of drugs and related compounds.

Bibliography: p.
Includes index.
1. Drugs--Metabolism. 2. Sulphates--Metabolism.
I. Mulder, Gerard J. [DNLM: Sulfates--Metabolism. 2. Drugs. QV280 S9497]
RM301.55.S9   615´.7   80-21862
ISBN 0-8493-5920-1

Direct all inquiries to CRC Press, Inc., 2000 N.W. 24th Street, Boca Raton, Florida 33431.

© 1981 by CRC Press, Inc.

International Standard Book Number 0-8493-5920-1
Library of Congress Card Number 80-21862
Printed in the United States

THE EDITOR

Gerard J. Mulder, Ph.D., is currently Associate Professor in the Department of Pharmacology of the State University of Groningen, The Netherlands. Dr. Mulder received his Ph.D. in biochemical pharmacology at the State University of Groningen with specialization on properties of UDP-glucuronyltransferase and its role in the elimination of its substrates in bile in the rat.

From 1975 to 1976 Dr. Mulder was a guest worker at the National Heart and Lung Institute of the National Institutes of Health, Bethesda, Maryland. He is a member of the Biochemical Society of London. Dr. Mulder has published numerous articles on glucuronidation and sulfation in vitro and in vivo.

His current research interests include the role of sulfation and glucuronidation in the detoxification and toxification of xenobiotics with special attention to the availability of the various co-substrates for conjugation.

CONTRIBUTORS

A. H. Olavesen, Ph.D.
Senior Lecturer in Biochemistry
Department of Biochemistry
University College
Cardiff, Wales
United Kingdom

G. M. Powell, Ph.D.
Reader in Biochemistry
Department of Biochemistry
University College
Cardiff, Wales
United Kingdom

A. B. Roy, Ph.D., D.Sc.
Senior Fellow
Department of Physical Biochemistry
Australian National University
John Curtin School of Medical Research
Canberra
Australia

TABLE OF CONTENTS

Chapter 1

INTRODUCTION

G. J. Mulder

Sulfate conjugation was discovered around 1875 by Baumann.[1-3] He isolated phenyl sulfate from the urine of a patient who had been treated with phenol; later he and his group demonstrated the presence of several sulfated phenols in urine, and studied some properties of sulfation.[4,5] These sulfate esters constituted the so-called "ethereal sulfate" fraction; they were considered to be "ethers" of the organic aryl group and the $-SO_3$ group: $Ar-O-SO_3H$. In fact, these compounds are half-esters of sulfuric acid and name "ethereal sulfate" is only used these days for historical reasons.

The chemical mechanism of the sulfate conjugation remained obscure at that time; it was believed that inorganic sulfate reacted directly with the substrate by enzymatic catalysis. However, between 1944 and 1956 the role of adenosine 3'-phosphate 5'-sulfatophosphate (PAPS), the cosubstrate of sulfation, was discovered by Lipmann's group and others. Only when the chemical structure of this cosubstrate had been elucidated, a clear picture of the mechanism of sulfation emerged.

In the meantime, R.T. Williams had started his work on the metabolism in vivo of foreign compounds (xenobiotics), of which many were excreted in bile or urine as sulfate conjugates, often after phase I metabolism (oxidation, reduction, or hydrolysis). The fate of numerous compounds in vivo was investigated by his group. Also, the mechanisms of their excretion in bile and urine were studied; in general, sulfate conjugates were more rapidly eliminated than the parent compounds, and usually were much less pharmacologically active. However, this was not always the case; several aromatic amines, for instance, become extremely reactive and potentially toxic upon sulfation.

Sulfate activation and conjugation received relatively little further interest once the main characteristics of PAPS synthesis and its role in sulfate transfer had been discovered. Probably this was due to the idea current at that time, that sulfation was a purely detoxifying reaction. Moreover, for sulfation of endogenous compounds, an ample supply of sulfate seemed to be available and, in the case of high doses of xenobiotics, usually glucuronidation with its much higher capacity could easily take over when sulfation capacity was insufficient, or inorganic sulfate depleted. The purification to homogeneity of the sulfotransferases had to wait until the late 1970s. This lack in interest in sulfation is further illustrated by the surprising fact that the second report on purification of APS kinase, one of the enzymes of sulfate activation, appeared only in 1973, 15 years after the first report in 1958; since then little has been reported on this enzyme. ATP-sulfurylase, the enzyme that catalyzes the first step of sulfate activation, has been extensively characterized, mainly, it seems, because its product APS is important in many bacterial strains as an electron acceptor. The second activation step is usually not necessary, since sulfate reduction in most of these microorganisms seems to require APS rather than PAPS.

The overall process of sulfation is shown in Figure 1. The supply of inorganic sulfate required for sulfation of both endogenous acceptor groups and xenobiotics comes mainly from the food under normal, nonfasting conditions; both absorption of inorganic sulfate and sulfoxidation of cysteine deliver inorganic sulfate to cells and tissues (Chapter 3). Under fasting conditions, inorganic sulfate can be supplied by catabolism of proteins and other macromolecules, especially the highly sulfated glycosaminoglycans.

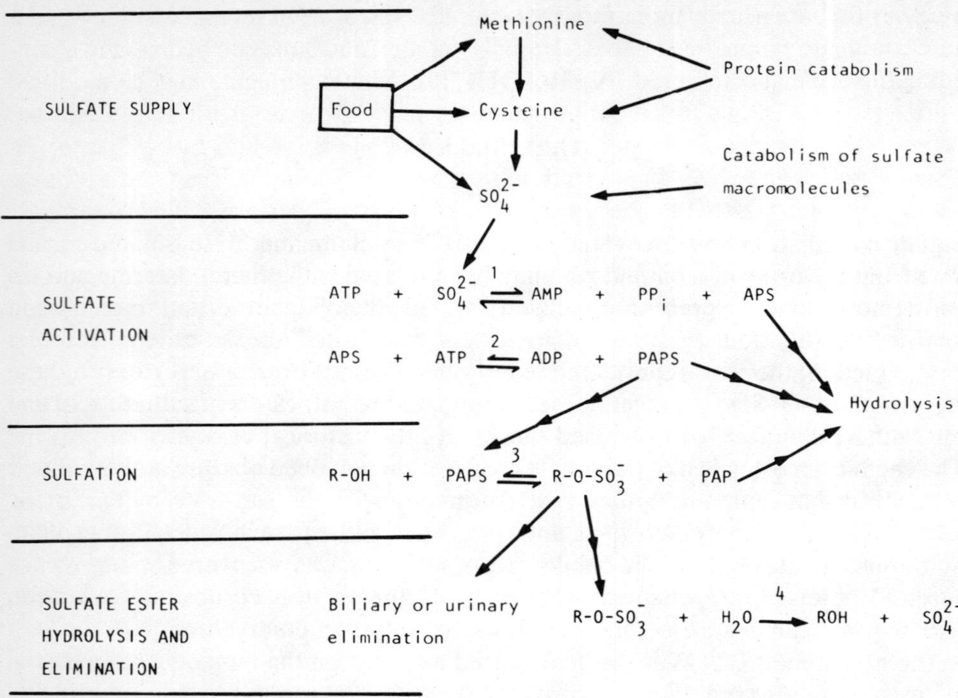

FIGURE 1. Sulfate metabolism and sulfation: 1. ATP-sulfurylase; 2. APS kinase; 3. Sulfotransferases; 4. Sulfatases.

Activation of inorganic sulfate to the group-donating cosubstrate, PAPS, takes place in a two-step reaction, catalyzed by ATP-sulfurylase and APS kinase. In higher animals PAPS seems to be used exclusively for sulfation, but in many microorganisms both APS and PAPS are electron acceptors; PAPS is required for the synthesis of cysteine. In most, if not all tissues of mammals, the sulfate activating system seems to be present (Chapter 4).

Sulfation of drugs and endogenous compounds occurs in most, probably all, animals and plants. A group of sulfotransferases catalyzes this transfer to various substrates; the specificity of these enzymes is derived from endogenous substrates, or xenobiotics from the natural environment. Purification and characterization of these sulfotransferases, as far as they use low-molecular weight substrates, is discussed in Chapter 5.

Under physiological conditions both sulfate activation and sulfate transfer take place in the same cell. When sulfation of a compound is studied in vivo therefore, the outcome is the result of complicated interactions in the cell. In order to study the factors that affect sulfation rate in vivo, in recent years isolated perfused organs and especially isolated cell preparations (mainly hepatocytes) have been used to elucidate the factors that determine the overall sulfation process in vivo. Availability of sulfate, substrate specificity and kinetics of the transferases, competition between glucuronidation and sulfation for the same substrate, and pharmacokinetic factors clearly all play a role. Selective inhibition of sulfation is an important tool to study the role of sulfation in detoxification and toxification (Chapter 6).

Once the sulfate conjugates are synthesized, they will be exposed to all the mechanisms that the body possesses to eliminate them. One of the main reasons why they are sulfated in the first place is that they could not be eliminated rapidly enough from the body. Thereby, sulfation gets a chance to convert them to the sulfate conjugates that are usually more rapidly excreted. However, in several cases, even the sulfate conjugate cannot be eliminated rapidly enough, and it may be hydrolyzed again, yielding the original compound. Alternatively, the sulfate conjugate may be modified by other enzymes (e.g., by oxidation and reduction) as occurs with several steroid sulfates. Final elimination from the body takes place in urine and bile (Chapter 7).

Usually, sulfation means detoxification; however, steroid sulfates may be a storage form for some steroids that can be kept as a "silent reserve," or be modified specifically (Chapters 6 and 7). In some cases the sulfate conjugates are very unstable, chemically extremely reactive compounds that may be involved as ultimate carcinogens in carcinogenesis of the parent compound (Chapter 8). Whether sulfate conjugation means detoxification or toxification therefore depends on the substrate used.

In this book the sulfation of macromolecules will not be covered because with these substrates very different factors play a role (e.g., the macromolecular nature of the substrate), and different physiological processes are involved. For similar reasons the sulfation of lipids is not covered. In the various chapters, references will be given where possible, to recent reviews on these subjects.

The only previous book about sulfation, by Roy and Trudinger,[6] appeared in 1970, and dealt with all aspects of sulfation. This book gives an excellent review of the literature up until 1969; since then many new data have become available. A more complete survey of all types of sulfur-containing biological compounds is given in a recent volume in the series *Metabolic Pathways*.[7] A recent Ciba symposium covers the same, wide field.[8] With the increasing interest in sulfation in respect to toxification and detoxification of xenobiotics in mind, we have concentrated on the aspects that are most intimately connected with drug metabolism.

REFERENCES

1. **Baumann, E.,** Ueber gepaarte Schwefelsäuren im Harn, *Arch. Gesammte Physiol.*, 12, 69, 1876.
2. **Baumann, E.,** Ueber Sulfosäuren im Harn, *Ber. Dtsch. Chem. Ges.*, 9, 54, 1876.
3. **Baumann, E.,** Ueber gepaarte Schwefelsäuren im Organismus, *Arch. Gesammte Physiol.*, 13, 285, 1876.
4. **Baumann, E.,** Ueber die Synthese von Aether-Schwefelsäuren ünd des Verhaltens einiger aromatischer Substanzen im Thierkörper, *Z. Physiol. Chem.*, 1, 244, 1877.
5. **Christiani, A. and Baumann, E.,** Ueber den Ort der Bildung des Phenolschwefelsäure im Thierkörper, *Z. Physiol. Chem.*, 2, 350, 1878.
6. **Roy, A. B. and Trudinger, P. A.,** *The Biochemistry of Inorganic Compounds of Sulphur,* Cambridge University Press, Cambridge, 1970.
7. **Grennberg, D. M.,** *Metabolic Pathways,* Vol. 7, *Metabolism of Sulfur Compounds,* 3rd ed., Academic Press, New York, 1975.
8. *Sulphur in Biology*, Ciba Foundation Symposia 72, Excerpta Medica, Amsterdam, 1980.

Chapter 2

THE CHEMISTRY OF SULFATE ESTERS AND RELATED COMPOUNDS

A. B. Roy

TABLE OF CONTENTS

I. INTRODUCTION

In biochemistry, the name sulfate ester is given to a mono ester of sulfuric acid and a hydroxyl-containing compound which is usually prepared as an alkali metal salt, $R.OSO_3^- M^+$. In solution these are fully ionized so that the nature of the cation may not be important, but this is by no means always the case, either in biochemical or chemical reactions, and instead of simply writing, for example, phenyl sulfate, one should write potassium phenyl sulfate, barium phenyl sulfate, etc., as the case may be. In a more chemical context this avoids confusion with the corresponding diesters, which do not occur naturally. For example, diphenyl sulfate, $C_6H_5.OSO_2O.C_6H_5$, may also incorrectly be called phenyl sulfate. In what follows, terms such as phenyl sulfate will be used to mean the mono ester, and the associated cation will only be mentioned where it is important or where confusion could occur.

Chemical Abstracts indexes these compounds in two ways: the esters of simple compounds are listed under "Sulfuric acid, esters: mono X ester Y salt" while those of more complex alcohols or phenols are listed under the parent compounds.

Some other types of compounds are fairly closely related to the sulfate esters; these are the thiosulfate esters or Bunte salts, $R.SSO_3^- M^+$; the sulfamates, $R.NHSO_3^- M^+$; and the sulfatophosphates which contain the grouping $-O.PO (OH).OSO_3^-$. All of these, like the sulfate esters themselves, yield SO_4^{2-} with varying ease on acid hydrolysis. The first two groups of compounds are presently listed in *Chemical Abstracts* under the headings thiosulfuric acid, mono X ester Y salt, and sulfamic acid, mono X ester Y salt, respectively. The biologically important sulfatophosphates are listed under the parent nucleotide, for example, adenylic acid, monoanhydride with sulfuric acid.

Representatives of all the above types of compounds are found in biological systems as can be seen from Table 1 which lists those substances whose chemistry will be considered in this chapter. Further details of their chemistry can be found in the appropriate chapters of References 1 to 4.

II. SULFATE ESTERS

As has already been pointed out, these are the mono esters of sulfuric acid and a hydroxyl-containing compound which may be aliphatic, alicyclic, aromatic, or heterocyclic and which may be a *C*-hydroxy or an *N*-hydroxy compound. Obviously, the properties of these esters will depend very much upon the structure of the organic part of the molecule, and here it will be possible to give no more than general indications of their chemistry.

A. Synthesis of Sulfate Esters

There are two general methods which have been used for the preparation of many different sulfate esters and a host of minor methods which have been used less frequently, often only for the preparation of specific compounds. Many of the methods can be adapted for the preparation of $[^{35}S]$-sulfate esters but, because of the commercial availability of the reagents, those using $H_2^{35}SO_4$ or $[^{35}S]$-chlorosulfonic acid are most convenient.

1. With Adducts of Sulfur Trioxide

This is the first of the general methods and uses the sulfur trioxide adduct of a Lewis base as the sulfate donor. The most common of these adducts are pyridine-sulfur trioxide and *N,N*-dimethylaniline-sulfur trioxide, but those of triethylamine, dimethylformamide and dioxan, to name only a few, have been quite widely used. In general

Table 1

TYPES OF SULFATE ESTER AND RELATED COMPOUNDS FOUND IN BIOCHEMICAL SYSTEMS

Characteristic group	Type of compound	Naturally occurring examples	Examples formed in vivo from a xenobiotic
$>$C.OSO$_3^-$	Alkyl sulfates	Propan-2-yl sulfate	Dimetridazole $\rightarrow$ Hydroxydimetridazole sulfate
	Aryl sulfates[a]	Indoxyl sulfate	Salicylamide $\rightarrow$ Salicylamide sulfate
	Steroid sulfates		
	Phenols	Oestrone sulfate	Most steroids must be assumed to form
	Primary alcohols	Cortisol 21-sulfate	sulfate esters in vivo.
	Secondary alcohols	Cholesteryl sulfate	
	Carbohydrate sulfates[b]		
	Primary alcohols	Galactosamine 6-sulfate	No example known
	Secondary alcohols	Galactose 3-sulfate	
$>$N.OSO$_3^-$	Hydroxamic acid sulfates	Sinigrin[c]	*N*-Acetyl-2-aminofluorene $\rightarrow$ *N*-Acetyl-*N*-hydroxy-2-aminofluorene sulfate
$>$C.SSO$_3^-$	Thiosulfates	*S*-Sulfocysteine	No example known
$>$C.NH.SO$_3^-$	Sulfamates	2-Sulfoamino-2-deoxyglucose[d]	2-Naphthylamine $\rightarrow$ 2-Naphthyl sulfamate
$-$O.PO(OH).OSO$_3^-$	Sulfatophosphates	Adenosine 5'-sulfatophosphate	No example known

[a] Tyrosine *O*-sulfate occurs in some peptides such as fibrinopeptide B and caerulein.

[b] In animals, carbohydrate sulfates usually occur in more complex molecules such as glycosaminoglycans, sulfolipids, and glycosides (e.g., holuthurin A).

[c] Sinigrin and related mustard oil glycosides are of widespread occurrence in plants but no naturally occurring hydroxamic acid sulfate has yet been found in animals.

[d] In animals, occurs only in glycosaminoglycans.

terms, the reactivity of the adduct varies inversely with the strength of the base so that it is possible to moderate the fundamental reaction, that of the hydroxyl group with SO$_3$, to any desired extent by the choice of a suitable reagent, from the very reactive dimethylformamide-sulfur trioxide, through pyridine-sulfur trioxide, to the rather stable triethylamine-sulfur trioxide. However, as pointed out by Gilbert,[5] base strength is not the only factor which governs the reactivity of the adduct. Two variants of this general method are available, and both require strictly anhydrous conditions.

In the first, the adduct is formed by the reaction at 0°C, or less, of chlorosulfonic acid with the base in an inert solvent such as CHCl$_3$ or CS$_2$ after which the acceptor is added to the reaction mixture and the temperature allowed to rise. This method is simple, but the products may be contaminated with Cl$^-$ which can be difficult to remove. Details can be found in the classical work of Burkhardt and Lapworth on the synthesis of aryl sulfates[6,7] and in more recent syntheses of the sulfates of hydroxypyridines.[8]

In the other general variant, the purified sulfur trioxide adduct is isolated and then used in the sulfation reaction. Obviously, in this case there is no possibility of contamination of the product with Cl$^-$ and that with SO$_4^{2-}$ is also generally less. The adducts are easily prepared[5] by the reaction of the base in an inert solvent, such as CHCl$_3$, with SO$_3$ or with chlorosulfonic acid; the latter method has the disadvantage that the hydrochloride of the base is produced in equivalent amounts, and although the major part of this can easily be removed, the traces which remain can sometimes cause problems (see Section IIA6). Some sulfur trioxide adducts are commercially available. Examples of this type of sulfation are to be found in the synthesis of many types of steroid sulfate using triethylamine-sulfur trioxide,[9] and of carbohydrate sulfates[10] or the rather unstable sulfates of *N*-acetyl-*N*-hydroxyarylamines using pyridine-sulfur trioxide.[11,12]

2. With H_2SO_4 and a Carbodiimide

This is the second of the general methods, and although it has not been as widely used, it is potentially valuable. It uses H_2SO_4 as a sulfating agent in the presence of dicyclohexylcarbodiimide as a condensing agent. Synthesis of alkyl sulfates,[13] aryl sulfates,[13] carbohydrate sulfates,[14] steroid sulfates,[15] and oxime *O*-sulfates[13] have been described. More complex products such as pyrosulfate diesters are sometimes produced by this method.[13]

3. Miscellaneous Methods

Many other methods of preparing sulfate esters are available. Direct sulfation with H_2SO_4 was classically used for the synthesis of simple alkyl sulfates,[1,2,16] but it is also useful for the preparation of the sulfate esters of amino compounds, for example, choline *O*-sulfate,[17] serine-*O*-sulfate,[18] tyrosine *O*-sulfate,[19] dopamine 3- and 4-*O*-sulfates,[20] and serotonin *O*-sulfate.[21] Chlorosulfonic acid has been used directly for the formation of hydroxylamine *O*-sulfate,[22] sulfamic acid for the synthesis of steroid sulfates[23] (see also Section IVD) and pyridinium sulfate plus acetic anhydride for the preparation of estrone sulfate.[24] The latter reaction has also been used in this laboratory for the preparation of a number of simple aryl sulfates. A sulfate group can also be transferred from a sulfate ester to an acceptor; steroid sulfates have been prepared by the oxidative transfer of the sulfate group from ascorbate 2-sulfate to the steroid,[25] while the Cu^{2+}-catalyzed transfer of sulfate from quinolinyl 8-sulfate has been used to prepare aryl sulfates and carbohydrate sulfates[26] (see also Section IIB2C).

4. Elb's Persulfate Oxidation

All of the above methods sulfate an existing hydroxyl group. In contrast, the Elb's persulfate oxidation introduces an $-O.SO_3^-$ group directly into an aromatic ring by treatment with peroxydisulfate under alkaline conditions. The oxidation of phenols has been most studied, and the reaction almost certainly involves an electrophilic attack of the phenoxide ion on the peroxide bond in the peroxydisulfate ion although earlier work suggested that the sulfate ion radical was the reactive species.[2] The method has been used for the synthesis of nitrocatechol[27] and nitroquinol[28] sulfates from 4- and 3-nitrophenol, respectively. Amines can also be oxidized, and methods have been described for the synthesis of several *o*-aminophenyl sulfates[29] as well as indoxyl sulfate.[30]

5. Indirect Methods

Some sulfate esters are best prepared by indirect methods, for example, the ketoxime *O*-sulfates by the reaction of hydroxylamine *O*-sulfate with the appropriate ketone.[31] Aminophenyl, aminocatechol, and aminoquinol sulfates are prepared by the reduction of the corresponding nitroaryl sulfates either by Fe^{2+} or by H_2/Pt.[7,32,33] More complex sulfate esters are obtained by reduction of nitroaryl sulfates in alkaline solution,[7] as is shown below for 2-nitrophenyl sulfate. This gives a mixture of azobenzene 2, 2′-disulfate and hydrazobenzene 2,2′-disulfate, and the latter can be rearranged in acid to give 4,4′-diaminodiphenyl 3,3′-disulfate.

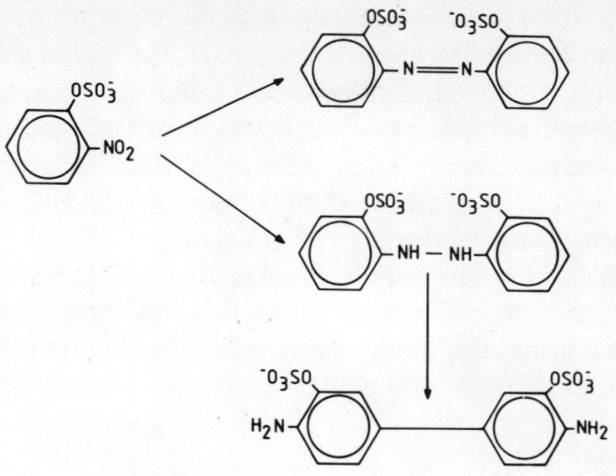

Reduction of nitroaryl sulfates with Zn gives a hydroxylamine, and this fact has recently been used[34] to prepare *N*-acetyl-*N*-hydroxy-4-aminophenyl sulfate by reduction of 4-nitrophenyl sulfate to the corresponding hydroxylamine which is then acetylated, as shown below.

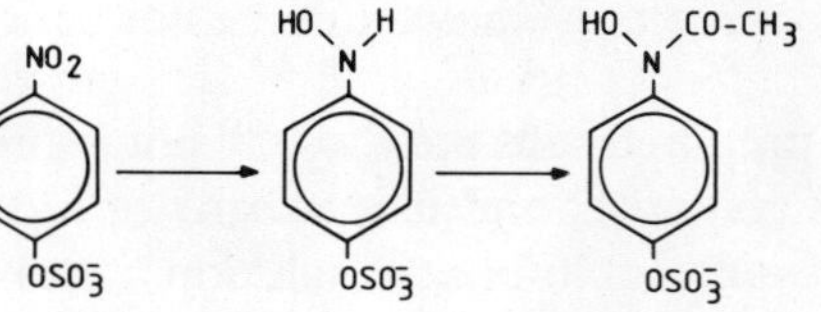

6. *Some Difficulties*

The synthesis of sulfate esters is generally straightforward, and the products usually have the expected structures, but difficulties can arise when the parent alcohol is optically active because racemization may occur. Burwell[35,36] was the first to show that the extent of the racemization varied with the method of sulfation: sulfation of butan-2-ol with pyridine-sulfur trioxide, dioxan-sulfur trioxide, or sulfamic acid gave essentially complete retention of configuration, whereas sulfation with H_2SO_4 or chlorosulfonic acid gave extensive racemization, probably because of the existence of a complex equilibrium mixture containing butene. More recently, Matcham and Dogson[37] have confirmed these findings using a number of secondary alcohols, and they have further shown that the nature of the product obtained after sulfation with pyridine-sulfur trioxide depended upon how that reagent had been prepared. When prepared from pyridine and sulfur trioxide, the reagent gave complete retention of configuration, but when prepared from pyridine and chlorosulfonic acid,[3] racemization occurred. It was suggested that the difference in behavior was caused by the traces of pyridinium chloride which the latter reagent contained.[37] So far no similar phenomenon has been noted during the sulfation of steroids or carbohydrates. Matcham and Dodgson[37] have also shown that during the sulfation of scondary alcohols with H_2SO_4, migration of the hydroxyl group may occur, again probably because of the existence of an unsaturated intermediate.

The sulfation of polyhydroxy compounds can also pose problems which reach their peak in the synthesis of authentic monosaccharide sulfates. These can only be obtained[38] by the sulfation of suitably protected derivatives. Even with simple dihydric alcohols or phenols, difficulties can arise, and simply restricting the amount of sulfating agent to one molar proportion does not necessarily ensure the formation of a monosulfate although some degree of selective sulfation may be possible by suitable choice of conditions[9,13] when the hydroxyl groups are of different types. On the other hand, despite these warnings, 2-hydroxy-5-nitrophenyl sulfate (nitrocatechol sulfate) and 4-chloro-2-hydroxyphenyl sulfate have been prepared by the direct sulfation of 4-nitrocatechol[39] and 4-chlorocatechol,[40] respectively. It is striking that in the synthesis of these two compounds the *para*-directing effect of the chlorine atom and the *meta*-directing effect of the nitro group are effective.

Finally, a point which should be kept in mind is the possible fortuitous formation of sulfate esters during other procedures, as exemplified by the formation of serine and threonine *O*-sulfates during the extensive drying of acid hydrolystates of histone sulfates[41] which must contain sulfuric acid.

B. Properties of Sulfate Esters

Sulfate esters are normally obtained as salts, internal salts in suitable cases.[8,26] The corresponding free acids, the X hydrogen sulfates, are generally unstable and cannot be isolated although alkyl hydrogen sulfates, including at least some carbohydrate sulfates, can be obtained in solution, most simply by passage of a solution of the salt through the H^+ form of a strong cation exchange resin. The free acids are strong acids, but their strengths have not been determined, although it was long ago suggested[42] that they were stronger than H_2SO_4 because they showed no buffer action in 0.25 M HCl, whereas K_2SO_4 did.

The most commonly prepared salts are those of potassium, but those of other metals are easily obtainable if required, and it is worthy of note that the barium salts are generally (but not always) soluble in acid solution, so providing a useful distinction between $R.OSO_3^-$ and SO_4^{2-}. Again in general, the alkali metal salts of sulfate esters are soluble only in polar solvents—water, lower alcohols, dimethylformamide, etc. A useful solvent is butan-l-ol because it can be used to extract many sulfate esters, especially aryl sulfates and steroid sulfates, from aqueous solution.

The salts of organic bases, unlike the alkali metal salts, frequently have sharp melting points and some are soluble in nonpolar solvents. The methylene blue salts of many sulfate esters are soluble in $CHCl_3$ and this is the basis of a quantitative method for their determination[3] and for their detection on paper[43] and thin-layer[44] chromatograms (see also Section VI). The pyridinium salts of several steroid sulfates are also soluble in $CHCl_3$.[45] Other commonly used bases are 4-toluidine,[46] the aminoacridines,[40] and, especially for carbohydrate sulfates, brucine.[38] This solubility in nonpolar solvents of the salts of sulfate esters with organic bases should be kept in mind when isolating sulfate esters from natural sources because ion pairs, soluble in say $CHCl_3$, may be formed with naturally occurring cations. For example, dehydroepiandrosterone sulfate, and so presumably other steroid sulfates, form complexes with cationic detergents and with phosphatides which are soluble in $CHCl_3$; obviously this phenomenon could, if unsuspected, cause a loss of sulfate ester.[47] It is of interest that the converse situation may also be important because there are indications of an interaction in vivo between the sulfolipid, cerebroside sulfate (containing galactose 3-sulfate residues) and biogenic amines.[48]

Because sulfate esters are generally prepared as the barium, potassium, or sodium salts, there is almost no information on any influence the cation might have on the behavior of the ester. This influence may not be negligible, as was shown by the early studies of Sobel et al. They showed[49] that while the calcium and ferrous salts of cholesteryl sulfate required heating at 80 to 110°C to form dicholesteryl ether, the aluminium salt slowly underwent the same reaction at room temperature.

There has been no tabulation of the properties of sulfate esters in general but a useful summary of the physical characteristics of steroid sulfates is available.[50]

1. Spectral Properties

The spectral properties of sulfate esters mainly reflect the structure of the organic part of the molecule. The visible and ultraviolet spectra usually show little of interest although they can be valuable for the identification and determination of specific esters. Almost the only generalization which can be made is that aryl sulfates show a decreased λ_{max} and a slightly decreased ϵ_{max} when compared with the parent phenol.[8,51] These differences are particularly obvious in alkaline solution, and the striking difference between, say, the yellow 4-nitrophenolate ion and the colorless 4-nitrophenyl sulfate has many analytical applications.

Measurements of specific rotation have been useful in characterizing carbohydrate sulfates[38] and secondary alkyl sulfates.[52] With the latter there are surprisingly large solvent effects: changing the solvent from water to 80% ethanol changed the sign of the rotation, a phenomenon which, until recognized, caused some confusion.

Infrared spectra can be informative because of the absorptions due to the sulfate group itself, principally those assigned to S–O bond stretching in the 1210- to 1250-cm^{-1} region and to C–O–S vibrations in the 800- to 850-cm^{-1} region. Both alkyl[53] and aryl[8,54] sulfates have been examined, and a considerable amount of interest has been shown in the carbohydrate sulfates because it was at one time considered[55] that the position of the absorption in the 1240-cm^{-1} region could be used to differentiate between the sulfate esters of primary, secondary axial, and secondary equatorial hydroxyl groups. This is not the case, and it is now obvious that any aglycone or substituent on the sugar may profoundly influence the position of the C–O–S absorption.[56]

Nuclear magnetic resonance spectra are again of interest primarily with regard to the structure of the organic part of the molecule, and particularly with the localization of the sulfate group in polyhydroxy compounds. The sulfate esters of polyhydroxy phenols[54] and of glycosides[56] have been examined by PMR, but much more useful information is available from ^{13}C–NMR spectra. In polyhydroxy phenols,[54] sulfation causes a downfield shift, with respect to tetramethylsilane, of 2.8 to 5.8 ppm in the signal from the carbon atom carrying the sulfate group and larger upfield shifts of 5.4 to 7.8 ppm in the signals from the carbon atoms *ortho* and *para* to this. In monosaccharide sulfates,[56-59] sulfation is accompanied by a marked downfield shift of between 6.2 and 9.5 ppm in the signal from the carbon atom carrying the sulfate group compared with up-field shifts of 1.1 to 2.5 ppm in the signals from the adjacent carbon atoms. Some data are given in Table 2, which also shows that it is possible to distinguish between the α and β anomers of the carbohydrate sulfates. It seems safe to say that in the future, ^{13}C–NMR will be the method of choice for the characterization of the sulfate esters of polyhydroxy compounds.

Mass spectrometry has been little used in studies of sulfate esters because of the involatility of the usual salts, but reports have appeared of the application of field desorption mass spectrometry to the alkali metal salts of some alkyl and steroid sulfates[37,60] and of electron impact mass spectrometry of aryl sulfates after their conversion to the corresponding alkylaryl diesters.[61] Usov et al[62] have used mass spectrometry to locate the substituent in a series of amidosulfates of D-galactose, and this suggests that a similar technique might be a useful adjunct to the ^{13}C–NMR methods described above for the characterization of monosaccharide sulfates. Some further information is to be found in Section IIB4.

2. Hydrolysis

Sulfate esters are hydrolyzed in acid, neutral, and alkaline solutions, but the rates of

Table 2
^{13}C-NMR CHARACTERISTICS OF MONOSACCHARIDE SULFATES: DOWN-FIELD SHIFTS (PPM) OF THE CARBON ATOMS OR CARRYING SULFATE GROUPS

Parent sugar

Position of sulfation	Xylose		Galactose		Glucose		Mannose		Methyl 3-*O*-methyl manno-pyrano-side		*N*-Acetyl-glucos-amine	
	α	β	α	β	α	β	α	β	α	β	α	β
2	5.2[a]	6.7[a]	7.3[b]	8.1[b]	—	—	7.1[a]	—	7.0[d]	—	—	—
3	—	—	8.4[b]	7.5[b]	9.3[b],9.5[c]	8.4[b],8.5[c]	—	—	—	—	—	—
4	—	—	8.2[b,e]	7.8[b,e]	—	—	—	—	8.2[d]	—	—	—
6	—	—	6.3[b]	6.2[b]	6.4[b],6.5[c]	6.2[b],6.6[c]	—	—	6.3[d]	—	6.4[b]	6.2[b]

[a] Turvey (personal communication).
[b] Reference 59.
[c] Reference 57.
[d] Reference 58.
[e] Tentative assignments.

these reactions are highly dependent upon the conditions and upon the structure of the ester. Different types of carbohydrate sulfate, for example, show different rates of acid hydrolysis.[63] In general, the acid hydrolysis of aryl sulfates is more rapid than that of alkyl sulfates, but exactly comparable data are difficult to find; it seems, however, that phenyl sulfate is hydrolyzed in acid some 100 times faster than is methyl sulfate. On the other hand, tertiary alkyl sulfates have been reported to be particularly labile.[64] Also in general, acid hydrolysis is more rapid than alkaline hydrolysis which is more rapid than neutral hydrolysis; values of the apparent first-order velocity constants, k_o, for the hydrolysis of 2-nitrophenyl sulfate at pH 1, 7, and 14 are 1.3×10^{-3}, 0.009×10^{-3} and 0.068×10^{-3} sec^{-1}, respectively, at 100°C.[65]

a. In Acid

Acid hydrolysis is an A-1 reaction[66,67] — that is, a first order reaction in which the reactive species is the protonated form of the reactant — with fission of the O–S bond and, with optically active secondary alkyl sulfates, no inversion of configuration. As shown many years ago by Burkhardt et al.,[42] the rate of acid hydrolysis of aryl sulfates is increased by the presence of electron-withdrawing substituents in the aromatic ring, there being a linear relationship between log k and the pK of the phenolic hydroxyl group. The hydroxypyridine sulfates do not seem to show this effect.[8] The proposed mechanism of the hydrolysis is shown below where the rate-liming step is the fission of the S–O bond.

$$R\text{-}O\text{-}SO_3^- \overset{H^+}{\rightleftharpoons} R\text{-}O\text{-}SO_3^- \rightleftharpoons \left[R\text{-}O\cdots SO_3 \right] \rightleftharpoons R\text{-}OH + SO_3$$

$$SO_3 + H_2O \longrightarrow H_2SO_4$$

This is consistent[67] with the observations that the rate of hydrolysis of an aryl sulfate, $R.OSO_3^-$, is related to the acid strength of the phenol, R.OH, and that aryl sulfates are more rapidly hydrolyzed than are alkyl sulfates. The latter follows from the possibility of the transition state being stabilized by interactions with the aromatic ring, interactions which are obviously not possible in the alkyl sulfates. A similar mechanism, involving protonation of the phenolic oxygen atom, is believed to occur in the intramolecular catalysis which occurs in the hydrolysis of 2-carboxyphenyl sulfate (salicyl sulfate)[68] and of 2-(4(5)-imidazolyl)-phenyl sulfate,[69] although the possible occurrence of more complex pathways has not been excluded.

Despite the generally accepted view that the acid hydrolysis of a sulfate ester gives the parent hydroxy compound, it should be noted that this is not always the case, as has been well documented for the hydrolysis of steroid sulfates. For example, it has long been known that the hydrolysis of dehydroepiandrosterone sulfate (3β-sulfooxyandrost-5-en-17-one) in hot HCl gives not only dehydroepiandrosterone (3β-hydroxyandrost-5-en-17-one) but also 3β-chlorandrost-5-en-17-one[70] and androst-3,5-dien-17-one.[71]

Both of these are derived from the cyclosteroid ion which gives, in neutral solution, *i*-androstanolone (see Section IIB2c). More recent studies[72] have shown that the hydrolysis of androsterone sulfate (3α-sulfooxy-5α-androstan-17-one) in boiling 1 *M* HCl gives a complex mixture of products including androsterone (3α-hydroxy-5α-androstan-17-one, 18%), 5α-androst-2-en-17-one (58%), 5α-androst-3-en-17-one (15%), 3β-hydroxy-5α-androstan-17-one (4%), 2α-hydroxy-5α-androstan-17-one (1%), and 2β-hydroxy-5α-androstan-17-one (1%). An even more drastic change occurs during the acid hydrolysis of 20-sulfooxy-5α-pregnan-3β-ol: this is accompanied by enlargement of the D ring to give 17α-methyl-D-homo-5α-androstane-3β,17aβ-diol (uranediol).[73] Obviously, all these reactions must involve fission of the C–O bond, despite their being carried out in acid. Further examples can be found in Reference 74.

b. In Alkali

Alkaline hydrolysis is generally slower and is also more complex because both C–O and S–O fission occur;[75] at pH values greater than about 12, the rate is directly proportional to the concentration of the hydroxyl ion.[76] With simple alkyl sulfates, alkaline hydrolysis seems to be an S_N2 reaction and, in the case of optically active secondary alkyl sulfates, the alcohol of inverted configuration is produced.[77]

Complications may arise because alkaline hydrolysis can be accompanied, or replaced, by elimination of SO_4^{2-}. This is particularly important with sugar sulfates. For example, the 6-sulfates of α- or β-methyl galactopyranoside or glucopyranoside are converted to the corresponding 3,6-anhydroglycosides upon treatment for a few minutes with 0.1 *M* NaOH at 100°C, whereas di-*O*-isopropylidenegalactopyranose 6-sulfate, which does not have a free hydroxyl in the 3 position, is stable to 2 *M* NaOH at 100°C for many hours.[78] A similar elimination of SO_4^{2-} to give the four-membered oxide ring characteristic of the anhydro bile alcohols occurs when a bile alcohol sulfate, such as scymnol 26-sulfate, is treated with alkali.[79]

c. In Neutral Solution

Hydrolysis in neutral solution is much slower and is usually only of importance with the more labile aryl sulfates, such as the nitrophenyl sulfates.[65,76] The fission of the O–S bond is the more important reaction, but kinetically the hydrolysis is complex and seems to be intermediate between an S_N1 and an S_N2 reaction.[76]

A rather different type of neutral hydrolysis occurs with quinolinyl 8-sulfate: this is catalyzed by Cu^{2+} so that at 40°C in 0.1 *M* KCl containing 1 m*M* Cu^{2+} the velocity constant for the hydrolysis is 0.11×10^{-3} sec^{-1} compared with that of 0.07×10^{-3} sec^{-1} for the hydrolysis in 3 M HCl at the same temperature.[26,80] The reaction involves chelation of the Cu^{2+} with the heterocyclic nitrogen atom, and it seems likely that the sulfate esters of other suitable heterocyclic compounds would undergo similar reactions.

Finally, neutral hydrolysis occurs with the 3β-sulfates of Δ^5 steroids such as dehydroepiandrosterone sulfate; in such cases the hydrolysis is accompanied by rearrangement so that the product is not dehydroepiandrosterone but *i*-androstanolone (6β-hydroxy-3,5-cycloandrosten-17-one).[81]

d. Effects of Micelles

The effects of micelles on the hydrolysis of sulfate esters are interesting, particularly in the case of the alkyl sulfates because the higher members themselves form micelles. In a series of alkyl sulfates of increasing chain length the incidence of micelle formation was accompanied by a 10- to 100-fold increase in the rate of acid hydrolysis.[82] Micellization gave a slight decrease in the rate of alkaline hydrolysis while the rate of neutral hydrolysis was scarcely affected.[82] More complicated effects were found in the hydrolysis of 2,4-dinitrophenyl sulfate in the presence of cationic (hexadecyltrimethyl-ammonium bromide), neutral (polyoxyethylenedinonylphenol), and anionic (sodium dodecyl sulfate) micelles.[83] In neutral solution, the cationic and neutral micelles increased the rates of hydrolysis by factors of 3.2 and 2.6, respectively, while in acid solution all three types of micelles increased the rate of hydrolysis. In alkaline solution the anionic micelles had an inhibitory effect. For a more detailed consideration of these kinetic effects, and the associated changes in thermodynamic parameters, the original work[83] must be consulted.

As detergent micelles may be present in biochemical systems used in studies of the metabolism of foreign compounds, their possible effects on the stability of sulfate esters should not be forgotten.

e. Enzyme Models

There has been some recent interest in the development of models for the enzymic hydrolysis of sulfate esters. The first of these studies[84] showed that β-cyclodextrin, containing seven glucose units, increased the rates of hydrolysis of a number of sulfate esters. The effects were small, with a maximum k_2/k_u (ratio of velocity constants of catalyzed and uncatalyzed reactions) of 18.7, and were explained by a binding of the esters to the cyclodextrin. Very much greater effects were obtained[85] with a highly branched polyethyleneimine (mol wt, 60,000) having 10% of its nitrogen atoms alkylated with dodecyl groups and 15% with methyleneimidazole. At a concentration of 34 μg/m*l* (60 μ*M* imidazole), pH 9.2, and a temperature of 20°C, this polymer gave a 10^{12} increase in the rate of hydrolysis of nitrocatechol sulfate.[85] Further, the kinetics of the reaction were consistent with a binding of the ester through the dodecyl groups of the polymer followed by its hydrolysis catalyzed by the imidazole groups. It would appear that such synthetic enzymes, or synzymes, could be very valuable for the mild hydrolysis of sulfate esters from natural sources.

Finally, there have been studies[86] of the fission of 2,4-dinitrophenyl sulfate catalyzed by the macrocyclic oxime, 10-hydroxy-11-hydroxyamino[20]-paracyclophane. At equimolecular concentrations of the oxime and the ester, in 0.1 M NaOH, the ratio of k_2/k_u was approximately 1600. The oxime was therefore a much less effective catalyst than the substituted polyethyleneimine. Again the mechanism appeared[86] to be a hydrophobic binding of the ester to the oxime followed in this case by the transfer of sulfate to give the oxime *O*-sulfate.

3. *Solvolysis*

Sulfate esters hydrolyze or solvolyze very rapidly in mixtures of certain organic solvents and water, the increase in rate over that in water sometimes being quite spectacular. For example, changing the solvent from water to moist dioxan gives an increase of 10^7 in the rate of the acid-catalyzed hydrolysis of methyl sulfate.[87] The increase occurs in neutral as well as in acid solvent-water mixtures, and the reactive intermediate is apparently the same as that in aqueous solution, $R.O^+H.SO_3^-$, and, again, as in water, it is the O–S bond which is split.[87,88] There is a similar difference between the rates of solvolysis of alkyl and aryl sulfates as there is for their hydrolysis, and it has been claimed[89] that solvolysis on thin-layer plates prior to chromatography can be used to distinguish between alkyl and aryl sulfates.

Although detailed kinetic studies have not been made, most practical information comes from the solvolysis of steroid sulfates, either in neutral[45] or acid[88] solution. Early studies,[45] for example, showed that solvolysis in a series of ethers under neutral conditions was facilitated by increasing basicity of the solvent: as the solvolysis was accompanied by the liberation of one equivalent of acid, it could hardly have been occuring under neutral conditions after the first few molecules had reacted. Solvolysis in alcohols, on the other hand, took place with no change in pH.[45] In a detailed study of the solvolysis of steroid sulfates in acid solution—that is, the solvolysis of steroid hydrogen sulfates—it was shown that the increase in rate over that in water was not simply a function of the decrease in the dielectric constant of the medium but that specific solvent effects were also involved.[88] Ethers were effective in proportion to the availability of the electrons on the oxygen atom so that aromatic ethers, such as furan, were not particularly effective, whereas tetrahydrofuran was. The mechanism of the solvolysis which has been proposed invokes the formation of a sulfur trioxide adduct, as shown below.

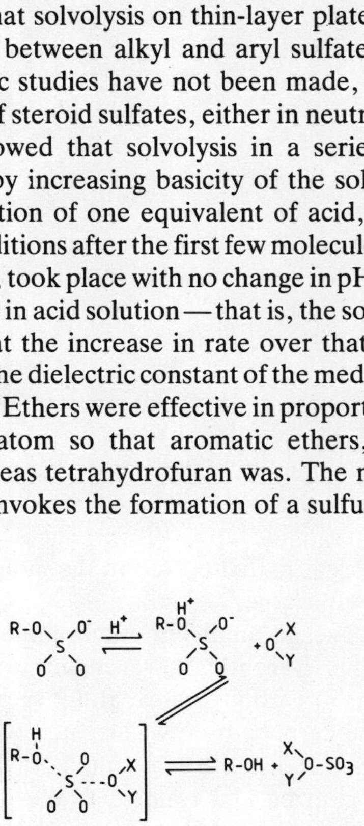

When X.O.Y is an ether, this is followed by hydrolysis,

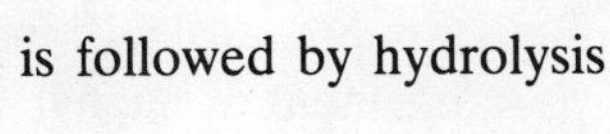

but when it is an alcohol (X.OH), it is followed by rearrangement of the sulfur trioxide adduct to the alkyl sulfate.

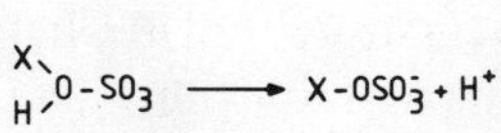

The overall reactions are therefore,

$$R.OSO_3^- + H_2O \xrightarrow{X.O.Y} R.OH + SO_4^{2-} + H^+$$

and

$$R.OSO_3^- + X.OH \longrightarrow R.OH + X.OSO_3^-$$

Whether or not these equations correctly represent the course of the solvolysis of sulfate esters is, from a practical point of view, unimportant. What is important is that such reactions provide a very gentle means of hydrolyzing sulfate esters, and thus of avoiding the formation of artefacts which so often accompanies the reaction in purely aqueous solution, because the solvolysis can be carried out at room temperature or below. It should be noted that although much of the interest in solvolysis has lain with steroid sulfates,[45,88] similar reactions occur with simple alkyl sulfates,[87] aryl sulfates,[90] and carbohydrate sulfates.[91]

Some recent work has shown[92] that the solvolysis of sulfate esters in "neutral" dioxan requires initiation by traces of electrophiles from, for example, glass; after this initiation, there is a very rapid hydrolysis brought about by the formation of increasing amounts of acid reaction products. In clean Teflon® vessels the potassium salts of octan-2-yl sulfate and cholestan-3β-yl sulfate were stable for prolonged periods in hot moist dioxan, but rapid solvolysis was initiated by the addition of traces of many acid contaminants likely to occur in a normal laboratory.

4. Some Chemical Reactions

One of the most important general reactions of sulfate esters is the formation of diesters, such as the methyl steroid sulfates,[93,94] by treatment with diazomethane. The propyl derivatives of aryl sulfates, which have been used for mass spectrometry (see Section IIB1), are formed by treatment of the sulfate ester with *n*-propyl iodide and silver perchlorate in sulfur dioxide at $-40°C$.[61] These diesters are fully covalent compounds which are rather easily hydrolyzed to the monoesters under conditions in which the latter are relatively stable.[95]

The simple alkyl sulfates, such as methyl or ethyl sulfates, are themselves alkylating agents, albeit rather poor ones. Recently, however, this property has been utilized in a method of coupling proteins to carbohydrates, and it seems that it could be of quite widespread application. The carbohydrate was treated with 2-[(4-aminophenyl)-sulfonyl]-ethyl hydrogen sulfate to form the substituted ethyl ether of the carbohydrate which was subsequently diazotized and coupled to the protein.[96]

Some sulfate esters rather readily undergo rearrangement. For example, potassium phenyl sulfate rearranges to potassium phenol 4-sulfonate on heating at 150 to 160°C, a reaction similar to the Fries rearrangement of phenyl carboxylate esters, although the latter requires the presence of $AlCl_3$, while ammonium methyl sulfate rearranges to *N*-methylammonium sulfate on heating at 220°C.[1] A more recently discovered rearrangement is the tris-catalyzed isomerization, at room temperature and neutral pH, of glucose 6-sulfate to fructose 6-sulfate.[97]

In general, the presence of a sulfate group does not confer any unexpected reactivity on other groups in the molecule, although some important exceptions to this are mentioned below and will be further considered in Chapter 8. Another example will be considered in Section IVC: this is the destabilizing effect of an *O*-sulfate group vicinal to a sulfoamino (sulfamate) group which greatly increases the lability of the latter to acid. Some other differences in behavior can be noted: for example, diazotization of 1-amino-2-naphthol gives 1,2-naphthoquinone, whereas diazotization of 1-amino naphthyl 2-sulfate gives naphthalene 1,2-diazooxide.[7] The converse situation may arise when reaction at another group in the molecule affects the sulfate ester bond; this is seen in the behavior of 2-aminophenyl sulfate and the 2-aminonaphthyl sulfates which lose sulfate during diazotization under the usual conditions to give any of a number of compounds whose precise nature depends upon the structure of the parent ester.[7] It is, therefore, surprising that 2-aminoestrone sulfate can be diazotized to give the quite stable 2-diazoestrone sulfate.[98]

One general point about the reactivity of sulfate esters must be made: nitroaryl sulfates are usually more reactive than the corresponding aryl sulfates. This reactivity should be kept in mind when such nitro compounds are used, as they frequently are, in biochemical systems. For example, amines readily undergo nucleophilic reactions with nitrophenyl sulfates, such as 4-nitrophenyl sulfate: tertiary amines react more rapidly than secondary amines which are more reactive than primary amines.[76] Two pathways are followed: there may be S–O cleavage to give a sulfamate or C–O cleavage to give a nitranilide, as follows:

$$R-NH_2 + \underset{OSO_3^-}{\overset{NO_2}{\bigcirc}} \longrightarrow \underset{OH}{\overset{NO_2}{\bigcirc}} + R-NH-SO_3^- \quad ; \quad \underset{NH-R}{\overset{NO_2}{\bigcirc}} + HSO_4^-$$

The former reaction usually predominates.[76] The apparent slow "hydrolysis" of 4-nitrophenyl sulfate in alkaline solutions of proline, or proline-containing proteins,[99] can almost certainly be explained by this reaction.

The reaction of 4-nitrophenyl sulfate with thiophenol, although much slower, may be analogous; the products here are 4-nitrophenol, diphenyl disulfide and SO_3^{2-}.[100] The formation of SO_3^{2-} was not shown directly but is particularly interesting because of the participation of thiols in the biological reduction of SO_4^{2-}. Again this reaction is probably responsible for the slow "hydrolysis" of 4-nitrophenyl sulfate in alkaline solutions of cysteine.[99]

The hydroxamic acid sulfates—for example, the sulfate esters of *N*-acetyl-*N*-hydroxy-2-aminofluorene, *N*-acetyl-*N*-hydroxy-2-naphthylamine, or *N*-hydroxyphenacetin—are very reactive; they decompose in water to a variety of products[11] and they rapidly form covalent derivatives with nucleic acids and proteins. This type of reaction is probably responsible, at least in part, for the carcinogenicity of *N*-acetyl-2-aminofluorene. The details of the reactions are not known, but in the case of the phenacetin derivative they seem to involve the formation of the quinone-imine from the sulfate ester.[101] These reactions will be considered further in Chapter 8.

A type of reaction which is becoming of increasing interest can be termed transesterification. As has already been pointed out (Section IIB1), the alkali metal salts of sulfate esters are not amenable to study by mass spectrometry, although the alkylaryl diesters derived from aryl sulfates have proven useful.[61] An alternative approach is to hydrolyze the sulfate ester to the parent alcohol or phenol and convert this to a suitable derivative, preferably in a single step. There have been reports of the formation of trimethylsilyl ethers by the direct reaction of a suitable reagent with galactose 3-sulfate (in sulfolipids),[102] with dopamine 3- or 4-*O*-sulfate,[103] and with morphine sulfate,[104] but only recently has a rather detailed study[105] been made of the reactions of a series of perfluoroacid anhydrides with sulfate esters. When treated overnight at room temperature with a 1:1 mixture of the anhydride and ethyl acetate, aryl sulfates gave a quantitative yield of the appropriate aryl ester. Other types of sulfate ester gave a mixture of products, apparently alkenes. The transesterification is catalyzed by acids and inhibited by pyridine, and so is quite different from the reaction of acid anhydrides with phenols. Two mechanisms have been proposed. It was suggested[105] that in dilute acid there was a nucleophilic attack of the aryl sulfate on a protonated form of the anhydride leading to the elimination of SO_3 and the formation of a complex which subsequently eliminated acetic acid to give the aryl ester. In more concentrated acid, on the other hand, it was suggested that the protonated form of the ester eliminated SO_3 to give the phenol which was then acylated. Whatever may be the detailed mechanism of the reaction, it seems likely to be a useful one for the characterization of aryl sulfates. The failure of the reaction with simple alkyl sulfates and with steroid sulfates, other than the rather reactive dehydroepiandrosterone sulfate, is unfortunate, but in these cases it may be possible to use an earlier transesterification technique which was devised for the preparation of steroid acetates. In this, the methylene green salt of the steroid sulfate (androsterone sulfate or dehydroepiandrosterone sulfate) was extracted into $CHCl_3$, taken to dryness, and then heated at 70 to 75°C for 30 min in acetic acid containing 0.02% of perchloric acid. More than 95% yields of androsterone and dehydroepiandrosterone acetates were obtained[106] so that this technique might prove a useful adjunct to that using the perfluoroacid anhydrides.

5. General Comments

Only a few general points can be made but they are of some practical importance. Many sulfate esters crystallize with solvent of crystallization—for example, pyridinium estrone sulfate with $CHCl_3$[45]—and particularly with water of crystallization. The latter can have a deleterious effect on the stability of the esters, as has been well shown with steroid sulfates where the triethylammonium salts, unlike the alkali metal salts, crystallize in an anhydrous form and are particularly stable.[9] All sulfate esters are more or less easily hydrolyzed, particulary in acid solution, so that they should generally be stored under anhydrous conditions in the cold, although even then decomposition can occur in certain, hopefully rare, cases.[49] If the esters must be stored in solution, this should be neutral and buffered because the hydrolysis of a sulfate ester is accompanied by the liberation of a proton (Equation 1) so that in the absence of a buffer the

$$R.OSO_3^- + H_2O \longrightarrow R.OH + SO_4^{2-} + H^+ \tag{1}$$

hydrolysis is autocatalytic. It therefore follows that when recrystallizing an old sample of a sulfate ester which may have been partly hydrolyzed, it is wise to ensure that the solvent contains enough base to keep the solution neutral and so prevent even more extensive hydrolysis occurring. Finally, at least in the case of some nitrophenyl sulfates, there is evidence[107] of photocatalytic decomposition so that it is wise to store sulfate esters in the dark.

In the case of $[^{35}S]$-sulfate esters the situation is different, and they should not be stored as solids because there is ample evidence that under such conditions $[^{35}S]$-sulfate esters of high specific activity undergo quite rapid radiochemical decomposition.[108,109] These esters should therefore be stored frozen, at about $-20°C$, in neutral solution.

The characterization of sulfate esters is not easy and, as has been discussed above, it appears that ^{13}C-NMR will prove to be the method of choice in future although, to judge by recent developments, the mass spectra of suitable derivatives may prove useful.

III. THIOSULFATE ESTERS

These can be regarded either as the sulfate esters of thiols or as *S*-alkyl and *S*-aryl derivatives of thiosulfate. Like sulfate esters, they are usually prepared as the alkali metal salts, the Bunte salts. Salts of organic bases can easily be obtained and, like those of sulfate esters, may have advantages of well-defined melting points, solubility in organic solvents, etc.

In general, thiosulfate esters can be prepared by the reaction under anhydrous conditions of a sulfur trioxide adduct[110] or of H_2SO_4 and a carbodiimide[13,111] with a thiol. Alkyl thiosulfates can be prepared by the reaction of thallous thiosulfate with an alkyl bromide[112] while a general method of considerable importance utilizes the nucleophilic attack of SO_3^{2-} on a disulfide[113] according to Equation 2. This is an equilibrium, the position of which varies very much with pH, but it has been much used for preparative purposes.[110,112,114] Many details are given in Reference 112.

$$SO_3^{2-} + R.SS.R \rightleftharpoons R.SSO_3^- + R.S.^- \tag{2}$$

Thiosulfate esters are quite readily hydrolyzed by acid, apparently by an A-1 reaction quite analogous to that for the hydrolysis of sulfate esters, to the parent thiol and sulfate. There are, however, important differences:[110] alkyl and aryl thiosulfates are hydrolyzed at comparable rates, and the introduction of an electron-withdrawing substituent into phenyl thiosulfate does not increase the rate of hydrolysis, quite contrary to the situation with phenyl sulfate. The differences probably arise because the transition state in the hydrolysis of the thiosulfate ester cannot be stabilized through interactions involving the aromatic ring. As with sulfate esters, the rate of the acid-catalyzed hydrolysis of thiosulfate esters is greatly increased in water-dioxan mixtures, the effect being even greater than with the former.[110]

Aryl thiosulfates are quite labile to alkali: treatment of phenyl thiosulfate with 0.3 *M* KOH for 5 min at 100°C converts it, via phenyl sulfenate, to diphenyl disulfide.[112] Phenyl sulfate is quite stable under these conditions.

Other chemical properties of the Bunte salts were summarized some years ago by Milligan and Swan.[113] No further comment is needed here because no thiosulfate ester derived from a thiol-containing xenobiotic has yet been isolated despite the early statement[115] that the administration of thiophenol to rabbits led to the increased urinary excretion of "ethereal sulfate." Thiosulfate esters are nevertheless important biochemically: alanine 3-thiosulfate (*S*-sulfocysteine) and its glutathione analogue occur naturally,[3] and similar thiosulfate esters play a fundamental role in the interconversions of SO_4^{2-} and SO_3^{2-} in vivo.[116]

IV. SULFAMATES

Although most types of amine can form sulfamates,[117] in a biochemical context interest is concentrated on the aminosugars, particularly 2-amino-2-deoxyglucose, and the arylamines. The sulfamate of the former occurs in heparin and related glycosaminoglycans, while those of the latter are metabolites of the parent arylamines.[118] Sulfamates are also of interest because of their use as artificial sweetening agents.

A. Synthesis of Sulfamates

Valuable accounts of early work on the preparation and properties of sulfamates are given in References 117 and 119, while more recent work is considered in Reference 120. Sulfamates are most conveniently prepared by treatment of the amine with a sulfur trioxide adduct.[2] The reaction may be carried out under anhydrous conditions[118] or in cold aqueous alkali; the latter type of reaction is particularly useful because it allows the selective sulfation of the amino group in aminoalcohols.[2] For example, 2-deoxy-2-sulfo-aminoglucose has been prepared by the direct sulfation of glucosamine in aqueous solution with pyridine-sulfur trioxide[121] or, better, with trimethylamine-sulfur trioxide,[122] the latter reagent having the advantage that it does not form the red pigment produced from pyridine-sulfur trioxide in aqueous alkali.

Like sulfate esters, sulfamates are usually prepared as alkali metal salts, but the salts of organic bases may have useful properties such as solubility in organic solvents[3] and sharp melting points.

B. Spectral Properties

There is little information on the spectral properties of sulfamates, but several seem to show a rather broad absorption at 1420 to 1450 cm^{-1}, not seen in sulfate esters, as well as that at 1200 to 1220 cm^{-1} which does occur in the latter.[123]

As with sulfate esters (Section IIB1), PMR spectra are useful for characterizing sulfamates.[123] The formation of an alkyl sulfamate gives a down-field shift of 0.21 to 0.48 ppm in the signal from the proton attached to the carbon atom bearing the amino group. In the case of glucosamine, formation of the sulfamate gives a down-field shift in the signal of the proton on carbon 2, 0.57 ppm for the α anomer and 0.47 ppm for the β anomer. These shifts have proven useful in the characterization of some 5′-sulfo-amino-5′-deoxyribonucleosides synthesized as analogues of nucleoside 5′-phosphates.[124]

C. Hydrolysis

Sulfamates are stable to alkali but are readily hydrolyzed in acid, in general terms their stability to acid being related to the basicity of the parent amine so that N-alkyl sulfamates are more stable than N-aryl sulfamates.[125] The latter may be hydrolyzed under the usual conditions for diazotizing an aromatic amine so that the formation of a diazonium salt does not necessarily distinguish between an amine and its sulfamate. This lability to acid of the sulfamate group has been particularly useful in the study of heparin which contains 2-deoxy-2-sulfoaminoglucose residues; these are particularly labile and are quantitatively hydrolyzed in 90 min in 0.04 M HCl at 100°C, conditions which scarcely affect the sulfate ester groups which are also present.[126] In fact, the sulfate ester groups may be stabilized through electrostatic shielding by the protonated amino groups which are formed on hydrolysis of the sulfamate.

Most of the detailed studies have been made with N-aryl sulfamates. The acid hydrolysis of N-phenyl[127] and N-1-naphthyl sulfamate[128] are A-2 reactions in which there is an initial protonation of the nitrogen atom followed by a nucleophilic attack of water on the sulfur, as shown below.

$$R-NH-SO_3^- \;\overset{H^+}{\rightleftharpoons}\; R-\overset{+}{N}H_2-SO_3^- \;\xrightarrow{H_2O}\; R-NH_3^+ + HSO_4^-$$

The hydrolysis of N-alkyl sulfamates follows the same course,[129] and the data for both sets of compounds can be correlated by the appropriate treatment.[130] The introduction of an electron-withdrawing substituent in the *para* position of *N*-phenyl sulfamate increased the rate of acid hydrolysis, as did the addition of increasing amounts of acetone to the solvent.[131]

The apparent first order rate constants for the hydrolysis of a series of substituted *N*-phenyl sulfamates in 0.09 M HCl, 10% acetone, at 50°C ranged [131] from 2.2 to 5.3 × 10^{-5} sec^{-1}, whereas the value for 2-deoxy-2-sulfoaminoglucose at 57°C in 0.1 M HCl was very much greater,[132] 1.2 × 10^{-3} sec^{-1}, despite the fact that *N*-alkyl sulfamates are generally more stable than *N*-aryl sulfamates.[125] It has been shown that the unexpected lability of 2-deoxy-2-sulfoaminoglucose is caused by the presence of vicinal hydroxyl groups in the molecule, and in model compounds an *O*-sulfate vicinal to a sulfoamino group has an even greater destabilizing influence than a vicinal hydroxyl group.[132] The 5′-sulfoamino-5′-deoxyribonucleosides, which do not have a hydroxyl group vicinal to the sulfoamino group have been stated[124] to be very stable in acid solution.

As with sulfate esters, sulfamates also undergo solvolytic reactions, especially in a polar solvent such as pyridine.[133]

D. Some Chemical Reactions

Only two reactions of sulfamates need comment. The first is the rearrangement of many *N*-aryl sulfamates to the corresponding aminoaryl sulfonates; for example, heating potassium *N*-phenyl sulfamate at 180°C gives potassium sulfanilate. Such rearrangements have generally been considered to be intramolecular, but this is not necessarily so.[120] At least in dioxan–H$_2$SO$_4$, in which the sulfamates are not soluble so that the reaction is a heterogeneous one, the rearrangement of *N*-phenyl sulfamate to sulfanilate is intermolecular, apparently involving a rapid splitting of the sulfamate to aniline and SO$_3$ followed by a slow sulfonation of the former by the latter.[134] Nevertheless, generalization may be unwise because under the same conditions the rearrangement of *N*-1-naphthyl sulfamate to 1-aminonaphthalene 4-sulfonate is only partly intermolecular.[135] Surprisingly, *N*-2-naphthyl sulfamate did not rearrange under these conditions.[135]

The second general reaction of some interest is the ability of sulfamates to act as sulfating agents. As already pointed out (Section IIA3), sulfamic acid itself is a useful sulfating agent, and it has been shown that substituted sulfamic acids can be even more useful.[136] There has been no extensive use of such methods for the synthesis of sulfate esters, but a number of carbohydrate sulfates and nucleotide sulfates have been prepared using *N*-piperidinyl sulfamate.[137] A sulfur trioxide adduct is likely to be an intermediate in these reactions which are the reverse of those between nitrophenyl sulfates and amines[76] (see Section IIB4).

V. SULFATOPHOSPHATES

The sulfatophosphates, or phosphosulfates, differ somewhat from the other derivatives of sulfuric acid considered in this chapter because they are anhydrides of sulfuric acid and phosphoric acid; of the other compounds so far mentioned only the sulfate esters of nitrophenols show some anhydride character. The existence of inorganic sulfatophosphates ($^-$O$_3$S.O.PO$_3^{2-}$) has been reported[138] and denied,[139] but there is no doubt about the biochemical importance of their esters in which the phosphate is esterified with the 5′-hydroxyl of adenosine or adenosine-3′-phosphate to give adenosine 5′-sulfatophosphate and adenosine 3′-phosphate 5′-sulfatophosphate, respectively. These very important nucleotides will be considered further in Chapter 4.

Aryl sulfatophosphates are relatively simple to prepare and have been obtained by the sulfation of the appropriate aryl phosphoric acid in anhydrous solution with pyridine-sulfur trioxide[140] or dimethylformamide-sulfur trioxide.[141]

The preparation of nucleoside sulfatophosphates is more difficult because of the likelihood of sulfating the hydroxyl groups of the sugar. Adenosine 5'-sulfatophosphate has been made by the sulfation of adenosine 5'-phosphoric acid with pyridine-sulfur trioxide in aqueous solution (about 5 percent yield),[142] with triethylamine-sulfur trioxide in anhydrous conditions (60 to 75 percent yield),[143] and with H_2SO_4 and a carbodiimide (20 to 25% yield).[144] The latter method gave extensive sulfation of the sugar hydroxyls. An anion-exchange method, in which a nucleoside diphenyl pyrophosphate is treated with SO_4^{2-} in pyridine has been developed[145] and has given good yields of adenosine 5'-sulfatophosphate and of other purine and pyrimidine sulfatophosphates.

The synthesis of adenosine 3'-phosphate 5'-sulfatophosphate is more difficult because of the relative inaccessibility of adenosine 3', 5'-bisphosphate or adenosine 2', 3'-cyclic phosphate 5'-phosphate as starting materials. It has, however, been prepared by similar methods to those used for the preparation of adenosine 5'-sulfatophosphate.[143,146-148] The method of choice would appear to be the last which provides as an intermediary product adenosine 2', 3'-cyclic phosphate 5'-sulfatophosphate; this can be hydrolyzed with ribonuclease-T_2 to give adenosine 3'-phosphate 5'-sulfatophosphate or by spleen phospho-diesterase to give adenosine 2'-phosphate 5'-sulfatophosphate. The former has been obtained in a yield of 68%.[148] The use of immobilized ribonuclease–T_2 to hydrolyze the cyclic nucleotide is a valuable innovation[149] because the enzyme can be used repeatedly over a period of many months.

Little is known of the chemistry of the sulfatophosphates except that they are very acid-labile compounds; the half-life of the sulfatophosphate group in adenosine 3'-phosphate 5'-sulfatophosphate in 0.1 M HCl at 37°C is only 6 min.[150] Conversely, they are relatively stable to alkali, and the same compound is only partly hydrolyzed after 2 hr in 0.1 M NaOH at 100°C.[146] They can apparently rather readily transfer a sulfate group to suitable acceptors such as aminosugars or simple hydroxyl-containing compounds;[151] the transfer occurs on standing with charcoal, and although it was only detected by the use of adenosine 3'-phosphate 5'-[^{35}S]-sulfatophosphate of very high specific activity the possibility of its occurrence should be kept in mind because charcoal is often used as an absorbent in the isolation of sulfatophosphates from biological material. Recently is has been shown[151a] that on storage for several months at $-18°C$ in 0.9 M NH_4HCO_3, adenosine 5'-sulfatophosphate and adenosine 3'-phosphate 5'-sulfatophosphates were almost quantitatively converted to the corresponding adenosine 5'-phosphoramidates with the simultaneous liberation of SO_4^{2-}.

There is more detailed information available about the hydrolysis of aryl sulfatophosphates, but the kinetics are rather complex because of the many possible ionic forms of these compounds. At 55°C, k_{obs} was about 2.8×10^{-3} sec^{-1} at pH 1 and 3×10^{-3} sec^{-1} between pH 6 and 10, respectively.[140] Rather more than 90% of the reaction occurred by fission of the O–S bond, the remainder by fission of the O–P bond, and it was considered that the acid-catalyzed hydrolysis of the sulfatophosphate group occurred by an A-1 reaction similar to that occurring with the aryl sulfates.[140,141]

Other anhydrides of sulfuric acid are known, but they need not be considered here except to point out that an interesting comparison has been made between acetyl sulfate and phenyl sulfatophosphate from the standpoint of the unique role of the sulfatophosphate group as the biological sulfate donor.[140]

VI. ANALYTICAL TECHNIQUES

No special analytical techniques are routinely used in the study of sulfate esters and related compounds. They are, as already discussed, the salts of strong acids and are amenable to methods developed for the separation of other such compounds and also of the much weaker acids, the phosphate esters. They are, therefore, usefully handled by ion-exchange chromatography and by electrophoresis; in the former, they usually require more drastic conditions for elution than do the phosphate esters, and in the latter conditions can be chosen such that they have a much higher mobility than do phosphate esters. The only naturally occurring acids of comparable strength with which they could be confused are the sulfonic acids (see Reference 3 for examples), but these are readily distinguished from the sulfate esters by the fact that they do not yield SO_4^{2-} on acid hydrolysis.

Their column chromatography need not be considered here; the only problem may be the detection of the desired compound in the eluate. Paper and thin-layer chromatography are useful, but the solvent systems required will depend entirely upon the nature of the organic part of the molecule so that no general information can be given except that acid conditions should be avoided to prevent possible hydrolysis or solvolysis. Some useful thin-layer systems have been described[152] and further information can be obtained in Reference 3. Recently, a useful method has been described[153] for the separation of the individual sulfated bile acid conjugates; this uses reversed-phase partition thin-layer chromatography of the calcium complexes of the esters. Again, the detection of the ester may pose problems unless the organic component has some suitable property, and the only general technique requires its hydrolysis to SO_4^{2-} and the localization of this. A suitable method is that of Schneider and Lewbart[154] which uses solvolysis for some hours in dioxan-HCl vapor to give SO_4^{2-} which is located by the barium rhodizonate method. This method was originally developed for paper chromatograms where the limit of detection was given as about 1 nmol of steroid sulfate,[152] but it should be equally applicable to thin-layer chromatograms. Some sulfate esters can be detected by the methylene blue method[3] either on paper[43] or thin-layer[44] chromatograms; for steroid sulfates the limits of detection have been given as 1 nmol and 0.2 nmol, respectively. Obviously these methods could be used equally well for the detection of sulfate esters after zone electrophoresis. Qualitative analysis of sulfate esters is more extensively discussed in Chapter 6, Section IIA.

The quantitative determination of sulfate esters and related compounds is not easy. Some can be determined spectrophotometrically or by methods based on the solubility in chloroform of their methylene blue salts.[3] Methods using high-performance liquid chromatography have recently been developed: 4-nitrophenyl sulfate has been determined, in the presence of the free phenol and its glucuronide, by reversed-phase high-performance liquid chromatography,[155] while adenosine 5'-sulfatophosphate and adenosine 3'-phosphate 5'-sulfatophosphate have been separated from contaminating nucleotides by paired-ion high-performance liquid chromatography,[156] with tetrabutyl-ammonium perchlorate as the pairing agent. The latter method is particularly useful because it allows the routine determination of adenosine 3',5'-bisphosphate in preparations of adenosine 3'-phosphate 5'-sulfatophosphate, a procedure of some importance because of the strong inhibitory action of the former on the sulfotransferases (see Chapter 5). Such high-performance chromatographic methods are likely to become the ones of choice for the determination of specific sulfate esters.

The only completely general method for their determination requires their quantitative hydrolysis to SO_4^{2-} which must then be determined. It should be noted that complete hydrolysis to SO_4^{2-} may be incompatible with the quantitative recovery of the organic part of the molecule in an unchanged form (see Section IIB2a). Methods for the determination of SO_4^{2-} in the nmol range fall into three main types, and none is entirely satisfactory; there is no method which has the simplicity and sensitivity of the colorimetric determination of phosphate. The first type depends upon the production, under highly standardized conditions, of a suspension of $BaSO_4$, the turbidity of which is then measured. Probably the most used method of this type is that of Dodgson[157] which requires about 1 μmol of SO_4^{2-} in a volume of 0.2 ml although more sensitive variants of the method are described in the same reference. The second group is based on the precipitation of SO_4^{2-} as benzidine sulfate and, after careful washing of the precipitate, the spectrophotometric determination of the benzidine therein either directly by dissolving the benzidine sulfate in HCl[158] or by coupling of its diazonium salt.[159] The two specified methods require about 100 nmol SO_4^{2-} in 0.5 ml and 500 nmol in 1 ml, respectively. Finally there are spectrophotometric methods utilizing the dissociation of barium rhodizonate in the presence of SO_4^{2-}. Two such methods have recently been described,[158,160] both of which require about 50 nmol of SO_4^{2-} in 0.6 ml, although a greater sensitivity can readily be obtained. It must be stressed that all these methods, and all other variants of them, are extremely sensitive to quite minor changes in conditions—changes in pH, presence of other ions, presence of organic molecules, to name only a few—so that strict adherence to the specified conditions is essential. Further, although the methods work well with pure solutions of SO_4^{2-}, they may not do so under all conditions; for example, the presence of sugars can interfere with the benzidine method by preventing the precipitation of benzidine sulfate. Of the methods which are available, those based on the precipitation of benzidine sulfate are in many ways the most satisfactory, but the carcinogenicity of benzidine must preclude its use in many laboratories in which case methods using rhodizonic acid are probably the second choice. A recent review of methods for determination of sulfate is available.[161] Sulfate may be detected by thin-layer chromatography.[162,163] Also a histochemical technique for the demonstration of sulfate in tissue slices has been reported.[164]

REFERENCES

1. **Suter, C. M.,** *The Organic Chemistry of Sulfur,* John Wiley & Sons, New York, 1944.
2. **Gilbert, E. E.,** *Sulfonation and Related Reactions,* Interscience, New York, 1965.
3. **Roy, A. B. and Trudinger, P. A.,** *The Biochemistry of Inorganic Compounds of Sulphur,* Cambridge University Press, Cambridge, 1970.
4. **Oae, S.,** *Organic Chemistry of Sulfur,* Plenum Press, New York, 1977.
5. **Gilbert, E. E.,** The reactions of sulfur trioxide, and of its adducts, with organic compounds, *Chem. Rev.,* 62, 550, 1962.
6. **Burkhardt, G. N. and Lapworth, A.,** Arylsulphuric acids, *J. Chem. Soc.,* p. 684, 1926.
7. **Burkhardt, G. N. and Lapworth, A.,** Nitroarylsulphuric acids and their reduction products, *J. Chem. Soc.,* p. 141, 1929.
8. **Jerfy, A. and Roy, A. B.,** Sulphated derivatives of some hydroxypyridines, *Aust. J. Chem.,* 23, 847, 1970.
9. **Dusza, J. P., Joseph, J. P., and Bernstein, S.,** Steroid conjugates IV. The preparation of steroid sulfates with triethylamine-sulfur trioxide, *Steroids,* 12, 49, 1968.
10. **Peat, S., Bowker, D.M., and Turvey, J. R.,** Sulphates of monosaccharides and derivatives VI. D-Glucose 2-sulphate, D-galactose 2- and 3-sulphates and D-galactose, *Carbohydr. Res.,* 7, 228, 1968.
11. **Boyland, E. and Manson, D.,** The biochemistry of aromatic amines. The metabolism of 2-naphthylamine and 2-naphthylhydroxylamine derivatives, *Biochem. J.,* 101, 84, 1966.
12. **Maher, V. M., Miller, E. C., Miller, J. A., and Szybalski, W.,** Mutations and decreases in density of transforming DNA produced by derivatives of the carcinogens 2-acetylaminofluorene and N-methyl-4-aminoazobenzene, *Mol. Pharmacol.,* 4, 411, 1968.

13. **Hoiberg, C. P. and Mumma, R. O.**, Preparation of sulfate esters. Reactions of various alcohols, phenols, amines, mercaptans, and oximes with sulfuric acid and dicyclohexylcarbodiimide, *J. Am. Chem. Soc.*, 91, 4273, 1969.

14. **Mumma, R. O., Hoiberg, C. P., and Simpson, R.**, Preparation of sulfate esters. *N,N'*-Dicyclohexyl-carbodiimide-mediated sulfation of carbohydrate derivatives, *Carbohydr. Res.*, 14, 119, 1970.

15. **Mumma, R.O., Hoiberg, C. P., and Weber, W. W.**, Preparation of sulfate esters. The synthesis of steroid sulfates by a dicyclohexylcarbodiimide-mediated sulfation, *Steroids*, 14, 67, 1969.

16. **Dodgson, K. S., Fitzgerald, J.W., and Payne, W. J.**, Chemically defined inducers of alkylsulphatases present in *Pseudomonas* C12B, *Biochem. J.*, 138, 53, 1974.

17. **Schmidt, E., Ueber Cholin**, Neurin and Verwandte Verbindungen, *Liebig's Ann. Chem.*, 337, 37, 1904.

18. **Dodgson, K. S., Lloyd, A. G., and Tudball, N.**, *O*-Sulphate esters of L-serine, L-threonine and L-hydroxyproline, *Biochem. J.*, 79, 111, 1961.

19. **Fitzgerald, J. W., Maca, W. H., and Rose, F. A.**, Physiological factors regulating tyrosine-sulphate sulphohydrolase activity in *Comomonas terrigena:* occurrence of constitutive and inducible enzymes, *J. Gen. Microbiol.*, 111, 407, 1979.

20. **Jenner, W. N. and Rose, F. A.**, Studies on the sulfation of 3,4-dihydroxyphenylethylamine (dopamine) and related compounds by rat tissues, *Biochem. J.*, 135, 109, 1973.

21. **Kishimoto, Y., Takahashi, N., and Egami, F.**, Synthesis and properties of serotonin O-sulfate, *J. Biochem. (Tokyo)*, 49, 436, 1961.

22. **Sommer, F., Schulz, O. F., and Nassau, M.**, Uber die Sulfoperamidsaure, *Z. Anorg. Allg. Chem.*, 147, 142, 1925.

23. **Joseph, J. P., Dusza, J. P., and Bernstein, S.**, Steroid conjugates. I. The use of sulfamic acid for the preparation of steroid sulfates, *Steroids*, 7, 577, 1966.

24. **Levitz, M.**, Synthesis of estrone-6,7-[^{3}H] sulfate-[^{35}S], *Steroids*, 1, 117, 1963.

25. **Mumma, R. O.**, Ascorbic acid sulfate as a sulfating agent, *Biochim. Biophys. Acta*, 165, 571, 1968.

26. **Nagasawa, K. and Yoshidome, H.**, A metal-catalyzed reaction of 8-quinolyl sulfate and its application to the preparation of biochemically related sulfate esters, *J. Org. Chem.*, 39, 1681, 1974.

27. **Roy, A. B.**, Comparative studies on the liver sulphatases, *Biochem. J.*, 68, 519, 1958.

28. **Jeffrey, H. J. and Roy, A. B.**, A spectrophotometric determination of arylsulphatase activity, *Anal. Biochem.*, 77, 478, 1977.

29. **Boyland, E., Manson, D., and Sims, P.**, The preparation of *o*-aminophenyl sulphates, *J. Chem. Soc.*, p. 3623, 1953.

30. **Boyland, E., Sims, P., and Williams, D. C.**, The oxidation of tryptophan and some related compounds with persulphate, *Biochem. J.*, 62, 546, 1956.

31. **Smith, P. A. S.**, Ketoxime-O-sulfonic acids, *J. Am. Chem. Soc.*, 70, 323, 1948.

32. **Smith, J. N.**, Some sulphate esters of nitroquinol and 4-nitrocatechol, *J. Chem. Soc.*, p. 2861, 1951.

33. **Bernstein, S. and McGilvery, R. W.**, Enzymatic conjugation of *m*-aminophenol, *J. Biol. Chem.*, 198, 195, 1952.

34. **Gemborys, M. W. and Gribble, G. W.**, Synthesis of *N*-hydroxyacetaminophen, a postulated toxic metabolite of acetaminophen, and its phenolic sulfate conjugate, *J. Med. Chem.*, 21, 649, 1978.

35. **Burwell, R. L.**, Racemization, alkylsulfuric acid formation and exchange in the reaction between sulfuric acid-d_2 and optically active 2-butanol, *J. Am. Chem. Soc.*, 67, 220, 1945.

36. **Burwell, R. L.**, The stereochemistry of the sulfation of optically active secondary butyl alcohol, *J. Am. Chem. Soc.*, 71, 1769, 1949.

37. **Matcham, G. W. J. and Dodgson, K. S.**, Preparation and characterization of substrates suitable for the study of stereospecific alkylsulphohydrolases of detergent-degrading micro-organisms, *Biochem. J.*, 167, 717, 1977.

38. **Turvey, J. R.**, Sulfates of the simple sugars, *Adv. Carbohydr. Chem.*, 20, 183, 1965.

39. **Flynn, T. G., Rose, F. A., and Tudball, N.**, Preparation of dipotassium 2-hydroxy-5-nitrophenyl [^{35}S] sulphate, *Biochem. J.*, 105, 1010, 1967.

40. **Dodgson, K. S., Rose, F. A., and Spencer, B.**, Studies on sulphatases. 10. The isolation and characterization of biosynthetic arylsulphates, *Biochem. J.*, 60, 346, 1955.

41. **Murray, K.**, The formation of *O*-sulphates of serine and threonine in protein hydrolysates, *Biochem. J.*, 110, 155, 1968.

42. **Burkhardt, G. N., Ford, W. G. K., and Singleton, E.**, The hydrolysis of arylsulphuric acids. I, *J. Chem. Soc.*, p. 17, 1936.

43. **Crépy, O. and Judas, O.**, Détermination quantitative et qualitative des sulfates de stéroides à l'aide de bleu de methylene II. Détection de sulfates de stéroides en chromatographie sur papier, *Rev. Fr. Etud. Clin. Biol.*, 5, 284, 1960.

44. **Crépy, O., Judas, O. and Lachaise, B.,** Méthodes de détection des stéroides conjugués séparés par chromatographie en couche mince, *J. Chromatogr.,* 16, 340, 1964.

45. **McKenna, J. and Norymberski, J. K.,** Steroid sulphates. I. Some solvolytic reactions of the salts of steroid sulphates, *J. Chem. Soc.,* p. 3889, 1957.

46. **Barton, A. D. and Young, L.,** *p*-Toluidine salts of monoaryl sulfates, *J. Am. Chem. Soc.,* 65, 294, 1943.

47. **Burstein, S.,** Interaction of [7α-^{3}H] androstenolone sulfate with cationic detergents and phophatides, *Biochim. Biophys. Acta,* 62, 576, 1962.

48. **Masek, K., Bensch, K., and Felsenfeld, H.,** Cerebroside sulfate-amine interaction in neoplastic mast cells, *FEBS Lett.,* 9, 337, 1970.

49. **Sobel, A. E., Owades, P. S., and Owades, J. L.,** Sulfate esters as intermediates in the formation of 7-dehydrocholesterol and dicholesteryl ether, *J. Am. Chem. Soc.,* 71, 1487, 1949.

50. **Bernstein, S., Dusza, J. P., and Joseph, J. P.,** *Physical Properties of Steroid Conjugates,* Springer-Verlag, New York, 1968.

51. **Hearse, D. J., Olavesen, A. H., and Powell, G. M.,** The preparation and characterization of a series of [^{35}S]-labelled aryl sulphate esters for metabolic studies, *Biochem. Pharmacol.,* 18, 173, 1969.

52. **Bartholomew, B., Dodgson, K. S., Matcham, G. W. J., Shaw, D. J., and White, G. F.,** A novel mechanism of enzymic ester hydrolysis. Inversion of configuration and carbon-oxygen bond cleavage by secondary alkylsulphohydrolases from detergent-degrading micro-organisms. *Biochem. J.,* 165, 575, 1977.

53. **Lloyd, A. G., Tudball, N., and Dodgson, K. S.,** Infrared studies on sulphate esters. III. *O*-Sulphate esters of alcohols, amino alcohols and hydroxylated amino acids, *Biochim. Biophys. Acta,* 52, 413, 1961.

54. **Ragan, M. A.,** Phenol sulfate esters: ultraviolet, infrared, [^{1}H] and [^{13}C] nuclear magnetic resonance spectroscopic investigation, *Can. J. Chem.,* 56, 2681, 1978.

55. **Lloyd, A. G. and Dodgson, K. S.,** Infrared studies on sulphate esters. II. Monosaccharide sulphates, *Biochim. Biophys. Acta,* 46, 116, 1961.

56. **Harris, M. J. and Turvey, J. R.,** Sulphates of monosaccharides and derivatives. VIII. Infrared spectra and optical rotation of some glycoside sulphates, *Carbohydr. Res.,* 15, 51, 1970.

57. **Honda, S., Yuki, H., and Takiura, K.,** Fourier transform [^{13}C]-nuclear magnetic resonance spectra of D-glucose 3- and 6–sulfates, *Carbohydr. Res.,* 28, 150, 1973.

58. **Usov, A. I., Yarotskii, S. V., and Vasyanina, L. K.,** Synthesis and investigation by the [^{13}C]-NMR method of sulfates of 3-*O*-methyl-α-D-mannopyranoside, *Bioorganicheskaya Khimiya,* 1, 1583, 1975.

59. **Archbald, P. J., Fenn, M. D., and Roy, A. B.,** ^{13}C-N.M.R. studies of glucose and galactose monosulphates, *Carbohydr. Res.,* 1981, in press.

60. **Games, D. E., Games, M. P., Jackson, A. H.,** Olavesen, A. H., Rossiter, M., and Winterburn, P. J., Field desorption mass spectrometry of sodium and potassium salts, *Tetrahedron Lett.,* p. 2377, 1974.

61. **Paulson, G., Simpson, M., Giddings, J., Bakke, J., and Stolzenberg, G.,** The conversion of aryl sulfate ester salts to alkyl aryl derivatives suitable for analysis by electron impact mass spectrometry, *Biomed. Mass Spectrom.,* 5, 413, 1978.

62. **Usov, A. I., Deryabin, V. V., Chizhov, O. S., Kadentsev, V. I., Zolotarev, B. M., and Kochetkov, N. K.,** Mass spectrometric study of acetylated amidosulfates of D-galactose, *Izv. Akad. Nauk SSSR, Ser. Khim.,* p. 1084, 1975.

63. **Rees, D. A.,** A note on the characterization of carbohydrate sulphates by acid hydrolysis, *Biochem. J.,* 88, 343, 1963.

64. **Fieser, L. F.,** Naphthoquinone antimalarials. XVI. Water-soluble derivatives of alcoholic and unsaturated compounds, *J. Am. Chem. Soc.,* 70, 3232, 1948.

65. **Fendler, E. J. and Fendler, J. H.,** Hydrolysis of nitrophenyl and dinitrophenyl sulfate esters, *J. Org. Chem.,* 33, 3852, 1968.

66. **Batts, B. D.,** Alkyl hydrogen sulphates. II. The hydrolysis in aqueous acid solution, *J. Chem. Soc. B,* p. 551, 1966.

67. **Kice, J. L. and Anderson, J. M.,** The mechanism of the acid hydrolysis of sodium aryl sulfates, *J. Am. Chem. Soc.,* 88, 5242, 1966.

68. **Benkovic, S. J.,** Studies on sulfate esters. II. Carboxyl group catalysis in the hydrolysis of salicyl sulfate, *J. Am. Chem. Soc.,* 88, 5511, 1966.

69. **Benkovic, S. J. and Dunikoski, L. K.,** Intramolecular catalysis of sulfate ester hydrolysis. A model for aryl sulfate sulfohydrolase, *Biochemistry,* 9, 1390, 1970.

70. **Venning, E. H., Hoffman, M. M., and Browne, J. S. L.,** Isolation of androsterone sulfate, *J. Biol. Chem.,* 146, 369, 1942.

71. **Dobriner, K., Rhoads, C. P., Lieberman, S., Hill, B. R., and Fieser, L. F.,** Abnormal α-keto steroid excretion in patients with neoplastic disease, *Science,* 99, 494, 1944.

72. **Ramseyer, J., Williams, J. S., and Hirschmann, H.,** Carbon-oxygen cleavage in the acid hydrolysis of androsterone sulfate, *Steroids,* 9, 347, 1967.

73. **Hirschmann, H. and Williams, J. S.,** The isolation of 5α–pregnane-3β,20β-diol 20-sulfate and its hydrolysis to uranediol (17α-methyl-D-homo-5α-androstane-3β,17aβ-diol), *J. Biol. Chem.,* 238, 2305, 1963.

74. **Bernstein, S., Dusza, J. P., and Joseph, J. P.,** Chemistry: synthesis and characterization, in *Chemical and Biological Aspects of Steroid Conjugation,* Bernstein, S. and Solomon, S., Eds., Springer-Verlag New York, 1970.

75. **Spencer, B.** Studies on sulphatases. 20. Enzymic cleavage of aryl hydrogen sulphates in the presence of $H_2{}^{18}O$, *Biochem. J.,* 69, 155, 1958.

76. **Benkovic, S. J. and Benkovic, P. A.,** Studies on sulfate esters. I. Nucleophilic reactions of amines with *p*-nitrophenyl sulfate, *J. Am. Chem. Soc.,* 88, 5504, 1966.

77. **Burwell, R. L.,** The hydrolysis of optically active secondary butyl hydrogen sulfate, *J. Am. Chem. Soc.,* 74, 1462, 1952.

78. **Percival, E. G. V.,** Carbohydrate sulphates, *Q. Rev. Chem. Soc.,* 3, 369, 1949.

79. **Haslewood, G. A. D.,** *Bile Salts,* Methuen, London, 1967.

80. **Hay, R. W. and Edmonds, J. A. G.,** The copper (II)-catalysed hydrolysis of 8-hydroxyquinoline sulphate, *Chem. Commun.,* p. 969, 1967.

81. **Teich, S., Rogers, J., Lieberman, S., Engel, L. L., and Davis, J. W.,** The origin of 3, 5-cycloandrostan-6β-ol-17-one (i-androsten-6β-ol-17-one) in urinary extracts, *J. Am. Chem. Soc.,* 75, 2523, 1953.

82. **Kurz, J. L.,** Effects of micellization on the kinetics of the hydrolysis of monoalkyl sulfates, *J. Phys. Chem.,* 66, 2239, 1962.

83. **Fendler, E. J., Liechti, R. R. and Fendler, J. H.,** Micellar effects on the hydrolysis of 2, 4-dinitrophenyl sulfate, *J. Org. Chem.,* 35, 1658, 1970.

84. **Congdon, W. I. and Bender, M. L.,** The β-cyclodextrin-accelerated hydrolysis of aryl sulfates: a model for enzymic catalysis through binding, *Bioorg. Chem.,* 1, 424, 1971.

85. **Kiefer, H. C., Congdon, W. I., Scarpa, I. S., and Klotz, I.,** Catalytic accelerations of 10^{12}-fold by an enzyme-like synthetic polymer, *Proc. Natl. Acad. Sci. U.S.A.,* 69, 2155, 1972.

86. **Sunamoto, J., Kondo, H., Okamoto, H., and Taira, K.,** A sulfotransferase model. Covalent participation of a macrocyclic oxime in the hydrolysis of 2,4-dinitrophenyl sulfate, *Bioorg. Chem.,* 6, 95, 1977.

87. **Batts, B. D.,** Alkyl hydrogen sulfates. I. Hydrolysis in moist dioxan solution, *J. Chem. Soc. B.,* p. 547, 1966.

88. **Burstein, S. and Lieberman, S.,** Kinetics and mechanism of solvolysis of steroid hydrogen sulfates, *J. Am. Chem. Soc.,* 80, 5235, 1958.

89. **Hurwitz, A. R.,** Differential sulfate ester hydrolysis, *Anal. Biochem.,* 46, 338, 1972.

90. **Benkovic, S. J. and Benkovic, P. A.,** Studies on sulfate esters. III. A comparison of the solvolyses of salicyl sulfate and sulfur trioxide, *J. Am. Chem. Soc.,* 90, 2646, 1968.

91. **Seib, P. A., Liang, Y.-T., Lee, C.-H., Hosenay, R. C., and Deyoe, C. W.,** Synthesis and stability of L-ascorbate 2-sulphate, *J. Chem. Soc. Perkin Trans. 1,* p. 1220, 1974.

92. **Goren, M. B. and Kochansky, M. E.,** The stringent requirement for electrophiles in the facile solvolytic hydrolysis of neutral sulfate ester salts, *J. Org. Chem.,* 38, 3510, 1973.

93. **McKenna, J. and Norymberski, J. K.,** Steroid sulphates. II. Cholestan-3β-yl methyl sulphate and cholesteryl methyl sulphate, *J. Chem. Soc.,* p. 3893, 1957.

94. **Emiliozzi, R.,** Esters sulfuriques mixtures du méthanol et d'hydroxystéroides dans la série de l'androstane, *Bull. Soc. Chim. Fr.,* p. 911, 1960.

95. **Kaiser, E. T.,** Reactions of sulfonate and sulfate esters, in *Organic Chemistry of Sulfur,* Oae, S., Ed., Plenum Press, New York, 1977.

96. **Himmelspach, K. and Wrede, J.,** Use of 2-[(4- aminophenyl)-sulfonyl] -ethyl hydrogen sulfate for the preparation of a dextran-specific immunogen, *FEBS Lett.,* 18, 118, 1971.

97. **Fitzgerald, J. W.,** The tris-catalysed isomerization of potassium D-glucose 6-*O*-sulfate, *Can. J. Biochem.,* 53, 906, 1975.

98. **Chin, C.-C. and Warren, J. C.,** Synthesis of 2-diazoestrone sulfate and use for affinity labeling of steroid binding sites, *Biochemistry,* 9, 1917, 1970.

99. **Dodgson, K. S. and Spencer, B.,** Studies on sulphatases. 15. The arylsulphatases of human serum and urine, *Biochem. J.,* 65, 668, 1957.

100. **Kurusu, T., Tagaki, W., and Oae, S.,** Reaction of *p*-nitrophenyl sulfate with thiophenol, *Bull. Chem. Soc. Jpn.,* 43, 1553, 1970.

101. **Mulder, G. J., Hinson, J. A., and Gillette, J. R.,** Conversion of the *N-O*-glucuronide and *N-O*-sulfate conjugates of *N*-hydroxyphenacetin to reactive intermediates, *Biochem. Pharmacol.,* 27, 1641, 1978.

102. **Karlsson, K.-A., Samuelsson, B. E., and Steen, G. O.,** Mass spectrometry of polar complex lipids. Analysis of a sulfatide derivative, *Biochem. Biophys. Res. Commun.,* 37, 22, 1969.

103. **Bronaugh, R. L., Hattox., S. E., Hoehn, M. M., Murphy, R. C., and Rutledge, C. O.,** The separation and identification of dopamine 3-*O*-sulfate and dopamine 4-*O*-sulfate in urine of Parkinsonian patients, *J. Pharmacol. Exp. Ther.,* 195, 441, 1975.

104. **Yeh, S. Y., Gorodetzky, C. W., and Krebs, H. A.,** Isolation and identification of morphine 3- and 6-glucuronides, morphine 3,6-diglucuronide, morphine 3-ethereal sulfate, normorphine and normorphine 6-glucuronide as morphine metabolites in humans, *J. Pharm. Sci.,* 66, 1288, 1977.

105. **Murray, S. and Baillie, T. A.,** Direct derivatization of sulphate esters for analysis by gas chromatography mass spectrometry, *Biomed. Mass Spectrom.,* 6, 82, 1979.

106. **Eberlein, W. R.,** Transesterification of urinary steroid sulfates, *J. Clin. Endocrinol. Metab.,* 22, 963, 1962.

107. **Havinga, E., de Jongh, R. O., and Dorst, W.,** Photochemical acceleration of the hydrolyses of nitrophenyl phosphates and nitrophenyl sulphates, *Rec. Trav. Chim.,* 75, 378, 1956.

108. **Lloyd, A. G., Balazs, E. A., Embery, G., and Wusteman, F. S.,** The self-irradiation of carbohydrate O-[^{35}S]-sulphate and N-[^{35}S]-sulphate esters, *Biochem. J.,* 98, 34p., 1966.

109. **Shapiro, S. S. and Poon, J. P.,** Apparent sulfation of glycosaminoglycans by ascorbic acid 2-[^{35}S] sulfate: an explanation, *Biochim. Biophys. Acta,* 385, 221, 1975.

110. **Kice, J. L., Anderson, J. M., and Pawlowski, N. E.,** The mechanism of the acid hydrolysis of Bunte salts (*S*-alkyl and *S*-aryl thiosulfates), *J. Am. Chem. Soc.,* 88, 5245, 1966.

111. **Mumma, R. O., Fujitani, K., and Hoiberg, C. P.,** Dicyclohexylcarbodiimide — mediated sulfation of alkanethiols. New method for preparation of organic thiosulfates, *J. Chem. Eng. Data,* 15, 358, 1970.

112. **Lecher, H. Z. and Hardy, E. M.,** Some new methods for preparing Bunte salts, *J. Org. Chem.,* 20, 475, 1955.

113. **Milligan, B. and Swan, J. M.,** Bunte salts (RSSO$_3$Na), *Rev. Pure Appl. Chem.,* 12, 72, 1962.

114. **Nakamura, T. and Sato, R.,** Synthesis from sulphate and accumulation of *S*-sulphocysteine by a mutant strain of *Aspergillus nidulans, Biochem. J.,* 86, 328, 1963.

115. **Williams, R. T.,** *Detoxication Mechanisms,* Chapman and Hall, London, 1959, 492.

116. **Siegel, L. M.,** Biochemistry of the sulfur cycle, in *Metabolic Pathways,* Vol. 7, 3rd ed., Greenberg, D. M., Ed., Academic Press, New York, 1975.

117. **Audrieth, L. F., Sveda, M., Sisler, H. H., and Butler, M. J.,** Sulfamic acid, sulfamide and related aquo-ammonosulfuric acids, *Chem. Rev.,* 26, 49, 1940.

118. **Boyland, E., Manson, D., and Orr, S. F. D.,** The biochemistry of aromatic amines. 2. The conversion of arylamines into arylsulphamic acids an arylamine *N*-glucosiduronic acids, *Biochem. J.,* 65, 417, 1957.

119. **Audrieth, L. F. and Sveda, M.,** Preparation and properties of some *N*-substituted sulfamic acids, *J. Org. Chem.,* 9, 89, 1944.

120. **Spillane, W. J.,** Sulfamic acid and its derivatives, *Int. J. Sulfur Chem.,* 8, 469, 1973.

121. **Lloyd, A. G., Wusteman, F. S., Tudball, N., and Dodgson, K. S.,** Preparation of potassium 2-deoxy-2-[^{35}S]-sulphoamino-D-glucose, *Biochem. J.,* 92, 68, 1964.

122. **Lloyd, A. G., Embery, G., and Fowler, L. J.,** Studies on heparin degradation. I. Preparation of [^{35}S]-sulphamate derivatives for studies on heparin degrading enzymes of mammalian origin, *Biochem. Pharmacol.,* 20, 637, 1971.

123. **Inoue, Y. and Nagasawa, K.,** Synthesis and spectral properties of *N*-sulfated and /or *O*-sulfated amino alcohols, *J. Org. Chem.,* 38, 1810, 1973.

124. **Mungall, W. S., Lemmen, L. J., Lemmen, K. L., Dethmers, J. K., and Norling, L. L.,** Nucleoside 5′-monophosphate analogues. Synthesis of 5′-sulfoamino-5′-deoxynucleosides, *J. Med. Chem.,* 21, 704, 1978.

125. **Hurd, C. D. and Kharasch, N.,** Reaction of the dioxane-sulfotrioxide reagent with aniline. Classification of the sulfamic acids, *J. Am. Chem. Soc.,* 69, 2113, 1947.

126. **Foster, A. B. and Huggard, A. J.,** The chemistry of heparin, *Adv. Carbohydr. Chem.,* 10, 335, 1955.

127. **Spillane, W. J., Goggin, C. B., Regan, N., and Scott, F. L.,** Kinetics and mechanism of the acid-catalyzed hydrolysis of *N*-phenylsulfamic acid, *Int. J. Sulfur Chem.,* 8, 565, 1976.

128. **Spillane, W. J., Regan, N., and Scott, F. L.,** Kinetics and mechanism of the acid-catalyzed hydrolysis of sodium *N*-1-naphthylsulphamate, *J. Chem. Soc. Perkin Trans. 2, p.* 445, 1974.

129. **Spillane, W. J., Scott, F. L., and Goggin, C. B.,** Kinetics and mechanisms of hydrolysis of *N*-alkyl and *N,N*-dialkylsulfamic acids, *Int. J. Sulfur Chem., Part A,* 1, 223, 1971.

130. **Spillane, W. J., Goggin, C. B., Regan, N., and Scott, F. L.,** Taft polar + steric equation as related to the hydrolysis of sulfamates, *Int. J. Sulfur Chem., Part A,* 3, 281, 1973.

131. **Scott, F. L. and Spillane, W. J.,** Mechanism of cleavage of the nitrogen-sulphur bond in *N*-arylsulphamates, *Chem. Ind., p.* 1999, 1967.

132. **Inoue, Y. and Nagasawa, K.,** Hydrolytic properties of *N*-sulfated compounds containing neighbouring hydroxyl or sulfate groups with reference to chemical properties of natural heparin, *Carbohydr. Res.,* 31, 359, 1973.

133. **Nagasawa, K. and Inoue, Y.,** Solvolytic desulfation of 2-deoxy-2-sulfoamino-D-glucose and D-glucose 6–sulfate, *Carbohydr. Res.,* 36, 265, 1974.

134. **Spillane, W. J. and Scott, F. L.,** The rearrangement of phenylsulphamic acid to sulphanilic acid in the presence of [^{35}S]-sulphuric acid, *J. Chem. Soc. B,* p. 779, 1968.

135. **Spillane, W. J., Scott, F. L., and Goggin, C. B.,** Studies on the rearrangement of 1- and 2-naphthylsulphamic acids, *J. Chem. Soc. B,* p. 2409, 1971.

136. **Nakano, K. and Yamaguchi, H.,** Sulfuration by use of *N*-substituted sulfamic acids, *Kogyo Kagaku Zasshi,* 67, 2055, 1964.

137. **Nagasawa, K. and Yoshidome, H.,** Alcoholysis reaction of sulfamic acids and its application to the preparation of biochemically related sulfate esters, *Chem. Pharm. Bull.,* 18, 2023, 1970.

138. **Fischer, J.-C., Palavit, G., Wartel, M., and Heubel, J.,** Préparation et caractérisation d'un sulfatophosphate, NaH$_2$PSO$_7$, *C. R. Acad. Sci., Ser. C,* 274, 867, 1972.

139. **Audrieth, L. F., Mills, J. R., and Netherton, L. E.,** Polymerization and depolymerization phenomena in phosphate-metaphosphate systems at higher temperatures. II. The thermal behavior of alkali metal monohydrogen sulfate—monohydrogen phosphate mixtures, *J. Phys. Chem.,* 58, 482, 1954.

140. **Benkovic, S. J. and Hevey, R. C.,** Studies in sulfate esters. V. The mechanism of hydrolysis of phenyl phosphosulfate, a model system for 3'-phosphoadenosine-5'-phosphosulfate, *J. Am. Chem. Soc.,* 92, 4971, 1970.

141. **Tagaki, W., Eiki, T., and Tanaka, I.,** The syntheses and hydrolyses of *p*-substituted phenyl phosphosulphates, *Bull. Chem. Soc. Jpn.,* 44, 1139, 1971.

142. **Baddiley, J., Buchanan, J. G., and Letters, R.,** Synthesis of adenosine-5' sulphatophosphate. A degradation product of an intermediate in the enzymic synthesis of sulphuric esters, *J. Chem. Soc.,* p. 1067, 1957.

143. **Cherniak, R. and Davidson, E. A.,** Synthesis of adenylyl sulfate and adenylyl sulfate 3'-phosphate, *J. Biol. Chem.,* 239, 2986, 1964.

144. **Reichard, P. and Ringertz, N. R.,** Chemical synthesis of adenosine 5'-phosphosulfates, *J. Am. Chem. Soc.,* 81, 878, 1959.

145. **Michelson, A. M. and Wold, F.,** Synthesis of some nucleotide anhydrides, *Biochemistry,* 1, 1171, 1962.

146. **Baddiley, J., Buchanan, J. G., Letters, R., and Sanderson, A. R.,** Synthesis of "Active sulphate" (Adenosine 3'-phosphate 5'-sulphatophosphate), *J. Chem. Soc.,* p. 1731. 1959.

147. **Melville, E. and Rutherford, F.,** A simple preparation of phospho-adenylyl sulphate labelled with ^{35}sulphur, *FEBS Lett.,* 37, 257, 1973.

148. **Horwitz, J. P., Neenan, J. P., Misra, R. S., Rozhin, J., Huo, A., and Phillips, K. D.,** Studies on bovine adrenal estrogen sulfotransferase. III. Facile synthesis of 3'-phospho and 2'-phosphoadenosine 5'-phosphosulfate, *Biochim. Biophys. Acta,* 480, 376, 1977.

149. **Sekura, R. D. and Jakoby, W. B.,** Phenol sulfotransferases, *J. Biol. Chem.,* 254, 5658, 1979.

150. **Robbins, P. W. and Lipmann, F.,** Isolation and identification of active sulfate, *J. Biol. Chem.,* 229, 837, 1957.

151. **Adams, J. B.,** Non-enzymic sulphation of hydroxy compounds by 3'-phosphoadenosine 5'-phosphosulphate, *Biochim. Biophys. Acta,* 62, 17, 1962.

151a. **Cooper, B. P., Baumgarten, F. E., and Schmidt, A.,** Two new reactions of the activated sulfates adenylylsulfate and 3'-phosphoadenylylsulfate, *Z. Naturforsch.,* 35c, 159, 1980.

152. **Wusteman, F. S., Dodgson, K. S., Lloyd, A. G., Rose, F. A., and Tudball, N.,** Thin-layer chromatography in the study of ester sulphates, *J. Chromatogr.,* 16, 334, 1964.

153. **Raedsch, R., Hofmann, A. F. and Tserng, K.-O.,** Separation of individual sulfated bile acid conjugates as calcium complexes using reversed-phase partition thin-layer chromatography, *J. Lipid Res.,* 20, 796, 1979.

154. **Schneider, J. L. and Lewbart, M. L.,** Enzymatic synthesis of steroid sulfates, *J. Biol. Chem.,* 222, 787, 1956.

155. **Diamond, G. and Quebbemann, A. J.,** Rapid separation of p-nitrophenol and its glucuronide and sulfate conjugates by reversed-phase high-performance liquid chromatography, *J. Chromatogr.,* 177, 368, 1979.

156. **Pennings, E. J. M. and Van Kempen, G. M. J.,** Analysis of 3'-phosphoadenylylsulfate and related compounds by paired-ion high-performance liquid chromatography, *J. Chromatogr.,* 176, 478, 1979.

157. **Dodgson, K. S.,** Determination of inorganic sulphate in studies on the enzymic and non-enzymic hydrolysis of carbohydrate and other sulphate esters, *Biochem. J.,* 78, 312, 1961.

158. **Ginsberg, L. C. and Di Ferrante, N.,** Sensitive methods for the determination of ester sulfate in biological systems, *Biochem. Med.,* 17, 80, 1977.

159. **Dodgson, K. S. and Spencer, B.,** Studies on the sulphatases. 5. The determination of inorganic sulphate in the study of sulphatases, *Biochem. J.,* 55, 436, 1953.
160. **Waheed, A. and Van Etten, R. L.,** A spectrophotometric determination of sulfate ion and its application in studies of substrate purity and of aryl sulfatase A kinetics, *Anal. Biochem.,* 89, 550, 1978.
161. **Belcher, T., Bogdanski, S. L., Rix, I. H. B., and Townshend, A.,** A review of methods for the determination of sulphate in urine, *Mikrochim. Acta,* 2, 81, 1977.
162. **Nader, H. B. and Dietrich, C. P.,** Determination of sulfate after chromatography and toluidine blue complex formation. *Anal. Biochem.,* 89, 550, 1978.
163. **Mitchell, S. C. and Waring, R. H.,** Detection of inorganic sulphate and other anions on paper and thin-layer chromatogram, *J. Chromatogr.,* 166, 341, 1978.
164. **Hadler, W. A., Da Cruz-Hoefling, M. A., and Ziti, L. M.,** The benzidine technique for the histochemical detection of the sulfate ion, *Acta Histochem.* 61, 197, 1978.

Chapter 3

SULFATE AVAILABILITY IN VIVO

G. J. Mulder

TABLE OF CONTENTS

I. INTRODUCTION

Sulfate availability to the organism may limit the role sulfation may play. In this chapter the various mechanisms by which sulfate is provided to the cell will be briefly discussed. In the next chapter the activation step, required for the synthesis of the donor of the sulfate group, adenosine 3′-phosphate 5′-sulfatophosphate (PAPS), will be discussed. Where possible, recent reviews will be referred to so that further information may be obtained from these sources.

Basically, there are two primary sources of inorganic sulfate: absorption of this anion from the gut and oxidation of the amino acid cysteine. Under some conditions, however, catabolism of sulfated macromolecules, especially glycosaminoglycans, may also provide inorganic sulfate.[1] Another possible route of administration is the absorption of inorganic sulfate from the airways, when it is applied as a spray.[2,3] In the isolated perfused rat lung it is rapidly absorbed after intratracheal administration, and causes bronchoconstriction due to local histamine release.

In some species inorganic sulfur may be converted by the microflora in the intestine to inorganic sulfate;[4] this occurs, for instance, in ruminants, but not in man or the rat and most other laboratory species.

II. ABSORPTION OF INORGANIC SULFATE FROM THE GUT

It would be expected that a primary source of inorganic sulfate in the body would be intake with the food and subsequent absorption from the gut. However, in many pharmacological handbooks the belief is expressed that inorganic sulfate salts tend to be absorbed minimally and hence, add water to the bowel, thus leading to diarrhea.[5] *Martindale's Pharmacopoeia*[6] states that sodium sulfate is "poorly absorbed from the gastronintestinal tract." This poor absorption is believed to explain the cathartic effect of oral administration of inorganic sulfate salts. Yet, the available data show that inorganic sulfate is excellently absorbed after oral administration, in spite of the supposedly poor membrane-permeating properties of this anion.[7] Therefore, the above explanation is apparently incorrect.

In the beginning of this century a strong controversy existed between those who contended that sulfate for sulfation only arose from sources other than absorbed inorganic sulfate (the sulfur-containing amino acids, for instance), and those that tried to prove that also inorganic sulfate in the food was available for sulfation.[8] At that time, of course, it was hard to prove that orally administered inorganic sulfate was used for sulfation, since no radioactive sulfate was available. Later it was shown that [35S]-labeled inorganic sulfate was absorbed from the intestinal tract, and was incorporated into many endogenous and exogenous substances.[9]

One of the first papers that conclusively showed absorption of inorganic sulfate and its utilization for sulfation of drugs was published in 1931 by Hele.[10] When he fed his dogs Patsy and Pansy nonradioactive inorganic sulfate, he measured a great increase in their urinary output of sulfate; upon addition of phenol, by stomach tube, the amount of free inorganic sulfate in urine decreased, and it was replaced by a big increase in the amount of ethereal sulfate, presumably phenyl sulfate. Similar results were obtained with indole showing that it was converted in vivo *(inter alia)* to indoxyl sulfate.

One of the problems at that time was the quantitative determination of inorganic sulfate and sulfate esters. Free inorganic sulfate was usually precipitated by barium chloride, and sulfur was determined in the precipitate. Total sulfur (without barium chloride precipitation) was also determined in the sample; subtraction yielded organic, presumably esterified, sulfur. This method, of course, gives inaccurate data because several other sources of sulfur (e.g., mercapturates) are measured as ethereal sulfate. Yet Hele's findings[10] however, were fairly conclusive, and indicated that inorganic sulfate was absorbed from the gastrointestinal tract in the dog. He found that about 22 to 66% of the sodium sulfate administered (0.8 mmol/kg daily) was utilized for synthesis of phenyl sulfate or indoxyl sulfate.

The first use of radiolabeled sulfate was reported in 1937.[11] Radioactive sodium [^{35}S]-sulfate was administered orally to a human volunteer, and urine was collected for several days. Of the dose of sodium sulfate (6.3 mmol) 15% was recovered within 9 hr. in the urine and a further 32% in the following 15 hr. This clearly showed that sodium sulfate was absorbed to a high degree. Much later, Bauer [12] showed the same for a tracer dose of [^{35}S]-sulfate that was administered orally to fasted volunteers (Figure 1). Eighty percent or greater was recovered in the 24-hr urine. Sixty to one hundred min after oral administration, [^{35}S]-sulfate attained equilibrium and achieved a plasma concentration equivalent to the intravenously administered tracer. This again proves rapid and almost complete absorption of a low dose of inorganic sulfate from the gut in man.

After the second world war more work with radiolabeled [^{35}S]-sulfate was reported, and it was firmly established (although not always accepted)[13] that inorganic sulfate fed to animals, was available in the body for incorporation into endogenous and exogenous substances. Within 24 hr, for instance, Dziewiatkowski[14] recovered more the 70% of the oral dose of sodium [^{35}S]-sulfate (1 mmol/kg) in the urine of the rat. Morrow et al.[15] recovered 41 to 64% of a tracer dose of sodium sulfate in urine within 8 hr after oral administration to 24 hr fasted cats; similar findings were obtained in an intestinal loop *in situ*. In the rat, [^{35}S]-labeled sodium and calcium sulfate were absorbed from the gut to a high degree:[16,17] in feeding experiments the sulfates were administered with the food at two levels, 0.10 and 0.42% (w/w), and 60 to 80% of the sulfate salts was absorbed. Subsequently, [^{35}S]-radioactivity was excreted in urine, or incorporated into endogenous compounds such as glycosaminoglycans in cartilage. These results confirmed the absorption of sulfate from the gut. A difference observed between the rats fed calcium sulfate and sodium sulfate[17] may be fictitious, since both diets contained calcium carbonate, and ionization in the stomach would yield both salts. Using unlabeled sulfate, Wellers[18] found a similar increase in the urinary output of inorganic sulfate after adding sodium sulfate to the food of rats.

In sheep, a rapid and fairly complete absorption of a tracer dose of sodium [^{35}S] sulfate was observed.[19,20] The radioactivity reached a peak in the plasma at 6 hr, and approximately 75% was excreted in urine. In baby pigs, more than 60% of the dose was recovered in urine.[21,22]

More detailed measurements were performed in adult pigs by Berry et al.[23] They studied absorption, excretion, placental transfer, and maternal-fetal tissue distribution of (presumably) a tracer dose of [^{35}S]-labeled sodium sulfate. The swine (gilts and barrows) were placed in metabolism crates, and blood, urine, and feces were collected. At the end of the collection period the animals were slaughtered and the tissue distribution of the radioactivity was determined. A peak in [^{35}S]-radioactivity in serum was found about 2 to 3 hr after an oral dose (Figure 1). Within 48 hr about 50% of the radioactivity had been excreted in urine; after intravenous (i.v.) administration, this was about 60%. Less than 2% had been excreted in feces after 48 hr, indicating almost complete absorption.

Similar experiments were done in dogs[24] that were dosed orally with ammonium sulfate (about 0.5 to 1.0 mmol/kg). The plasma sulfate concentration, determined 3½ hr after administration, had increased from 1.4 mM in controls to 2.2 mM after ammonium sulfate administration. At the same time there was a strong increase in the urinary output of inorganic sulfate. Within 4 hr about 50% of the dose had already been absorbed from the gut; the remainder was still in the intestine.

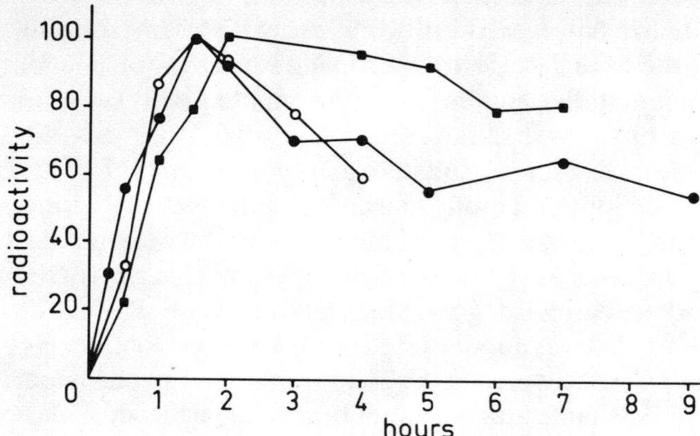

FIGURE 1.   Absorption of a tracer dose of [35S]-labeled sodium sulfate after oral administration in man, rat, and swine: plasma concentrations of radioactivity. The data for man[12] (○ − ○); for swine[23] (■ − ■); and for the rat[26] (● − ●). The highest value in each set of data has been taken to be 100, and the other values were calculated as percentage of this. The tracer dose was administered orally at t = 0.

In man, Meier and Schmidt-Kessen[25] also observed a rapid absorption of an orally administered mixture of (unlabeled) sodium-, magnesium-, and calcium-sulfate given in a total dose of 15 mmol (5 mmol of each salt). Their data suggest that the greater part of the dose is absorbed and ultimately excreted in urine in agreement with the results of Bauer.[12]

Finally in the rat, fairly complete data were obtained by Krijgsheld et al.[26] In the conscious, freely moving rat they administered various oral doses of sodium [35S]-sulfate. At a relatively low dose (3 mmol/kg), over 80% of the radioactivity was recovered in urine, indicating almost complete absorption of the dose. At a higher dose, however, the recovery in urine decreased because of diarrhea, and sodium sulfate was lost in the watery feces. Approximately 2 hr following oral administration, a peak in the [35S]-concentration in plasma was found (Figure 1). When 8 to 15 mmol/kg sodium sulfate were given, the serum concentration of inorganic sulfate increased from the normal level of 0.8 mM to 2.0 mM at the peak (Table 1). Interestingly, in control groups that received isoosmotic doses of sodium chloride a decrease in the serum level of sulfate was observed, for which as yet no explanation has been given.

The results described above permit several conclusions to be drawn. First, sodium sulfate and several other sulfate salts are rapidly absorbed from the gut in all species studied so far; since biological membranes are believed to be almost impermeable to sulfate, at least by diffusion, this passage would presumably require a carrier (facilitated diffusion?). The absorption of sulfate from the gut is almost quantitative, unless diarrhea occurs, preventing absorption. The serum sulfate concentration may increase two- to three-fold following oral administration of inorganic sulfate; further increases will presumably be prevented by renal excretion (see below).

The cathartic effect of sulfate solutions is probably not the result of a lack of absorption of sulfate from the gut. More likely however, the rapid transport of water into the gut, which is more rapid that that of sulfate from the gut into blood, causes accumulation of water in the gut, and thereby diarrhea.

Ammonia, calcium, potassium, and sodium salts of sulfate are used as food additives, The U.S. Food and Drug Administration (FDA) has proposed to give these food additives a generally recognized as safe (GRAS) status.[27] The inorganic sulfate content

Table 1

**EFFECT OF ORAL ADMINISTRATION OF SODIUM SULFATE AND SODIUM
CHLORIDE ON SERUM SULFATE IN THE RAT**

Orally administered	Serum sulfate concentration (mM)
Nothing	0.77 ± 0.04
Sodium sulfate	
0.5 mmol	1.34 ± 0.06[a]
2.5 mmol	1.95 ± 0.15[a]
5.0 mmol	2.13 ± 0.09[a]
Sodium chloride	
0.15 mmol	0.66 ± 0.03[b]
2.5 mmol	0.57 ± 0.02[a]
7.5 mmol	0.58 ± 0.02[a]

Note: The dose was administered in a volume of 2 ml water to rats of 300-g body weight. Serum sulfate was determined 2 hr after the administration of the dose, by a turbidimetric method. Blood was withdrawn under ether anaesthesia. The mean ± S.E.M. for 6 rats per group is given.

[a] Significantly different from control at $p < 0.005$ (Wilcoxon's test).
[b] The same at $p < 0.05$.

From Krijgsheld, K. R., Frankena, H., Scholtens, E., Zweens, J., and Mulder, G. J., *Biochim. Biophys. Acta,* 586, 492, 1979. With permission.

in most food products is unknown, presumably because it seemed of marginal nutritional importance (but see Section V).

III. INTESTINAL CARRIER TRANSPORT OF INORGANIC SULFATE

Since the sulfate anion is not very lipid soluble, a carrier most likely is involved in the transport of this ion across biological membranes as has been reported for erythrocytes (see section VI). The first indication of such a carrier transport in the intestine was reported by Deyrup in 1963, [28] who found in vitro a sodium-dependent accumulation of [^{35}S]-sulfate in the lower ileum of the rat. These findings were confirmed by Anast et al. [29] using the everted sac technique with intestine from rat, rabbit, and hamster. Their results suggest that sulfate transport is energy-dependent. Dziewiatkowski[7] confirmed this in a study on the properties of the sulfate transport system in everted sacs from rat intestine; metabolic inhibitors such as sodium azide inhibited the transport. Whereas transport from mucosal side to serosal side was highest in the ileum, the reverse transport was highest in the jejunum. Batt,[30] using mouse intestinal ring segments, similarly observed highest activity of the carrier in the terminal ileum of the adult mouse. In the very young mouse sulfate transport was very active along the whole small intestine and in the colon; 3 weeks after birth, however, the adult pattern had established itself, with the highest transport activity in the ileum. No sex differences were observed for sulfate transport. Prior hypophysectomy decreased the activity of the sulfate carrier in the rat intestinal everted sac;[29] this could be counteracted by injection of bovine growth hormone. The rate of transport in everted sacs from guinea pig intestine was higher than that in the rat preparation.[31]

More evidence on the carrier-mediated sulfate transport in the intestine came from work of Cardin and Mason.[32,33] Using the everted sac technique with rat lower ileum, they observed that a concentration gradient of [^{35}S]-sulfate was established across the sac wall: the [^{35}S]-concentration inside (serosa side) increased by as much as nine times over the concentration outside (mucosa side) at low concentration of sulfate. At higher sulfate concentrations (applied at the mucosa side) the gradient was less steep; this proved that sulfate accumulated against a concentration gradient. The apparent K_m of sulfate for the carrier was 0.4 to 0.6 mM, and the transport was saturable. Between the gut tissue and the solution inside in the sac there was no sulfate concentration gradient, indicating that sulfate could freely diffuse, once it had passed the mucosa cells. The sulfate transport was inhibited competitively by chemically related anions such as molybdate, tungstate, selenate, thiosulfate, and sulfite. Conversely, the transport of molybdate and tungstate was inhibited competitively by sulfate, and similarly was highest in the lower ileum of the rat. K_m values for the transport of these ions were of the same order of that for sulfate, but the V_{max} values were slightly lower. Similar transport phenomena were observed by Mason and Cardin in pieces from sheep intestine.[34] Recently, the sulfate transport in a marine gastropod, *Aplysia californica* intestine has been studied.[35]

The existence of sulfate transport across frog gastric mucosa has been suggested but has not been further substantiated.[36] Other sulfate carrier systems, such as occur in the erythrocyte, will be discussed in Section VI.

IV. GENERATION OF INORGANIC SULFATE FROM CYSTEINE AND METHIONINE

Most, if not all, of the sulfate requirements of mammals can be met with methionine and cysteine, ingested with the food in the form of proteins.[37] To this end, the -SH group of cysteine is oxidized, resulting in the release of SO_4^{2-}. Methionine can be converted into cysteine by transsulfuration. Reviews on the various aspects of conversion of sulfur in the amino acids into inorganic sulfate are available.[38-40] Here, the relevant data will be discussed only briefly.

The transsulfuration pathway, converting methionine into cysteine, proceeds according to the scheme shown in Figure 2.[39] Influences of the diet, hormones, age, and many other details on this pathway can be found in a review by Finkelstein.[38] Patients with a genetically deficient cystathionine synthesis have been described (see Finkelstein [41] for a review).

Through oxidation, cysteine is converted into alanine 3-sulfinate (Figure 3), presumably by cytosolic enzymes;[40] a dioxygenase incorporates both atoms of molecular oxygen into the substrate. Subsequently the sulfinate is transferred to the mitochondria and reacts with 2-oxoglutarate or oxaloacetate by transamination.[42] The 3-sulfinopyruvate spontaneously decomposes to sulfite. In the rat nicotinamide, hydrocortisone, and cysteine enhanced the cytosolic dioxygenase activity by an as yet unknown mechanism (Reference 43 and references therein).

In the rat, deprivation of sulfur-containing amino acids causes a dramatic decrease in the urinary excretion of inorganic sulfate, decreasing to near zero, shortly after beginning the sulfur-free diet.[44,45] The excretion of "ethereal" sulfate, though also decreases, continued long after free sulfate had virtually disappeared from the urine. At least 50 mg of methionine-sulfur per kilogram per day was required to sustain a positive growth rate and a positive sulfur balance. At that level however, inorganic sulfate in urine was still much below control. Yet, the urinary excretion of sulfate esters was about normal. Not only methionine, but also homocysteine could be used to provide sufficient sulfur to the rats. Further studies on methionine utilization have been reported by Almquist.[46] Uren et al.[47] have tried to decrease cysteine availability in vivo by injection of cyst(e)ine degrading enzymes in the rat; an i.v. injection of γ-cystathionase was briefly effective, and the γ-cystathionase inhibitor propargylglycine prevented this.

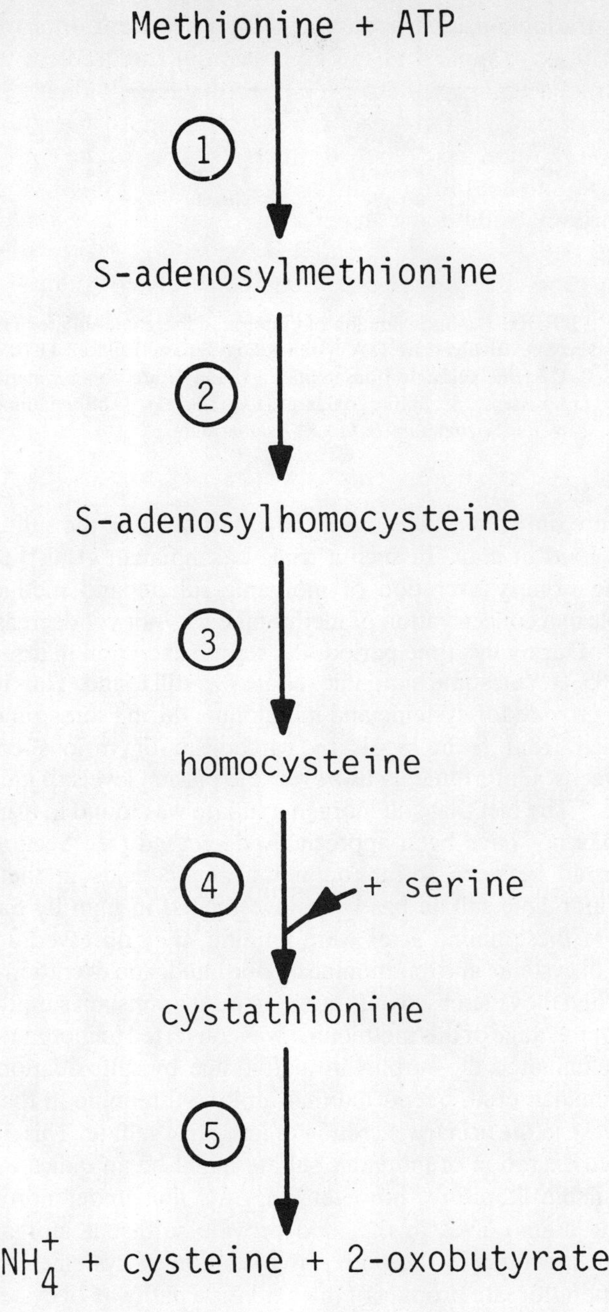

FIGURE 2. The cystathionine pathway. Enzymes in the scheme: 1. ATP : L-methionine *S*-adenosyltransferase (EC 2.5.1.6). 2. *S*-adenosyl-L-methionine : L-homocysteine *S*-methyltransferase (EC 2.1.1.10.). 3. *S*-adenosyl-L-homocysteine hydrolase (EC 3.3.1.1.). 4. Cystathionine β-synthetase (EC 4.2.1.22) (L-serine hydrolyase, adding homocysteine). 5. L-Cystathionine cysteine-lyase, deaminating (EC 4.4.1.1.).

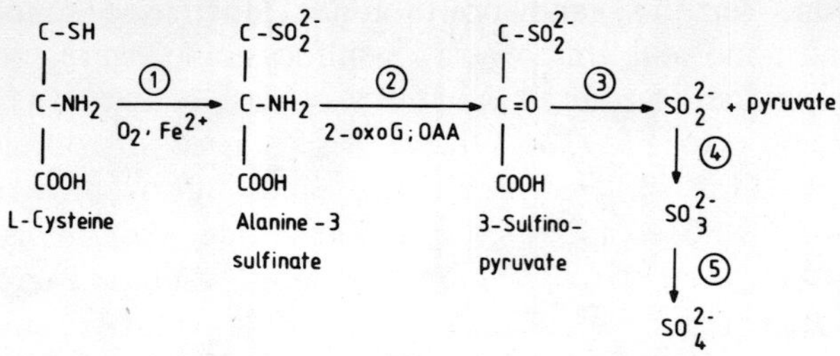

FIGURE 3.   Sulfoxidation of cysteine to inorganic sulfate. The enzymes involved are 1. A cysteine dioxygenase (EC 1.13.11.20.), 2. Cysteine sulfinate transaminase, 3. and 4. are nonenzymatic, rapid steps, 5. Sulfite oxidase (EC 1.8.3.1). Abbreviations: 2-oxoG, 2-oxoglutarate; OAA, oxaloacetate.

So far there are only few studies on the effect of deleting the sulfur-containing amino acids from the food in man. In such a trial, Lakshmanan et al.[48] found the expected decrease of the urinary excretion of inorganic sulfate and methionine; surprisingly however, the plasma concentration of methionine was not yet decreased 8 days after the start of the diet. During this time period, the sulfate excretion in urine was decreased by approximately 65%. Yet, some inorganic sulfate was still found. Thus it seems that protein catabolism can provide for cysteine and methionine during some time; inorganic sulfate may be released from tissue pools by catabolism of various compounds such as glycosaminoglycans. Unfortunately however, the plasma levels of inorganic sulfate were not determined.[48] The fact that still inorganic sulfate was found in urine suggests that the plasma level may not have been appreciably decreased (see Section VI).

The relationship between sulfur-containing amino acids in the food and urinary elimination of inorganic sulfate has been investigated in man by Sabry et al.[49] Under conditions where these amino acids were limiting, they observed a linear relationship between intake of cysteine and methionine on one hand, and excretion of inorganic sulfate on the other. When they increased only methionine at a constant supply of the other amino acids, a higher percentage of this methionine was converted to inorganic sulfate, indicating that the body eliminated the surplus in methionine by sulfoxidation. Parallel to these findings, Lakshmanan et al.[50] reported that limiting threonine in the diet, resulted in a significant increase in the urinary excretion of inorganic sulfate. This finding thus suggests that an increased excretion of inorganic sulfate might be an indicator of an unbalanced diet.[51] The available literature, however, suggests that under normal conditions, the sulfur-containing amino acids in the food provide sufficient inorganic sulfate for the various sulfation reactions in the body, by oxidation of cysteine.[52,53]

Sulfite is the penultimate product of the oxidation pathway of cysteine to sulfate. The pharmacokinetics of (i.v. administered) sulfite have been investigated in several mammalian species.[54,55] In most species it is rapidly converted to sulfate; the sulfite oxidase activity however, may be rate limiting at high doses of sulfite. An inverse correlation between sulfite oxidation and bisulfite toxicity in rabbit, hamster, guinea pig, mouse, and rat has been found:[56] the highest rate of the oxidase is observed in the rat, which is least sensitive to sulfite toxicity. Superoxide anions may be involved in sulfite oxidation.[57]

Recently, two patients with an inherited disease of sulfite oxidation have been described, in whom the sulfite oxidase activity was extremely low or not present. Mudd et al.[58-61] clearly demonstrated a defective sulfite oxidase in a patient that died at 2½ years of age. The child had many neurological abnormalities at birth, such as severe mental retardation, seizures, and opisthotonos. Increased amounts of sulfite, thiosulfate, and an abnormal amino acid, S-sulfocysteine, were found in urine. In post-mortem liver, kidney, and brain no sulfite oxidase activity was observed.[61] Two more patients were reported in 1977.[62] When a diet low in sulfur-containing amino acids was introduced, there was some physical and mental improvement. In retrospect, it might have been worthwhile to add some inorganic sulfate, to ensure a sufficient supply for sulfation reactions; then even less sulfur-containing amino acids might have been given. It seems that the latter patients had a less complete block of sulfite oxidase than the patient reported by Mudd et al.,[58] because about 50% of total sulfur in urine was in the form of inorganic sulfate, whereas Mudd's patient excreted almost no sulfate at all. This genetic defect in sulfur metabolism has been extensively reviewed by Finkelstein,[41] who also discussed several more genetic deficiencies in sulfur metabolism in man. Despite the occurrence of this genetic deficiency in the handling of sulfite, inorganic sulfite salts have been considered relatively safe as food additives.[63]

Finally it should be mentioned that methionine in the food is an important source of "activated" methyl groups, and that cysteine is required for glutathione synthesis, and in many species is the only precursor of taurine. An early review on many aspects discussed in this and the following section appeared in 1966.[64]

V. NUTRITIONAL ASPECTS OF INORGANIC SULFATE FEEDING

The potential growth-promoting effect of sulfate feeding in chickens, sheep, and several other species has extensively been investigated (see for reviews References 4 and 65). The assumption is that a sufficient supply of inorganic sulfate in the food might decrease the need for sulfoxidation of cysteine; thereby, more cysteine and methionine would be available for protein synthesis, resulting in increased growth. Therefore, the effect of various dietary sulfate salts on growth rates has been determined in a variety of species. In the chicken, both a growth-promoting and a growth-inhibiting effect was observed, depending on the sulfate salt used and other conditions.[66-68] In sheep a positive sulfur balance is of economic importance, since wool contains a high percentage of sulfur-containing amino acids. Sulfate feeding promotes growth in sheep.[69-71] A similar effect has been observed in pigs and cattle;[72,73] 2500 mg sodium sulfate per liter is well tolerated by cattle in the drinking water for a period of at least 90 days.[74] Also in young men, the addition of inorganic sulfate to a diet of soybean protein caused an increase in the nitrogen retention, most likely by a sparing effect on growth-limiting sulfur-containing amino acids.[75]

In the rat, some more detailed experiments have been performed in order to determine the mechanism of the growth-promoting effect. Smith[76] has determined the production of $^{14}CO_2$ from [1-^{14}C]-labeled methionine in the food of rats, in the presence and absence of 0.02% (w/w) inorganic sulfate. A significant decrease in $^{14}CO_2$ production was observed when sulfate was fed, as compared to controls, indicating a decreased demethylation of methionine, presumably because less sulfoxidation was required. Thus, more methionine might be available for protein synthesis. Indeed a small increase in feeding efficiency has been observed in the rat by the addition of sodium sulfate to the food.[17] Of course such a growth-promoting effect can only be seen if the basic diet has a very low natural nonprotein sulfur or inorganic sulfate content. James and Hove[77] found only growth promotion by sodium sulfate in the food in rats when a commercial casein diet was extensively washed with water at pH 8.5; by this procedure they decreased the inorganic sulfate content from 0.074 to 0.003%, and only then did they observe the growth-promoting effect. Since in many of the studies on the efficiency of inorganic sulfate feeding the inorganic sulfate content of the various diets was not reported (and since data on sulfate utilization and absorption usually are lacking),[16] it is often hard to evaluate the effects in terms of sulfate availability in blood in the animals. In conclusion however, the available data show that under conditions in which sulfur-containing amino acids are growth-limiting, inorganic sulfate feeding may have a growth-promoting effect, most likely because it increases the availability of the sulfur-containing amino acids for protein synthesis by decreasing the need for sulfoxidation. Although inorganic sulfate salts are relatively nontoxic and may be fed for prolonged periods of time, other changes may occur. For example sheep on a 1.27% (w/w) sodium sulfate monohydrate diet acquired bacteria in the ruminal fluid that produced more propionic-, butyric-, and higher fatty acids and less lactic acid than the gut flora in controls.[78]

Gut bacteria especially in ruminants may use inorganic sulfate for the synthesis of cysteine.[64,79-83] The gut bacteria reduce inorganic sulfate to sulfide, which subsequently is converted with *O*-acetylserine to cysteine.[84] Methionine can be synthesized from cysteine by further metabolism to cystathionine.[84,85] This reduction of inorganic sulfate requires the intermediary synthesis of adenosine 3′-phosphate 5′-sulfatophosphate (PAPS), which is further reduced.

Mammalian tissues lack a sulfate reducing system.[86] In germ-free rats therefore, no incorporation of sulfite or sulfate into amino acids or protein takes place. When in normal rats inorganic sulfate is fed, some sulfur may be incorporated into protein as a result of bacterial action. If sufficient sulfur-containing amino acids are present, however, the bacteria utilize these instead of synthesizing them from inorganic sulfate.

VI. SERUM CONCENTRATION, DISTRIBUTION, AND ELIMINATION OF INORGANIC SULFATE

There are wide variations in serum concentration of inorganic sulfate in various species[87] (Table 2), as measured by the turbidimetric method, according to Berglund and Sorbö.[88] In man, serum concentrations have been reported between 0.15 and 0.5 mM, with a mean of about 0.3 mM, clearly lower than in most other mammalian species.[25,88-92] Genetic factors may be involved in the species differences, but also large variations in serum sulfate concentration are to be expected, due to different feeding habits in animals and man. When rats are fed a standard diet, the variations are rather small.[87]

Meier and Schmidt-Kessen[25] have reported a circadian rhythm in the serum sulfate concentration in man with slightly higher levels at night than during daytime. A rather steep rise occurred between 3 and 5 p.m. Krijgsheld et al.[87] observed a circadian rhythm also in rats; a peak in the serum sulfate concentration occurred in the afternoon (Figure 4), and a rapid fall between 6 and 10 p.m. was coincident with the turning off of the light and resuming of the activity of the animals.

The serum sulfate concentration is a balance between absorption of inorganic sulfate and its production from cysteine, and sulfate elimination by (mainly) urinary excretion and incorporation into low molecular-weight substrates of sulfation. The serum sulfate concentration is primarily regulated by the kidneys, because below a certain threshold inorganic sulfate is completely reabsorbed from the primary urine in the proximal tubule.[93] If the sulfate concentration in serum increases above that threshold, urinary excretion will be increased. For that reason, high i.v. infusion rates of sodium sulfate result in an osmotic diuresis. Tubular secretion of sulfate has been considered[93] but seems of little importance in those species where it has been investigated. The urinary excretion mechanisms for sulfate have been reviewed by Mudge.[93]

In view of the above findings it is not very surprising that a great variation in urinary

Table 2
SERUM SULFATE CONCENTRATIONS IN VARIOUS SPECIES

Species	Sex	Inorganic sulfate[a] (mM)	Ref.
Man	m/f	0.3	See text, 87, 152
Monkey	m/f	0.46 ± 0.10	87
Rat			
Wistar	m	0.77 ± 0.04	87
Brown Norway	m	0.82 ± 0.02	87
WAG	m	0.72 ± 0.02	87
Mouse			
Swiss	m	1.26 ± 0.12	87, 152
C57 B1/6J	?	1.00 ± 0.09	152
Guinea pig	m/f	0.84 ± 0.04	87
Rabbit	m	2.01 ± 0.13	87
Cat	f	0.68 ± 0.03	87
Dog	f	1.39 ± 0.12	24
Sheep	f	1.24 ± 0.10	87
Goat	f	2.43	87
Shetland pony	f	1.06	87
Pig	f	0.75 ± 0.03	87
Cow	f	1.80	87
Hen	f	1.82 ± 0.32	87
Rooster	m	2.41 ± 0.13	87

[a] Mean ± S.E.M. or S.D.

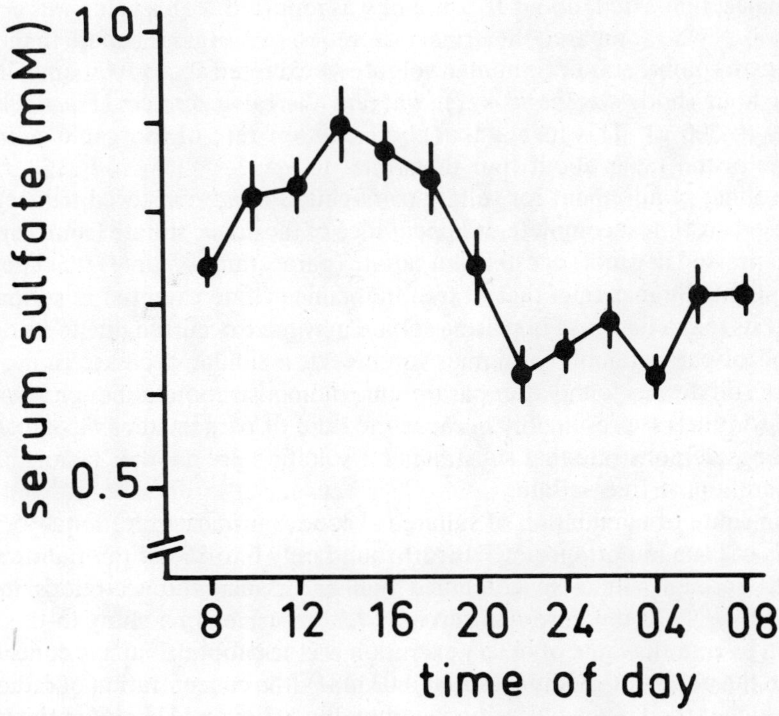

FIGURE 4. Circadian rhythm of serum sulfate in fed rats. Serum sulfate was determined turbidimetrically in blood collected from the aorta or the heart of rats anaesthesized with ether.[87] The rats had free access to food and water. Means ± S.E.M. are given of 10 rats at each point. The lights-on period was from 7 a.m. till 7 p.m.

output of inorganic sulfate is observed. First of all, it will be dependent on sulfate consumption and production. Secondly, the "sulfo-stat" in the kidneys will determine the rate of sulfate excretion in urine. Finally the blood flow to the kidneys is important: the lower the blood flow, the lower the urinary elimination. In man, the urinary inorganic sulfate excretion rate is about 20 to 25 mmol sulfate per 24 hr; [25,51,53,95-99] slightly lower values were reported for women than for men.[98] In children lower values were found:[100] about 18 mmol/24 hr for boys of 6 to 14 years of age, and 7 to 10 mmol/24 hr for girls of the same age. Considering the body weight of the children as compared to adults, it seems that their urinary excretion rate of inorganic sulfate is rather high. No data are available on age-dependent fluctations in serum sulfate levels and urinary excretion of inorganic sulfate. Upon fasting, the urinary excretion of inorganic sulfate tended to increase.[96]

Sabry et al.[49] observed a linear relationship between intake of sulfur-containing amino acids and urinary excretion of inorganic sulfate in man. Their results suggest that a surplus of cysteine or methionine is oxidized to inorganic sulfate. In agreement with these findings, Simmons[101] observed very low urinary inorganic sulfate levels in African children in a rural area as compared with an urban area. These findings correlated with a methionine-deficient diet in the rural area.

Very little data have been reported on the urinary excretion of inorganic sulfate in animals, and with the data that are available one has to keep in mind that there may be large variations because of differences in diet. For example, O'Connor and Summerill[24] found a basal excretion level of 300 μmol inorganic sulfate per hour in dogs (11 to 16 kg body weight). If these dogs were fed 10 g of meat per kilogram, however, this increased to 2400 μmol/hr, illustrating the effect of the diet. In fasted rabbits Bray et al.[102] measured an excretion rate of about 60 μmol/hr per rabbit. In the rat (body weight 250 to 300 g, males, nonfasted) about 18 μmol/hr was reported.[13] This value was confirmed by Büch et al.,[95] who compared the urinary excretion of inorganic sulfate in the rat and in male human volunteers. Their human volunteers excreted about 1000 μmol inorganic sulfate per hour (body weight 70 kg?), whereas the rats excreted 15 μmol/hr (body weight 250 to 300 g). This means that the excretion rate of inorganic sulfate on a weight-base in the rat is about four times that in man.

A high sulfate requirement for sulfate conjugation of administered paracetamol in the rat caused an almost complete disappearance of inorganic sulfate from urine.[95] The amount (expressed in μmol) of esterified sulfate (paracetamol sulfate) that appeared in urine was slightly higher than that of free inorganic sulfate excreted in controls. The latter suggests that a decrease in plasma sulfate may have occurred due to its depletion by sulfation of paracetamol. In human volunteers, a similar decrease in the urinary excretion of sulfate was found after paracetamol administration, although it was not as complete as in the rat presumably because the dose of paracetamol was much lower. These findings demonstrate that substrates for sulfation are another factor that affect urinary excretion of free sulfate.

The main route of elimination of sulfate in blood is urinary excretion;[9,12,14,103] biliary excretion is of little importance.[104,105] Bird[106] found only 6 to 8% of the radioactivity of [35S]-labeled sodium sulfate in combined bile and pancreatic secretions in sheep, whereas 63 to 76% of the dose was recovered from urine. In a study in the isolated perfused rat liver, a slow rate of biliary excretion was also found:[107] at low concentration of sulfate in the perfusion medium (about 0.03 mM), the concentration of radioactivity in bile was higher than in the perfusion medium, but at 0.6 and 1.3 mM in the medium, the concentrations of radioactivity of inorganic sulfate in bile and in medium were equal. In an autoradiographical study[108] however, a significant amount of radioactivity was found in the intestinal lumen of the mouse after intravenous injection of

[35S]-sodium sulfate. Kennedy et al.[109] established that some of intravenously administered [35S]-sodium sulfate in sheep was excreted in the stomach and metabolized by the ruminal flora. Would secretion by the stomach mucosa into the gut play a role?

The distribution volume of inorganic sulfate in the body ("sulfate space" or "radiosulfate space") is an important parameter in studies on the pharmacokinetics of administered sulfate, and may be used to determine the physiological, endogenous sulfate pools. In addition, physiologists have used the radiosulfate space as a measure of the distribution volume of extracellular water. Different types of pharmacokinetics will be obtained with unlabeled and a tracer dose of [35S]-labeled sulfate because of at least two reasons. In the first place an i.v. injection of a large dose of unlabeled sulfate, required to increase the serum concentration sufficiently in order to make this type of study possible, will increase the plasma concentration considerably above the absorption threshold in the kidney tubuli. Therefore, a rapid initial elimination will take place and this will lead to a correspondingly short halflife component in the eliminatory pattern of sulfate. A tracer dose of [35S]-sulfate, labeled at high specific radioactivity, on the other hand, does not increase the total serum concentration of inorganic sulfate, and therefore will lack this rapid component. In the second place, if radio-labeled sulfate is used, the [35S]-labeled sulfate will exchange with various (e.g., cellular) unlabeled sulfate pools. If unlabeled ions exchange with unlabeled ions, there is no net shift of sulfate from serum to cells or vice versa, but if a labeled ion in blood exchanges with unlabeled sulfate in cells, the radioactivity in blood decreases. Therefore, this effect will add a component to the elimination of [35S]-sulfate as compared with unlabeled sulfate, where this self-exchange is not measured. Furthermore, in studies with [35S]-labeled sulfate, usually no distinction has been made between inorganic sulfate and conjugated sulfate in the plasma samples: radioactivity in plasma has been counted indiscriminately. Of course most of the radioactivity will usually be present in the form of free sulfate, but under certain unfavorable conditions this may be different, for instance in patients with a high consumption of drugs that are metabolized by sulfate conjugation. If the pharmacokinetics of these conjugates are much different from that of free sulfate, the results in these patients must be misleading. In practice, so far only the pharmacokinetics of [35S]-sulfate have been studied in several species, including man, where it has some clinical value. Usually, the tracer dose is injected intravenously, but it may also be administered orally.[12] Since a tracer dose of [35S]-sulfate is not very rapidly excreted as long as plasma sulfate remains below the threshold for resorption, it may reach equilibrium and give a good estimate of the radiosulfate space. An indication of the time required for equilibrium may be the finding that after approximately 5 hr, the concentration in ascites fluid in man had equilibrated with the plasma concentration of [35S]-sulfate.[110] Clearance of [35S]-sulfate in man was 35 ml/min (per 1.73 m^2 surface area) and the distribution volume was 14.6% of body weight, with a range of 11.5 to 20.9%.[111] In dogs a higher distribution volume was found: 20.1% of body weight, with much less variation, probably because only a small proportion of their body weight is fat tissue. This value for the dog was confirmed, using nephrectomized dogs.[112] The distribution volume of radiosulfate slowly increases as a function of time after injection.[111] This may be due to slow penetration into cells, exchange of radiosulfate with unlabeled sulfate in cells, and incorporation into endogenous macromolecular compounds. These findings were confirmed in man by Ryan et al.[110] who used a slightly different method and found distribution volumes of 19.1 and 16.7% of body weight, respectively, for young soldiers and sedentary young males, and about 15% for elderly men and women. As is to be expected, various diseases affect this volume of distribution: during severe dehydration it may be decreased to 7% of body weight, and in patients with ascites, values of 23 to 26% have been reported.[110] In healthy human volunteers, Bauer[12] found a radiosulfate space of 15.3% after oral administration of radiosulfate, and 16.8% after its i.v. administration.

In the rat, the radiosulfate space was calculated to be 34% of body weight by Sheatz and Wilde.[113] In the liver, the same percentage of the tissue was available to radiosulfate, but in muscle only 12%. The blood cells equilibrated very rapidly with plasma [35S]-sulfate, and the ratio between the concentration inside and outside blood corpuscles was 0.44. Barratt and Walser reported a ratio of 0.35 for erythrocytes.[105] Later it was shown that in calves[114] and in the rat, the volume of the sulfate space was time-dependent: in the rat it was $23.6 + (1.2 \times t)$ percent of body weight, where t indicates hours after i.v. injection of the radiosulfate.[105] This may explain why much higher volumes have been reported, such as 34.6% of body weight in the rat; this was calculated from a single blood sample taken 3 hr after injection of [35S]-sulfate in nephrectomized rats.[115] The radiosulfate space in various tissue in the rat is given in Reference 105; an unknown part of the radioactivity in each tissue may have been incorporated in small conjugates or in macromolecules. The fractional distribution of total body sulfate has been calculated by Barratt and Walser[105] from the radiosulfate distribution at equilibrium.

Finally, Douglas et al.[116] have pointed out the importance of obtaining the complete plasma disappearance curve for radiosulfate, and not just the final phase, because analysis of the entire curve allows separation and measurement of each component of the elimination process. In the dog, both with intact and ligated kidneys, they observed the same sulfate space, namely about 17% of body weight. Further detailed analysis have been made in man with various diseases.[117]

VII. AVAILABILITY OF INORGANIC SULFATE IN BLOOD FOR INTRACELLULAR SULFATE POOLS; CARRIER TRANSPORT OF INORGANIC SULFATE

Since sulfation processes probably occur in all tissues in the body, sulfate must be available in the cells in each of them. Apart from the possibility that in some of the tissues this sulfate is provided exclusively by oxidation of cysteine, the possibility that inorganic sulfate in blood is used should be considered. It is generally assumed that membranes are virtually impermeable to sulfate ions by diffusion. This idea is supported by studies on sulfate permeation in erythrocyte ghosts, in which only a carrier-mediated transport of sulfate has been observed. In this experimental model the kinetics of sulfate transport have extensively been studied; the question remains, of course, whether the conclusions from these studies can be extended to other cell types.

In brief, the results indicate the involvement of a carrier protein embedded in the cell membrane, that catalyzes the self-exchange of sulfate, and its exchange with chloride.[118-128] Many other anions, for instance chloride, compete for the same transport process. The rate of chloride self-exchange, however, was about 20,000 times larger than sulfate self-exchange.[129] Differences in properties and affinities of both chloride and sulfate transport have been found for the inner and outer membrane surface in erythrocyte ghosts, suggesting asymmetry of the transport system.[128,130]

The sulfate transport system can be saturated with sulfate, and the rate of transport is pH-dependent: the flux decreases when the pH of the medium is increased from 6.5 to 8.5.[122] Several sulfonic acids irreversibly inhibit sulfate self-exchange in erythrocytes. Zaki et al.[119] analyzed proteins of the red cell membrane after solubilization by SDS polyacrylamide gel electrophoresis after these had been labeled with radioactive dinitrofluorobenzene (DNFB). When they incubated the cells with DNFB in the presence of 4,4′-diacetamide-stilbene-2,2′-disulfonic acid, they prevented labeling with DNFB of only one protein band. At the same time, the irreversible inhibition of sulfate transport by DNFB was prevented. Thus it was postulated that this protein band might be associated with the sulfate carrier. This carrier protein is only digested by trypsin when this protease is included internally in erythrocyte ghosts,[120] or when inside-out vesicles were prepared.[131] Its amino acid sequence is under investigation.[132] Even when the carrier protein is split into two major peptides, sulfate exchange is not completely lost.[120] Erythrocytes from every species studied were sensitive to the action of the protease pronase, and lost their sulfate transport activity.[133]

By treatment of erythrocyte ghosts with the detergent Triton® X-100, smaller vesicles can be prepared which still contain the carrier protein and can accumulate anions.[121] The carrier protein has been purified and incorporated into vesicles prepared from egg phosphatidylcholine; when erythrocyte lipid, cholesterol, and glycophorin were added, the reconstituted band 3-protein catalyzed sulfate transport into these vesicles. This transport was sensitive to pyridoxal phosphate-NaBH$_4$, a potent inhibitor of anion transport in red blood cells.[123] For further characterization of this carrier and its properties, a series of sulfonic acid derivatives of some isocyanates has been used with human red cells. These compounds competitively inhibited sulfate exchange initially, whereas upon incubation for a longer period of time, irreversible inhibition occurred.[125] Depending on the sulfonic acid used, from approximately 4 to 34% of the sulfate efflux was resistent to this inactivation for some as yet unknown reason. The mechanism of this irreversible inhibition is supposedly covalent binding of the sulfonic acid derivatives to the sulfate carrier system or to some protein in its immediate environment. The presence of a "transport site" and a "modifier site" has been suggested to explain the competitive and noncompetitive inhibition characteristics by a number of compounds. Recently, reversible inhibition of anion transport in human erythrocytes by tetrathionate has been reported; this inhibitor was only effective from the outside.[126] The authors suggest that it is bound to the "modifier site." This inhibitor is of interest because it is not an amphiphilic compound as the other sulfonic acid inhibitors are. Recently, Grinstein et al.[134] presented some evidence that the band-3 carrier protein might contain a mobile transport element that moves from the extracellular surface to the cytoplasmic face.

The sulfate exchange is strongly inhibited by relatively low intracellular calcium concentration,[127] whereas extracellular calcium does not affect the transport rate. Magnesium weakly activated sulfate exchange, but did not interfere with the calcium binding site. The K$_i$ for intracellular calcium was only about 6 μM, whereas the apparent dissociation constant for magnesium was 4 μM. Since the free calcium concentration in erythrocytes is only of the order of 0.2 to 0.7 μM, the inhibition by calcium may be of doubtful physiological significance, and may be only relevant under some pathological conditions.[127] A number of anions inhibit sulfate self-exchange in red cells;[122] the order of potency is $NO_3^- > Cl^- >$ acetate and oxalate $> HPO_4^{2-}$ A recent review on the properties of the anion transport system of red blood cells is available.[135]

Much less work has been done with other cell types. Some data, however, are available on ascites tumor cells.[136-139] The findings with these cells are very similar to those with red cells: a carrier system catalyzes the sulfate exchange with a K$_m$ of 2 mM for sulfate. In incubations with [^{35}S]-labeled sulfate at the outside of the cells, and unlabeled sulfate inside, the uptake of [^{35}S]-sulfate is enhanced when the ascites cells are preloaded with high sulfate concentrations, presumably because of a high exchange rate. High chloride concentrations inside the cells also stimulate sulfate uptake, probably through sulfate-chloride exchange. The Cl^-/SO_4^{2-} exchange has a stoichiometry of 1:1.[138] If chloride is present at the same surface as sulfate, it inhibits sulfate uptake by the cells, and sulfate can inhibit Cl^- self-exchange. This carrier is apparently relatively unimportant for chloride transport, since 94% of chloride uptake is provided by sulfate-independent transport; later findings, however, were interpreted by Levinson such that Cl^- and SO_4^{2-} share a common transport mechanism which is separately and differently influenced for Cl^- and SO_4^{2-} respectively.[139] The same pH-dependence of sulfate exchange was observed as was found with red cells: the flux decreased at higher pH values. Moreover, the pH seemed to determine the steady state ratio between intracellular and extracellular sulfate concentrations in the ascites cells: at pH 8 this ratio was about 0.5, whereas at pH 6 this ratio was about 0.85. The extracellular chloride concentration also affected this ratio with higher values at low chloride (30 to 35 mM) than at high chloride (130 to 150 mM): differences were 20 to 40% between these extremes. In studies on pH and chloride dependence of sulfate exchange, these effects should be kept in mind because they influence the steady-state intracellular sulfate concentration, and thereby, the sulfate exchange rate indirectly.

Sulfate transport by vesicles isolated from the brush-border membrane of rat-kidney cortex has been studied by Lücke et al.[140] They conclude that an electroneutral Na^+/SO_4^{2-} cotransport is catalyzed by these vesicles. Sodium ion was the only monovalent ion that catalyzed the sulfate transport. This carrier transport evidently is much different from that in erythrocytes. It is not inhibited by chloride, or known inhibitors of the erythrocyte anion transport system. Low concentrations of $HgCl_2$ almost completely inhibited this transport.

It is quite clear that intravenously or intraperitoneally injected inorganic sulfate (for which [^{35}S]-labeled sulfate conveniently has been used) is taken up by many tissues since it is incorporated in many tissues into cellular macromolecules or small molecules. However, usually the rate of uptake and the extent of uptake in these tissues has not been determined. Only in the case of the liver are some data available. Mulder and Scholtens[141] determined the rate of incorporation of intravenously injected [^{35}S]-labeled sodium sulfate into harmol sulfate, a low molecular-weight sulfate ester that is mainly synthesized in the liver and excreted in bile and urine in the rat. No lag-phase for the incorporation of [^{35}S]-sulfate was found, suggesting that sulfate in blood is immediately (i.e., within 1 min) available for sulfation in the liver. Moreover, their data also suggest that the specific radioactivity with which sulfate is incorporated into harmol sulfate follows the specific radioactivity of sulfate in blood. This confirms that there is (almost) no barrier for uptake of inorganic sulfate by the hepatocytes, as suggested by earlier results of Herbai[142] in mice where a rapid equilibration of sulfate in blood with the hepatic pool was found.

Often more detailed data on uptake of sulfate by a tissue are lacking because these data are best obtained using isolated cells, which cannot be obtained from every tisuse as easily as from liver (although even with isolated hepatocytes this type of study has not yet been performed). An alternative preparation in which rates of uptake can be determined is the isolated perfused organ. When the isolated perfused rat liver is provided with various concentrations of inorganic sulfate in the perfusion medium,[107] there is no first pass effect for sulfate. It seems that sulfate rapidly equilibrates with the hepatic intracellular sulfate pool. Even at extremely low concentration (about 0.03 mM) it is only slowly eliminated from the perfusion medium by the liver through excretion in bile and presumably, incorporation into compounds in the liver. Mulder and Keulemans[107] calculated from their data that the sulfate concentration in the liver (of the sulfate pool available for sulfation of drugs like harmol) was of the same order of magnitude as the plasma concentration, i.e., about 0.8 mM. In this calculation it has been assumed that the sulfate space in the liver was 50% of its weight. If the value determined by Barratt and Walser[105] is correct, namely 36% of liver weight, the concentration in that compartment would be slightly higher than in serum.

In a study in the dog, an extracorporeal system has been used to perfuse the cerebral circulation *in situ*,[143] and the unidirectional flux of sulfate and various other substances into brain was measured. Only slow uptake of sulfate was found, which confirmed the finding by Dziewiatkowski.[7] This author determined that only after 20 hr the concentrations of radioactivity in plasma and brain tissue in the rat were about the same. Ovine brain synaptosomes take up sulfate by a saturable mechanism with a K_m of 4.4 mM that is inhibited by p-hydroxymercuribenzoate.[144]

The placenta offers no barrier to sulfate passage, which is not surprising since sulfate is required for the synthesis of many substances needed for growth and regulation of the fetus. Several investigations have shown that [^{35}S]-sulfate is rapidly passed to the fetus, and is incorporated into various tissues, such as cartilage.[23,145-148]

Intracellular sulfate may be taken up by subcellular organelles. Rat-liver mitochondria rapidly take up inorganic sulfate, catalyzed by the dicarboxylate carrier;[149,150] similar findings were reported for corn mitochondria.[151] As yet it is not clear whether some organelle(s) may accumulate inorganic sulfate.

ACKNOWLEDGMENT

I am very much indebted to Dr. Jack A. Hinson, National Heart, Lung and Blood Institute, NIH, Bethesda, Md. (U.S.A.) for his critical review of the manuscript.

REFERENCES

1. **Perry, M. A., Powell, G. M., Wusteman, F. S., and Curtis, C. G.,** The catabolism of intravenously injected heparan N-[^{35}S] sulphate in the rat, *Biochem. J.,* 166, 373, 1977.
2. **Charles, J. M., Anderson, W. G., and Menzel, D. B.,** Sulfate absorption from the airways of the isolated perfused rat lung, *Toxicol. Appl. Pharmacol.,* 41, 91, 1977.
3. **Charles, J. M., Gardner, D. E., Coffin, D. L., and Menzel, D. B.,** Augmentation of sulfate ion absorption from the rat lung by heavy metals, *Toxicol. Appl. Pharmacol.,* 42, 531, 1977.
4. **Tisdale, S. L.,** Sulphur in forage quality and ruminant nutrition, *Technical Bulletin* No. 22, Sulphur Institute, Washington, D.C., 1977.
5. **Fingl, E.,** Cathartics and laxatives, in *The Pharmacological Basis of Therapeutics,* 5th ed., Goodman, L. S. and Gilman, A., Eds., MacMillan, New York, 1976, 806.
6. *Martindale's Pharmacopoeia,* 26th ed., Blacon, N.W. and Wade, A., Eds., Pharmaceutical Press, London, 1972, 1725.
7. **Dziewiatkowski, D. D.,** Metabolism of sulfate esters, in *Symposium: Sulfur in Nutrition,* Muth, O. H. and Oldfield, J. E., Eds., AVI Publishing, Westport, Conn., 1970, 97.
8. **Hele, T. S.,** Studies in the sulphur metabolism of the dog. I. The synthesis of ethereal sulphate, *Biochem. J.,* 18, 110, 1924.
9. **Laidlaw, J. C. and Young, L.,** A study of ethereal sulphate formation *in vivo* using radioactive sulphur, *Biochem. J.,* 54, 142, 1953.
10. **Hele, T. S.,** Studies in sulphur metabolism of dogs, synthesis of phenyl sulphate and indoxyl sulphate, *Biochem. J.,* 25, 1736, 1931.
11. **Borsook, H., Keighley, G., Yost, D. M., and McMillan, E.,** Urinary excretion of ingested radioactive sulfur, *Science,* 86, 525, 1937.
12. **Bauer, J. H.,** Oral administration of radioactive sulfate to measure extracellular fluid space in man, *J. Appl. Physiol.,* 40, 648, 1976.
13. **Binkley, F.,** The source of sulfate in the formation of ethereal sulfates, *J. Biol. Chem.,* 178, 821, 1949.
14. **Dziewiatkowski, D. D.,** On the utilization of exogeneous sulfate sulfur by the rat in the formation of ethereal sulfates as indicated by the use of sodium sulfate labeled with radioactive sulfur, *J. Biol. Chem.,* 178, 389, 1949.

15. **Morrrow, P. E., Hodge, H. C., Neuman, W. F., Maynard, E. A., Blanchet, H. J., Fassett, D. W., Birk, R. E., and Manrodt, S.,** The gastrointestinal nonabsorption of sodium cellulose sulfate labeled with S^{35}, *J. Pharmacol. Exp. Ther.,* 105, 273, 1952.
16. **Michels, F. G. and Smith, J. T.,** A comparison of the utilization of organic and inorganic sulfur by the rat, *J. Nutr.,* 87, 217, 1965.
17. **Button, G. M., Brown, R. G., Michels, F. G., and Smith, J. T.,** Utilization of calcium and sodium sulfate by the rat, *J. Nutr.,* 87, 211, 1965.
18. **Wellers, G., Boëlle, G., and Chevan, J.,** Recherches sur le métabolisme du soufre. IV. Couverture partielle de la dépense soufré endogène par la sulfate de sodium chez le rat blanc adulte, *J. Physiol. Paris,* 52, 903, 1960.
19. **Kulwich, R., Struglia, L., and Pearson, P. B.,** The metabolic fate of sulfur[35] in sheep, *J. Nutr.,* 61, 113, 1957.
20. **Bird, P. R. and Moir, R. J.,** Sulphur metabolism and excretion studies in ruminants. I. The absorption of sulphate in sheep after intraruminal or intraduodenal infusion of sodium sulphate, *Aust. J. Biol. Sci.,* 24, 1319, 1971.
21. **Heath, H., Rimington, C., Glover, T., Mann, T., and Leone, E.,** Studies using radioactive sulphur on ergothioneine formation in the pig, *Biochem. J.,* 54, 606, 1953.
22. **Kulwich, R., Struglia, L., and Pearson, P. B.,** Metabolic fate of [^{35}S]-labeled sulfate in baby pigs, *Proc. Soc. Exp. Biol. Med.,* 97, 408, 1958.
23. **Berry, R. K., Hansard, S. L., Ismail, R. J., and Wysocki, A. A.,** Absorption, deposition and placental transfer of sulfate sulfur by gilts, *J. Nutr.,* 97, 399, 1969.
24. **O'Connor, W. J. and Summerill, R. A.,** Sulphate excretion by dogs following ingestion of ammonium sulphate or meat, *J. Physiol.,* 200, 597, 1976.
25. **Meier, M. S. and Schmidt-Kessen, W.,** Untersuchungen über den Stoffwechsel des anorganischen Sulfates, *München. Med. Wochenschr.,* 120, 357, 1978.
26. **Krijgsheld, K. R., Frankena, H., Scholtens, E., Zweens, J., and Mulder, G. J.,** Absorption, serum levels and urinary excretion of inorganic sulfate after oral administration of sodium sulfate in the conscious rat, *Biochim. Biophys. Acta,* 586, 492, 1979.
27. *Federal Register (Washington, D.C.),* 43 (60), p. 12947, March 28, 1978.
28. **Deyrup, I. J.,** *In vitro* transport of radiosulfate by the lower ileum of the rat, *Fed. Proc.,* 22, 332, 1963.
29. **Anast, C., Kennedy, R., Volk, G., and Adamson, L.,** *In vitro* studies of sulfate transport by the small intestine of the rat, rabbit and hamster, *J. Lab. Clin. Med.,* 65, 903, 1965.
30. **Batt, E. R.,** Sulfate accumulation by mouse intestine: influence of age and other factors, *Am. J. Physiol.,* 217, 1101, 1969.
31. **Robinson, J. W.,** Species differences in the intestinal response to sulfate ions, *FEBS Lett.,* 5, 157, 1969.
32. **Cardin, C. J. and Mason, J.,** Sulphate transport by rat ileum: effect of molybdate and other anions, *Biochim. Biophys. Acta,* 394, 46, 1975.
33. **Cardin, C. J. and Mason, J.,** Molybdate and tungstate transfer by rat ileum: competitive inhibition by sulfate, *Biochim. Biophys. Acta,* 455, 937, 1976.
34. **Mason, J. and Cardin, C.J.,** The competition of molybdate and sulphate ions for a transport system in the ovine small intestine, *Res. Vet. Sci.,* 22, 313, 1977.
35. **Gerencser, G. A.,** Metabolic dependence of active sulfate transport in *Aplysia californica* intestine, *Comp. Biochem. Physiol.,* 63, 519, 1979.
36. **Holloman, T. L., Schwartz, M., Dinno, M. A., and Carrasquer, G.,** Ionic pathways of secretory membrane of frog gastric mucosa in Cl^--free media, *Am. J. Physiol.,* 231, 1649, 1976.
37. **Wellers, G.,** Quelques aspects du problème des besoins en soufre des animaux supérieures, *Ann. Nutr. Aliment.,* 18, 19, 1964.
38. **Finkelstein, J. D.,** Control of sulfur metabolism in mammals, in *Symposium: Sulfur in Nutrition,* Muth, O. H. and Oldfield, J. E., Eds., AVI Publishing, Westport, Conn., 1970, 46.
39. **Greenberg, D. M.,** Biosynthesis of cysteine and cystine, in *Metabolic Pathways,* Vol. 7, *Metabolism of Sulfur Compounds,* 3rd ed., Greenberg, D. M., Ed., Academic Press, New York, 1975, chap. 12.
40. **Singer, T. P.,** Oxidative metabolism of cysteine and cystine in animal tissues, in *Metabolic Pathways,* Vol. 7, *Metabolism of Sulfur Compounds,* 3rd ed., Greenberg, D. M., Ed., Academic Press, New York, 1975, chap. 14.
41. **Finkelstein, J. D.,** Enzyme defects in sulfur amino acid metabolism in man, in *Metabolic Pathways,* Vol. 7, *Metabolism of Sulfur Compounds,* 3rd ed., Greenberg, D. M., Ed., Academic Press, New York, 1975, chap. 15.
42. **Recasens, M., Benezra, R., Gabellec, M., Delaunoy, J., and Mandel, P.,** Purification and some properties of cysteine sulfinate transaminase, *FEBS Lett.,* 99, 51, 1979.
43. **Stipanuk, M. H.,** Effect of excess dietary methionine on the catabolism of cysteine in rats, *J. Nutr.,* 109, 2126, 1979.

44. **Wellers, G. and Chevan, J.,** Recherches sur le métabolism de sourfre. I. La dépense soufrée endogène chez le rat adulte au cours du jeûne hydrique et des inanitions azotée, soufrée et azotée et soufrée, *J. Physiol. Paris,* 51, 723, 1959.

45. **Wellers, G.,** Recherches sur le métabolism du soufre. II. Couvertures de la dépense endogène chez le rat adulte par la methionine et l'homocysteine. Le besoin soufré minimum, *J. Physiol. Paris,* 51, 999, 1959.

46. **Almquist, H. J.,** Sulfur nutrition of non-ruminant species, in *Symposium: Sulfur in Nutrition,* Muth, O. H. and Oldfield, J. E., Eds., AVI Publishing, Westport, Conn., 1970, chap. 13.

47. **Uren, J. R., Ragin, R., and Chay Kovsky, M.,** Modulation of cysteine metabolism in mice. Effects of propargylglycine and L-cyst(e)ine-degrading enzymes, *Biochem. Pharmacol.,* 27, 2807, 1978.

48. **Lakshmanan, F. L., Perera, W. D. A., Scrimshaw, N. S., and Young, V. R.,** Plasma and urinary amino acids and selected sulfur metabolites in young men fed a diet devoid of methionine and cystine, *Am. J. Clin. Nutr.,* 29, 1367, 1976.

49. **Sabry, Z. I., Shadarevian, S. B., Cowan, J. W., and Campbell, J. A.,** Relationship of dietary intake of sulphur amino acids to urinary excretion of inorganic sulphate in man, *Nature (London),* 206, 931, 1965.

50. **Lakshmanan, F. L., Vaughan, D. A., and Barnes, R. E.,** Urinary inorganic sulfate excretion in human subjects fed purified amino acid mixtures with and without threonine, *Fed. Proc. Abstr.,* 37, 359, 1978.

51. **Bodwell, C. E., Schuster, E. M., Brooks, B., and Womack, M.,** Biochemical indices in humans of protein nutritive value. 1. Urinary inorganic sulfate excretion at a high protein intake level, *Nutr. Rep. Int.,* 18, 125, 1978.

52. **Clark, H. E., Howe, J. M., Shannon, B. M., Carlson, K., and Kolski, S. M.,** Requirements of adult human subjects for methionine and cysteine, *Am. J. Clin. Nutr.,* 23, 731, 1970.

53. **Swenseid, M. E. and Wang, M.,** Sulfur requirements of the human, in *Symposium: Sulfur in Nutrition,* Muth, O. H. and Oldfield, J. E., Eds., AVI Publishing, Westport, Conn., 1970, chap. 14.

54. **Gibson, W. B. and Strong, F. M.,** Accumulation of ingested sulfite- and sulfate-sulfur and utilization of sulfites proteins by rats, *Food Cosmet. Toxicol.,* 12, 625, 1974.

55. **Gunnison, A. F. and Palmes, E. D.,** A model for the metabolism of sulfite in mammals, *Toxicol. Appl. Pharmacol.,* 38, 111, 1976.

56. **Tejnorova, I.,** Sulfite oxidase activity in liver and kidney tissue in five laboratory animal species, *Toxicol. Appl. Pharmacol.,* 44, 251, 1978.

57. **Inouye, B., Ikeda, M., Ishida, T., Ogata, M., Akiyama, J., and Utsumi, K.,** Participation of superoxide free radical and Mn^{2+} in sulfite oxidation, *Toxicol. Appl. Pharmacol.,* 46, 29, 1978.

58. **Mudd, S. H., Irreverre, F., and Laster, L.,** Sulfite oxidase deficiency in man: demonstration of the enzymatic defect, *Science,* 156, 1599, 1967.

59. **Irreverre, F., Mudd, S. H., Heizer, W. D., and Laster, L.,** Sulfite oxidase deficiency: studies of a patient with mental retardation, dislocated ocular lenses, and abnormal urinary excretion of S-sulfo-L-cysteine, sulfite and thiosulfate, *Biochem. Med.,* 1, 187, 1967.

60. **Percy, A. K., Mudd, S. H., Irreverre, F., and Laster, L.,** Sulfite oxidase deficiency: sulfate esters in tissues and urine, *Biochem. Med.,* 2, 198, 1968.

61. **Rosenblum, W. I.,** Neuropathologic changes in a case of sulfite oxidase deficiency, *Neurology,* 18, 1187, 1968.

62. **Shih, V. E., Abrams, I. F., Johnson, J. L., Carney, M., Mandell, R., Robb, R. M., Cloherty, J. P., and Rajagopalan, K. V.,** Sulfite oxidase deficiency. Biochemical and clinical investigations of a hereditary metabolic disorder in sulfur metabolism, *N. Engl. J. Med.,* 297, 1022, 1977.

63. Special report on sulfite as food additive, *Nutr. Rev.,* 34, 58, 1976.

64. **Dodgson, K. S. and Rose, F. A.,** Some aspects of the biochemistry of sulphur compounds, *Nutr. Abstr. Rev.,* 36, 327, 1966.

65. **Muth, O. H. and Oldfield, J. E., Eds.,** *Symposium: Sulfur in Nutrition,* AVI Publishing, Westport, Conn., 1970.

66. **Sibbald, I. R. and Cave, N. A.,** The response of chicks to ammonium, calcium, magnesium, potassium and sodium sulfate and to ammonium and potassium carbonates, *Poult. Sci.,* 55, 2209, 1976.

67. **Baker, D. H.,** Nutritional and metabolic interrelationships among sulfur compounds in avian nutrition, *Fed. Proc.,* 35, 1917, 1976.

68. **Motzok, I., Rasper, J., McCuaig, L. W., and Verma, R. S.,** Utilization of inorganic sulfate by the chick, *Nutr. Rep. Int.,* 19, 715, 1979.

69. **Bird, P. R.** Sulphur, nitrogen and energy utilization by sheep fed a sulphur-deficient and a sulphate-supplemented roughage-based diet, *Aust. J. Biol. Sci.,* 25, 1073, 1972.

70. **White, C. L. and Somers, M.,** Sulfur-selenium studies in sheep. 1. The effects of varying dietary sulfate and selenomethionine on sulfur, nitrogen and selenium metabolism in sheep, *Aust. J. Biol. Sci.,* 30, 47, 1977.

71. **Hidiroglou, M., Ho, S. K., Williams, C. J., and Ivan, M.,** Effects of level of dietary sulfur on the growth performance and blood mineral profile of sheep fed urea-supplemented corn silage, *Int. J. Vitam. Nutr. Res.,* 47, 284, 1977.

72. **Robel, E. J.,** Effects of different levels of methionine and sulfate on collagen metabolism and growth of young pigs, *Nutr. Rep. Int.,* 14, 147, 1976.

73. **Bouchard, R. and Conrad, H. R.,** Sulfur requirement of lactating dairy cows. III, *J. Dairy Sci.,* 56, 1435, 1973.

74. **Digesti, R. D. and Weeth, H. J.,** A defensible maximum for inorganic sulfate in drinking water of cattle, *J. Anim. Sci.,* 42, 1498, 1976.

75. **Zezulke, A. Y. and Calloway, D. H.,** Nitrogen retention in men fed isolated soybean protein supplemented with L-methionine, D-methionine, *N*-acetyl-L-methionine or inorganic sulfate, *J. Nutr.,* 106, 1286, 1976.

76. **Smith, J. T.,** An optimal level of inorganic sulfate for the diet of a rat, *J. Nutr.,* 103, 1008, 1973.

77. **James, K. A. C. and Hove, E. L.,** Effect of inorganic sulfate supplements on the growth of rats fed sulfur amino acid-deficient diets, *Can. J. Anim. Sci.,* 58, 49, 1978.

78. **Whanger, P. D. and Matrone, G.,** Effect of dietary sulfur upon the fatty acid production in the rumen, *Biochim. Biophys. Acta,* 98, 454, 1965.

79. **Huisingh, J., Gomez, G. G., and Matrone, G.,** Hypothesis that molybdate inhibits sulfate reduction by bacteria in rumen, *Fed. Proc.,* 32, 1921, 1973.

80. **Huisingh, J., McNeill, J. J., and Matrone, G.,** Sulfate reduction by a *desulfovibrio* species isolated from sheep rumen, *Appl. Microbiol.,* 28, 489, 1974.

81. **Siegel, L. M.,** Biochemistry of the sulfur cycle, in *Metabolic Pathways,* Vol. 7, *Metabolism of Sulfur Compounds,* 3rd ed., Greenberg, D. M., Ed., Academic Press, New York, 1975, chap. 7.

82. **McMeniman, N. P.,** Ben-Ghedalia, D., and Elliott, R., Sulfur and cysteine incorporation into rumen microbial protein, *Br. J. Nutr.,* 36, 571, 1976.

83. **Elliott, R.,** The Significance of the Dietary Nitrogen: Sulphur Ratio in Relationship to Microbial Protein Synthesis in the Rumen of Adult Sheep, Ph.D. thesis, Newcastle upon Tyne University, U.K., 1977.

84. **Umbarger, H. E.,** Amino acid biosynthesis and its regulation, *Annu. Rev. Biochem.,* 47, 533, 1978.

85. **Flavin, M.,** Methionine biosynthesis, in *Metabolic Pathways,* Vol. 7, *Metabolism of Sulfur Compounds,* 3rd ed., Greenberg, D. M., Ed., Academic Press, New York, 1970, chap. 11.

86. **Huovinen, J. A. and Gustafsson, B. E.,** Inorganic sulphate, sulphite and sulphide as sulphur donors in the biosynthesis of sulphur amino acids in germ-free and conventional rats, *Biochim. Biophys. Acta,* 136, 441, 1967.

87. **Krijgsheld, K. R., Scholtens, E., and Mulder, G. J.,** Serum concentration of inorganic sulfate in mammals: species differences and circadian rhythm, *Comp. Biochem. Physiol.,* 67A, 683, 1980.

88. **Berglund, F. and Sörbo, B.,** Turbidimetric analysis of inorganic sulphate in serum, plasma and urine, *Scand. J. Clin. Lab. Invest.,* 12, 147, 1960.

89. **Speier, F., quoted in Diem, K. and Lentner, C.,** *Wissenschaftliche Tabellen,* Ciba-Geigy A. G., Basel, Switzerland, 1971, 659.

90. **Miller, E., Hlad, C. J., Levine, S., Holmes, J. H., and Elrick, H.,** The use of radioisotopes to measure body fluid constituents. 1. Plasma sulfate, *J. Lab. Clin. Med.,* 58, 656, 1961.

91. **Kleeman, C., Taborsky, E., and Epstein, F.,** Improved method for determination of inorganic sulfate in biological fluids, *Proc. Soc. Exp. Biol. Med.,* 91, 480, 1956.

92. **Leskovar, R. and Weidmann, G.,** Flammenphotometrische Bestimmung der freien Sulfationen im Serum, *Z. Klin. Chem. Klin. Biochem.,* 12, 98, 1974.

93. **Mudge, G. H., Berndt, W. O., and Valtin, H.,** Tubular transport of urea, glucose, phosphate, uric acid, sulphate and thiosulphate, in *Handbook of Physiology,* American Physiological Society, Bethesda, Md., 1973, chap. 19.

94. **Berglund, F.,** Transport of inorganic sulphate by the renal tubules, *Acta Physiol. Scand. Suppl.,* 172, 1, 1960.

95. **Büch, H., Rummel, W., Pfleger, K., Eschrich, C. and Texter, N.,** Ausscheidung freien und konjungierten Sulfates bei Ratte und Menschen nach Verabreichung von *N*-Acetyl-*p*-Aminophenol, *Naunyn-Schmiedebergs Arch. Pharmakol.,* 259, 276, 1968.

96. **North, K. A. K., Lascelles, D., and Coates, P.,** The mechanisms by which sodium excretion is increased during a fast but reduced on subsequent carbohydrate feeding, *Clin. Sci. Mol. Med.,* 46, 423, 1974.

97. **Anderson, C.,** Ion chromatography: a new technique for clinical chemistry, *Clin. Chem. (N.Y.),* 22, 1424, 1976.

98. **Liappis, N. and Bantzer, P.,** Sex-specific differences in free inorganic sulfate excretion in 24 hour urine of healthy adults, *Aertzl. Lab.,* 24, 180, 1978.

99. **Dieu, J. P.,** Automated determination of urinary inorganic sulfate with the autoanalyzer, *Clin. Chem. (N.Y.),* 17, 1183, 1971.

100. **Liappis, N.,** Geschlechtsspezifische Unterschieder er Ausscheidung von freiem anorganischem Sulfat im 24-h-Harn von gesunden Kindern, *Klin. Paediatr.,* 189, 248, 1977.

101. **Simmons, W. K.,** Variations in urinary inorganic sulfate sulfur and urea nitrogen excretion in children on a rural African diet, *Arch. Latinoam. Nutr.,* 22, 403, 1972.

102. **Bray, H. G., Humphris, B. G., Thorpe, W. V., White, K., and Wood, P. B.,** Kinetic studies of the metabolism of foreign organic compounds. 4. The conjugation of phenols with sulphuric acid, *Biochem. J.,* 52, 419, 1952.

103. **Oldham, J. D., Mathison, G. W., and Milligan, L. P.,** Urinary excretion of intravenously injected [^{35}S] sulphate and [^{14}C] urea in sheep, *Can. J. Anim. Sci.,* 55, 207, 1975.

104. **Kent, P. W., Whitehouse, M. W., Jennings, M. A., and Florey, H. W.,** Observations on the incorporation of [^{35}S] in duodenal mucosubstances, *Q. J. Exp. Physiol.,* 41, 230, 1956.

105. **Barratt, T. M. and Walser, M.,** Extracellular fluid in individual tissues and in whole animals: distribution of radiosulfate and radiobromide, *J. Clin. Invest.,* 48, 56, 1969.

106. **Bird, P. R.,** Sulphur metabolism and excretion studies in ruminants. 7. Secretion of sulphur and nitrogen in sheep pancreatic and bile fluids, *Aust. J. Biol. Sci.,* 25, 817, 1972.

107. **Mulder, G. J. and Keulemans, K.,** The metabolism of inorganic sulfate in the isolated perfused rat liver. Effect of sulphate concentration on the rate of sulphation by phenolsulphotransferase, *Biochem. J.,* 176, 959, 1978.

108. **Rico, A. G., Godfraind, J. C., Bénard, P., Burgat-Sacare, V., and Braun, J. P.,** Metabolism of sodium sulfate isotopically marked with [^{35}S] in the mouse. 1. Autoradiographic study, *Ann. Rech. Vet.,* 4, 235, 1973.

109. **Kennedy, P. M., Hogan, J. P., Lindsay, J. R., and Hogan, R. M.,** Transfer of sulphur to the digestive tract of sheep, *Aust. J. Biol. Sci.,* 29, 525, 1976.

110. **Ryan, R. J., Pascal, L. R., Inoye, T., and Bernstein, L.,** Experiences with radiosulfate in the estimation of physiologic extracellular water in healthy and abnormal man, *J. Clin. Invest.,* 35, 1119, 1956.

111. **Walser, M., Seldin, D. W., and Grollman, A.,** An evolution of radiosulfate for the determination of the volume of extracellular fluid in man and dogs, *J. Clin. Invest.,* 32, 299, 1953.

112. **Swan, R. C., Madisso, H., and Pitts, R. F.,** Measurement of extracellular fluid volume in nefrectomized dogs, *J. Clin. Invest.,* 33, 1447, 1954.

113. **Sheatz, G. C. and Wilde, W. S.,** Transcapillary exchange rate and volume of distribution of sulfate and sodium as indicated by S^{35}O$_4$ and Na^{24} in the rat, *Am. J. Physiol.,* 162, 687, 1950.

114. **Thornton, J. R. and English, P. B.,** Radiosulphate: its metabolism and use in measurement of extracellular fluid volume in calves, *Res. Vet. Sci.,* 22, 298, 1977.

115. **Bauer, J. H., Burt, R. W., Whang, R., and Grim, C. E.,** Simultaneous determination of extracellular fluid and total body water. 1, *J. Lab. Clin. Med.,* 86, 1003, 1975.

116. **Douglas, G. J., Shklar, J. O., Forstner, G. D., and Mathews, R. E.,** Evaluation of radiosulfate as a measure of functional and total extracellular fluid, *Surg. Forum,* 20, 35, 1969.

117. **Galambos, J. T. and Cornell, R. G.,** Mathematical models for the study of the metabolic pattern of sulfate, *J. Lab. Clin. Med.,* 60, 53, 1962.

118. **Steck, T. L.,** The organization of proteins in the human red blood cell membrane. A review, *J. Cell Biol.* 62, 1, 1974.

119. **Zaki, L., Fasold, B., Schuhmann, B., and Passow, H.,** Chemical modification of membrane proteins in relation to inhibition of anion exchange in human red blood cells, *J. Cell. Physiol.,* 86, 471, 1975.

120. **Lepke, S. and Passow, H.,** Effects of incorporated trypsin on anion exchange and membrane proteins in human red blood cell ghosts, *Biochim. Biophys. Acta,* 455, 353, 1976.

121. **Wolosin, J. M., Ginsburg, H., and Cabantchik, Z. I.,** Functional characterization of anion transport system isolated from human erythrocyte membranes, *J. Biol. Chem.,* 252, 2419, 1977.

122. **Schnell, K. F., Gerhardt, S., and Schöppe-Fredenburg, A.,** Kinetic characteristics of the sulfate self-exchange in human red blood cells and red blood cell ghosts, *J. Membr. Biol.,* 30, 319, 1977.

123. **Ross, A. H. and McConnell, H. M.,** Reconstitution of band 3, the erythrocyte anion exchange protein, *Biochem. Biophys. Res. Commun.,* 74, 1318, 1977.

124. **Knauf, P. A., Fuhrmann, G. F., Rothstein, S., and Rothstein, A.,** The relationship between anion exchange and net anion flow across the human red blood cell membrane, *J. Gen. Physiol.,* 69, 363, 1977.

125. **Rakitzis, E. T., Gilligan, P. J., and Hoffmann, J. F.,** Kinetic analysis of the inhibition of sulphate transport in human red blood cells by isothiocyanates, *J. Membr. Biol.,* 41, 101, 1978.

126. **Deuticke, B., v.Bentheim, M., Beyer, E., and Kamp, D.,** Reversible inhibition of anion exchange in human erythrocytes by an inorganic disulfonate, tetrathionate, *J. Membr. Biol.,* 44, 135, 1978.

127. **Low, P. S.,** Specific cation modulation of anion transport across the human erythrocyte membrane, *Biochim. Biophys. Acta,* 514, 264, 1978.

128. **Ormos, G. and Manyai, S.,** Anion transport of the red cell under nonequilibrium conditions, *J. Physiol.*, 276, 501, 1978.
129. **Schnell, K. F., Besl, E., and Manz, A.** Asymetry of the chloride transport system in human erythrocyte ghosts, *Pfluegers Arch.*, 375, 87, 1978.
130. **Ku, C., Jennings, M. L., and Passow, H.,** A comparison of the inhibitory potency of reversibly acting inhibitors of anion transport on chloride and sulfate movements across the human red cell membrane, *Biochim. Biophys. Acta,* 553, 132, 1979.
131. **Grinstein, S., Ship, S., and Rothstein, A.,** Anion transport in relation to proteolytic dissection of band 3 protein, *Biochim. Biophys. Acta,* 507, 294, 1978.
132. **Williams, D. G., Jenkins, R. E., and Tanner, M. J. A.,** Structure of the anion-transport protein of the human erythrocyte membrane. Further studies on the fragments produced by proteolytic digestion, *Biochem. J.,* 181, 477, 1979.
133. **Kitao, T., Hattori, K., and Takeshita, M.,** Species differences in the effects of proteolytic enzymes on red cell membranes, *Experientia,* 33, 675, 1977.
134. **Grinstein, S., McCulloch, L., and Rothstein, H.,** Transmembrane effects of irreversible inhibitors of anion transport in red blood cells. Evidence for mobile transport sites, *J. Gen. Physiol.,* 73, 493, 1979.
135. **Cabantchik, Z. I., Knauf, P. A., and Rothstein, A.,** The anion transport system of the red blood cells. The role of membrane protein evaluated by the use of probes, *Biochim. Biophys. Acta,* 515, 239, 1978.
136. **Levinson, C. and Villereal, M. L.,** The transport of sulfate ions across the membrane of the Ehrlich ascites tumor cell, *J. Cell. Physiol.,* 85, 1, 1975.
137. **Levinson, C. and Villereal, M. L.,** Interaction of the fluorescent probe, 1-anilino-8-naphthalene sulfonate, with the sulfate transport system of Ehrlich ascites tumor cells, *J. Cell. Physiol.,* 86, 143, 1975.
138. **Villereal, M. L. and Levinson, C.,** Chloride-stimulated efflux in Ehrlich ascites tumor cells: evidence for 1:1 coupling, *J. Cell. Physiol.,* 90, 553, 1977.
139. **Levinson, C.,** Chloride and sulfate transport in Ehrlich ascites tumor cells: evidence for a common mechanism, *J. Cell. Physiol.,* 95, 23, 1978.
140. **Lücke, H., Stange, G., and Murer, H.,** Sulphate-ion/sodium-ion cotransport by brush-border membrane vesicles isolated from rat kideny cortex, *Biochem. J.,* 182, 223, 1979.
141. **Mulder, G. J. and Scholtens, E.,** The availability of inorganic sulphate in blood for sulphate conjugation of drugs in rat liver in vivo. [^{35}S] sulphate incorporation into harmol sulphate, *Biochem. J.,* 172, 247, 1978.
142. **Herbai, G.,** A double isotope method for determination of the miscible inorganic sulfate pool of the mouse applied to *in vivo* studies of sulfate incorporation into costal cartilage, *Acta Physiol. Scand.,* 80, 470, 1970.
143. **Drewes, L. R. and Gilboe, D. D.,** Nutrient transport systems in dog brain, *Fed. Proc.,* 36, 166, 1977.
144. **White, C. J. B.,** Some characteristics of sulfate uptake into synaptsomes, *Z. Naturforsch. Teil C,* 34, 487, 1979.
145. **Denko, C. W. and Priest, R. E.,** Utilization of maternal sulfate by the embryo and suckling rat, *Arch. Biochem. Biophys.,* 79, 252, 1959.
146. **Hansard, S. L. and Mohammed, A. S.** Maternal-fetal utilization of sulfate sulfur by the gravid ewe, *J. Nutr.,* 96, 247, 1968.
147. **Knight, E., Van Wart, J., and Roe, D. A.,** Effect of salicylamide on the placental transfer and fetal tissue distribution of sodium [^{35}S] sulfate in the rat, *J. Nutr.,* 108, 216, 1978.
148. **Thornburg, K. L., Binder, N. D., and Faber, J. J.,** Distribution of ionic sulfate lithium and bromide across the sheep placenta, *Am. J. Physiol.,* 236, C 58, 1979.
149. **Crompton, M., Palmieri, F., Capano, M., and Quagliariello, E.,** The transport of sulphate and sulphite in rat liver mitochondria, *Biochem. J.,* 142, 127, 1974.
150. **Crompton, M., Palmieri, F., Capano, M., and Quagliariello, E.,** A kinetic study of sulphate transport in rat liver mitochondria, *Biochem. J.,* 146, 667, 1975.
151. **Abou-Khalil, S. and Hanson, J. B.,** Energy-linked sulfate uptake by corn mitochondria via the phosphate transporter, *Plant Physiol.,* 63, 635, 1979.
152. **Cole, D. E. C., Mohyuddin, F., and Scriver C. R.,** A microassay for analysis of serum sulfate, *Anal. Biochem.,* 100, 339, 1979.

Chapter 4

SULFATE ACTIVATION

G. J. Mulder

TABLE OF CONTENTS

I. INTRODUCTION

Between 1950 and 1958 the chemical structure and biosynthesis of the cosubstrate for sulfate transfer, adenosine 3'-phosphate 5'-sulfatophosphate (PAPS) was investigated and clarified. After the initial discovery by De Meio and Tkacz[1] that a rat-liver homogenate could conjugate phenol with sulfate to form phenyl sulfate when inorganic sulfate, 2-oxoglutarate, and AMP were present, it was soon found out that the latter substrate was converted by the mitochondria in the homogenate into ATP: when mitochondrial ATP synthesis was inhibited by 2, 4-dinitrophenol or compounds with a similar action on mitochondrial oxidative phosphorylation, sulfation of phenolic compounds was inhibited.[2-4] ATP, inorganic sulfate, and Mg^{2+}, incubated without mitochondria but with a cytosolic preparation from rat liver (in the absence of a substrate for sulfation) formed an intermediate which could be used subsequently for sulfate transfer if a substrate for sulfation was added. This indicated that the formation of the cosubstrate for sulfation was independent of the sulfate transfer.[5] At first this cosubstrate was suggested to be adenosine 5'-sulfatophosphate (APS; Figure 1), synthesized in a single step.[6,7] But soon thereafter it was established that the active principle was PAPS, synthesized in a two-step synthesis, catalyzed by two cytosolic enzymes, ATP-sulfurylase and APS-kinase, as discovered by the work of Wilson et al.[8] and Robbins and Lipmann.[9,10] The two activating reactions are

$$ATP + SO_4^{2-} \rightleftharpoons APS + PP_i \tag{1}$$

$$APS + ATP \rightleftharpoons PAPS + ADP \tag{2}$$

The first reaction is catalyzed by ATP-sulfurylase (ATP: Sulfate Adenylyltransferase; EC 2.7.7.4.) and the second by APS-kinase (ATP: Adenylylsulfate 3'-phosphotransferase; EC 2.7.1.25). The sulfate activating system has been found present in most mammalian tissues,[11-14] has been demonstrated in several invertebrates,[11,12,15,16] crustaceans,[17] molluscs,[16] echinoderms,[18,19] insects,[20,21] higher plants, algae and fungi,[22,23] and microorganisms.[22] Several bacteria contain only the first step, leading to APS.[22]

Most studies on the properties of the activating enzymes have been performed on enzyme preparations from microorganisms. In these organisms often no sulfotransferase is present, because (P)APS is used here for assimilatory and dissimilatory sulfate reduction.[22-29] This of course, poses the question whether the findings with the bacterial enzymes may be extended to the mammalian situation. In this chapter, work on the bacterial enzymes will be reviewed when insufficient data are available on the mammalian enzymes.

In many tissues, studied either in vivo or in vitro [^{35}S]-labeled inorganic sulfate is incorporated into tissue macromolecules, especially glycosaminoglycans;[30-32] if it is assumed (a very likely assumption) that this incorporation occurs only after conversion of the added inorganic sulfate into PAPS, then it seems that most, if not all, mammalian tissues contain the sulfate-activating enzymes. As yet there are no indications that PAPS may be synthesized in one organ, and be transported to another via the blood. Further, one can only speculate about the reasons why PAPS is used as cosubstrate for sulfate transfer, rather than APS.

II. ADENOSINE 3'-PHOSPHATE 5'-SULFATOPHOSPHATE (PAPS)— SYNTHESIS AND PROPERTIES

The chemical structure of "activated sulfate" was established by Robbins and Lipmann.[33,34] After isolation of the cosubstrate of sulfation by Dowex®-1 chromatog-

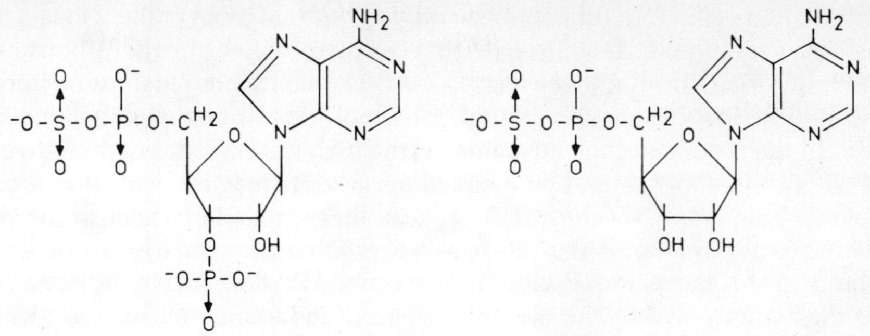

55

FIGURE 1. Chemical structure of PAPS (left) and APS (right).

raphy, they found a ratio of 2:1 for phosphate and adenosine; using a 3'-nucleotidase, they showed that one of the phosphate groups was in the 3'-position. Further studies with ATP labeled in the pyrophosphate end-group with [32P], and various nucleotidases proved that the sulfatophosphate group was in the 5'-position. The sulfatophosphate link is unstable at acidic pH, but stable at neutral or alkaline pH.

The identity of PAPS as sulfate donor was confirmed by chemical synthesis:[35] the synthetic PAPS was active as sulfate donor in the sulfotransferase reaction.[36] This latter was an important criterium because initially the "activated sulfate" isolated by Hilz and Lipmann[6] from *Neurospora sitophila* and lamb liver was thought to be APS. De Meio and Wizerkaniuk[7] at that time reached similar conclusions about the chemical nature of activated sulfate. When APS was synthesized chemically, however, it was shown not to donate its sulfate group in the sulfotransferase reaction, and therefore could not be the "activated sulfate." Around 1957 the cosubstrate of sulfation had been fully characterized as PAPS.

The systematic name for PAPS is adenosine 3'-phosphate 5'-sulfatophosphate, but several other names are in use, such as 3'-phospho-adenylyl sulfate and 3'-phosphoadenosine 5'-phosphosulfate. At present both unlabeled and [35S]-labeled PAPS are commercially available. Several methods for the synthesis of PAPS have been published, both biosynthetic and purely chemically synthetic ones.

A biosynthetic method on a preparative scale was first described by Brunngraber,[37] using PAPS-synthesizing enzymes from rat liver. Later modifications have employed preparations of the activating enzymes from a number of sources such as yeast, *Chlorella,* chicken liver, hen oviduct, or Furth-mouse mastocytomas.[37-45] Obviously, the method can be used to prepare [35S]-labeled PAPS.[38,43] The yield of these procedures is about 5 to 10% from the ATP used. Separation of PAPS from the other components after the enzymatic synthesis is achieved by column chromatography, using Dowex,® DEAE-Sephadex A25, or ECTEOLA as column material. A charcoal adsorption step in the original procedure may lead to variable losses and can be avoided.[40,46]

Chemical synthetic procedures have been published[47-49] and are discussed in Chapter 2, Section V.

The halflife of PAPS in 0.1 *N* HCl at 37°C is 6 to 9 min,[16,34] but no detectable hydrolysis was observed in 0.1 *N* NaOH at 37°C in 2 hr.[34] Even 2 hr at 100°C in the latter solution caused only incomplete hydrolysis.[36] The molar absorption of PAPS was 14,500 at 260 nm.[38,47] Data on the separation of PAPS from several other nucleotides by electrophoresis,[36,43,49] paper chromatography,[16,36,47] and thin-layer chromatography[49] are available. Recently, a separation by high performance liquid chromatography was reported.[50]

Determination of PAPS is most conveniently performed by an indirect assay, namely by measuring the amount of sulfate ester that can be formed by phenolsulfotransferase (preferably purified) from a given sample of PAPS-containing material. Procedures have been described using 2-naphthol,[11] harmol,[51] or 4-methylumbelliferone[52] as substrate. In the latter case, the advantage is the high fluorescence of 4-methylumbelliferone. 4-Nitrophenol[34] should be avoided because its reaction with PAPS is freely reversible[11] (Chapter 5, Section II.D.). Another procedure makes use of the luciferin-luciferase system of the sea pansy *Renilla reniformis,* which is sensitive to adenosine 3′, 5′-bisphosphate (PAP).[53] In this method PAPS is first hydrolyzed to PAP, which is then determined by the bioluminiscence it induces in this luciferin-luciferase system (see Chapter 5, Section VIII).

Only very limited data are available on concentrations of PAPS in various tissues of animals, most likely because PAPS is rather labile in biological material, and because the assay methods for PAPS are relatively complicated. Wong and Yeo[51] determined in boiled liver extracts from guinea pig, rat, mouse, and rabbit, respectively, 33 ± 4, 29 ± 2, 7.8 ± 1.5, and 5.3 ± 0.5 (means $\pm$ S.D.) μmol PAPS per kilogram tissue. No PAPS could be found in monkey and dog liver, nor in other tissues of the rat and guinea pig such as kidney, small and large intestines, heart, and brain. It is not yet known whether PAPS is stable enough to completely survive the time between killing the animal and transferring the liver into liquid air; these figures, therefore, are minimum levels. Indirect evidence in vivo confirmed that the PAPS concentration in the liver is very low, since [^{35}S]-labeled inorganic sulfate, injected intravenously, equilibrated within 1 to 2 min with the PAPS-sulfate pool in the liver, responsible for sulfation of the phenolic drug harmol.[54] The group of Kurup[55-57] reports that in rats fed an atherogenic diet the PAPS level in the liver decreased. In guinea pigs both on a normal and on an atherogenic diet, ascorbic acid increased the PAPS level somewhat. Low levels of pyridoxine gave a decrease in the rat, whereas high levels caused an increase. In the rabbit the same group evaluated the effect of thyroid hormones and thiouracil.[58]

III. ATP-SULFURYLASE

A. Assay Methods
The first step in the activation of sulfate is catalyzed by ATP-sulfurylase (ATP: Sulfate Adenyltransferase, EC 2.7.7.4):

$$ATP + SO_4^{2-} \rightleftharpoons APS + PP_i \tag{3}$$

The equilibrium of this reaction lies far to the left, and the forward reaction proceeds at an appreciable rate only when the products of the reaction are taken away, e.g., by inorganic pyrophosphatase activity, or by the second enzyme of sulfate activation, APS-kinase. Therefore, the activity of this enzyme is usually measured by an indirect assay, or by the reverse reaction, i.e., PP_i-dependent ATP synthesis from APS. Recently, however, a convenient assay for the forward reaction has become available. Four different types of assay have been developed.

In the first place the forward reaction, the production of APS from ATP and inorganic sulfate can be measured. Until recently the generation of APS by ATP-sulfurylase could only be demonstrated by isolating APS through electrophoresis or chromatography, but these procedures are too lengthy for routine measurements. Methods in which the APS formed was absorbed to charcoal proved to be unreliable.[59-61] A rapid method was recently devised by Reuveny and Filner,[62] who made use of the differential solubility of the salts of APS and inorganic sulfate. When the

ATP-sulfurylase incubation in the forward direction is stopped with five parts of ethanol, inorganic sulfate is completely insoluble in the mixture. The radioactivity remaining in solution in the supernatant was shown to be only [^{35}S]-APS because PAPS is also insoluble in the ethanol/water mixture. A high concentration of inorganic pyrophosphatase was included in the incubation to remove PP_i and thereby enhance the rate of the forward reaction. Obviously, the APS formed should not be further metabolized to PAPS, since this would lead to an underestimation of the rate. A very high ATPase activity in the enzyme preparation might also affect the rate of the reaction, by taking away ATP. This assay has been developed with an ATP-sulfurylase preparation from tobacco plant, but it has also been used with the rat-liver enzyme.[63] It is clear that the development of any other ethanol-soluble compound derived from $^{35}SO_4^{2-}$ will cause an overestimation of the reaction rate.

The reverse reaction, i.e., the PP_i-dependent production of ATP and inorganic sulfate from APS, can easily be measured because the ATP formed can be determined very sensitively by the luciferin-luciferase system.[56,57] Also the APS-dependent disappearance of PP_i has been used to assay the enzyme.[66] Methods for the chemical synthesis of APS are available.[47,67,68] Limitations of the method are obvious: any further metabolism of ATP will lead to underestimation of the activity of ATP-sulfurylase. Only purified enzyme preparations will give sufficiently reliable results because, besides ATPases, also any enzyme affecting APS (APS-kinase; APS-sulfohydrolase), and inorganic pyrophosphatase may decrease the observed rate of ATP formation. The addition of fluoride in the incubation may inhibit the endogenous inorganic pyrophosphatase and ATPase activities in the enzyme preparation.[69]

In a third assay method, the sulfate-dependent exchange of radioactive [^{32}P]-PP_i with the pyrophosphate end-group of ATP has been employed, especially in studies with the purified enzyme.[8,59,69,70]

$$\text{ATP} + [^{32}\text{P}] - \text{PP}_i \underset{\text{SO}_4^{2-}}{\rightleftharpoons} [^{32}\text{P} - \text{PP}_i] - \text{ATP} + \text{PP}_i \tag{4}$$

Again, with impure enzyme preparations, contaminating inorganic pyrophosphatase and ATPase may affect the assay; these enzymes may be inhibited by the addition of fluoride in the incubation.[69]

The most frequently used, but also most indirect, assay is the "molybdolysis" of ATP to AMP and PP_i (Equation 5), i.e., the

$$\text{ATP} + \text{H}_2\text{O} \xrightarrow[\text{MoO}_4^{2-}]{} \text{AMP} + \text{PP}_i \tag{5}$$

molybdate-catalyzed hydrolysis of ATP by ATP-sulfurylase.[8,71] When inorganic pyrophosphatase is added, the resulting PP_i is rapidly hydrolyzed to inorganic phosphate which can be conveniently measured. The control incubation measures phosphate production in the absence of molybdate. One has to take into consideration that at acidic pH, relatively high nonenzymatic hydrolysis of ATP by molybdate occurs,[72] which is much less severe with tungstate or vanadate. In the presence of ATPase activity, high blank values may be expected. A further complication is that molybdate may inhibit ATPase,[73] causing an underestimation of the ATP-sulfurylase activity in this method (because in the control incubation without molybdate, ATPase is not inhibited and yields too high control values). The mechanism of this molybdolysis is not quite clear; a highly unstable molybdate analogue of APS may be formed, which decomposes immediately upon synthesis.[71] Alternatively, one might speculate that proximity effects at the active site of ATP-sulfurylase might enhance the hydrolysis of

ATP by molybdate as was observed to occur nonenzymatically at acid pH.[72] Since the molybdolysis assay became available very early in the short history of ATP-sulfurylase and it is very easy to perform, it has been a very popular assay for the enzyme so far.

A method to detect ATP-sulfurylase in acrylamide gels using molybdolysis has been described by Skyring et al.[74]

B. Purification

The considerations above make it obvious that the degree of purification of an ATP-sulfurylase preparation is highly ambiguous and subject to errors which depend on the assay method employed. In the starting material, usually an homogenate, many interfering enzyme activities will be present and the measured activity in that fraction will be least reliable. During the various purification steps these contaminants will be removed differentially; therefore all claims about an "x-fold" purification should be viewed with caution and, maybe, some skepticism.

The first purification of ATP-sulfurylase was by Robbins and Lipmann in 1958 from yeast.[10,75] By ammonium sulfate fractionation and Geon electrophoresis, they obtained a 1400-fold purified enzyme (as judged by the results of the molybdolysis method), which sedimented as a single peak during ultracentrifugation. Since then, many more attempts at purification have followed, employing the more sophisticated methods that became available later. Only rarely, however, a mammalian source has been used, since mostly microorganisms were used such as yeast,[10,71,75-77] *Nitrobacter*,[78] *Clostridium*, or *Desulfovibrio*.[79] Further, the filamentous fungus *Penicillium chrysogenum*,[61,80,81] the blue-green alga *Spirulina platensis*,[82] and the red alga *Rhodella*[83] have been used. Of the higher plants, spinach and corn have been investigated.[59,84] Finally, in mammals the enzyme has been purified from mouse mastocytoma[60,85] and the liver of rat[63,86] and sheep.[66] Most of the data in this section, therefore, originate from experiments on the ATP-sulfurylase from nonmammalian sources. One general comment on the purification of ATP-sulfurylase is the following. So far, the molecular weights of the various ATP-sulfurylase preparations are of the order of 400,000 or higher, with only one exception: the enzyme from corn root had a molecular weight of only 42,000.[84] Because of this high molecular weight, a Sephadex G-200 step is often used as a first purification, since then many low-molecular weight proteins are removed and ATP-sulfurylase is eluted in the void volume.

So far, only three papers have reported a more extensive purification of ATP-sulfurylase from mammalian liver. Panikkar and Bacchawat[66] purified the enzyme from sheep liver by ammonium sulfate precipitation and Sephadex G-200 column chromatography, using the APS-dependent disappearance of PP_i as assay (the reverse reaction). They obtained a 200-fold purified enzyme preparation that was devoid of a number of interfering activities such as APS-kinase, inorganic pyrophosphatase, and ATPase. The preparation, however, was not further investigated as to its purity by physical methods such as polyacrylamide gel electrophoresis.

ATP-sulfurylase from rat liver has been purified 1000-fold by Levi and Wolf;[86] they have measured the reverse reaction by following ATP generation with the luciferin-luciferase system, as assay of the enzyme. The 100,000 g × 60-min rat-liver supernatant in 0.25 M sucrose/0.025M KC1 was used as starting material, and subjected to ammonium sulfate fractionation (40 to 65% fraction), acid precipitation (pH 6.5), and hydroxyapatite batch adsorption. The final product had a specific activity of 0.75 μmol ATP generated per minute per milligram protein. No physical characterization of the enzyme and its purity was done. This had to wait until almost 10 years later when Burnell and Roy[63] in 1978 gave many details of the physical properties of ATP-sulfurylase from rat liver. They used as starting preparation a rat-liver nonparticulate supernatant. The 35 to 65% ammonium sulfate precipitate was dialyzed and further treated by ethanol precipitation and a second ammonium sulfate step. After column chromatography on DEAE-Sephadex A-50 and hydroxyapatite, with gradient elution using KCl and phosphate, respectively, the purified enzyme preparation was subjected to Sepharose 4B column chromatography. A 2500-fold purified enzyme was obtained with a final specific activity of 2 μmol ATP formed per minute per milligram protein, measured as APS-dependent incorporation of $^{32}PP_i$ into ATP. No ATPase, APS-kinase, ADP-sulfurylase, or inorganic pyrophosphatase were present in the final preparation. Polyacrylamide gel electrophoresis revealed two major and one minor protein band; the major bands with molecular weights of about 500,000 and 1,000,000 daltons contained ATP-sulfurylase activity, whereas it could not be established with certainty whether there was activity in the minor band. Ultracentrifugation showed a complex Schlieren pattern of resolved and partly resolved peaks, which have to be characterized still further as to their nature. This is the purest preparation reported so far from rat liver. The heterogeneous composition is possibly due to different aggregation forms of the enzyme, as discussed by the authors.

The enzyme from another mammalian source, Furth mastocytoma, was extensively investigated by the group of Shoyab and Marx.[60,85,87] Two forms of the enzyme could be separated by DEAE-cellulose chromatography after initial purification by ammonium sulfate fractionation and Sepharose-4B chromatography. The difference between the forms seemed to be a difference in charge because the forms could also be separated by electrophoresis on Geon resin. No difference in enzymatic properties was found. In a later paper,[60] inconsistent behavior of ATP-sulfurylase on electrophoresis was reported, and the authors were unable to separate two peaks as before. The enzyme was purified 545-fold by a combination of column chromatography and electrophoresis; it was assayed by the formation of ATP from APS and PP_i (reverse reaction). The unreliable nature of this and similar assays in highly impure enzyme preparations was clearly demonstrated by the authors: the total amount of enzyme activity increased fivefold during the first ammonium sulfate fractionation, which may have been due to the removal of inhibitors or of interfering enzyme activities. Although in the final preparation no inorganic pyrophosphatase, ATPase, and APS-kinase were present, again it has not been characterized as to its contamination by other proteins.

Basically similar methods have been used to purify the enzyme from plant and microbial sources. ATP-sulfurylase from spinach leaves is associated with the chloroplast fraction; it was purified 53-fold from extracts of spinach leaves, using the luciferin-luciferase assay to measure ATP generated from APS and PP_i (reverse reaction).[64] Shaw and Anderson[59] purified ATP-sulfurylase 1000-fold from the same source by DEAE-cellulose chromatography. They included fluoride in their incubation system ($^{32}PP_i$-exchange with ATP) in order to inhibit inorganic pyrophosphatase that was present at high activity in the initial fractions. The ATP-sulfurylase from corn root has been purified 33-fold using DEAE-Sephadex chromatography.[84]

The purified enzyme from *Nitrobacter agilis* (DEAE-cellulose-32 column chromatography) gave a single band in starch-gel electrophoresis.[78] Many details are given by Tweedie and Segel[80] and Farley et al.[81] on their purified ATP-sulfurylase from *Penicillium chrysogenum*, which was purified to homogeneity as shown by electrophoresis on gels of various acrylamide concentrations. After heat treatment of the initial extract,[80] the supernatant was fractionated with ammonium sulfate. The 25 to 45% fraction was dialyzed and chromatographed on a column of Bio-gel^R agarose A-5, which binds the enzyme with very high affinity. Several further steps yielded a preparation that was purified 528-fold as judged by the $^{32}PP_i$ exchange reaction with ATP,[81] or 945-fold as judged by the molybdolysis assay.[80]

C. Properties and Substrate Specificity

ATP-sulfurylase (in its completely aggregated form) has a high molecular weight; when it is chromatographed on Sephadex G-200, it is usually recovered in the void volume.[60,66,86] Levi and Wolf[86] suggested a molecular weight of 800,000 to 900,000 from the behavior of their purified enzyme from rat liver on agarose Bio-gel® A-15m (with a reported fractionation capacity of 40,000 to 15,000,000 daltons). Varma and Nicholas[78] similarly reported a high molecular weight, 700,000 for the enzyme from *Nitrobacter agilis* as determined on Sephadex G-200, which certainly is not the most adequate column to determine the molecular weight of such a high-molecular weight protein. It seems therefore, that the later estimations (see below) of a molecular weight around 450,000 are more reliable than these very high values. The sedimentation coefficient of the *Nitrobacter agilis* enzyme determined on a sucrose gradient at 4°C was 12.8 S.[78] A slightly higher value was observed for the *Penicillium chrysogenum* enzyme,[81] namely 13.0 ($S_{20,w}$), calculated from extrapolation to zero protein concentration. Other physical characteristics of the enzyme were a Stokes radius of 72 Å, a free diffusion coefficient $D_{20,w}$ of 2.94×10^{-7} cm^3/sec, and a partial specific volume[81] of 0.733 cm^3/g. The molecular weight was between 425,000 and 440,000 as determined on a Sephadex G-200 column. This was confirmed by disc-gel electrophoresis on gels of varying pore size, which yielded a molecular weight of 440,000; a similar value could be calculated from the physical parameters of the enzyme. Discontinuous gel electrophoresis of carboxy-methylated ATP-sulfurylase in the presence of sodium dodecyl sulfate suggested that the *Penicillium* enzyme is composed of eight subunits of molecular weight 56,000. Binding studies revealed that the enzyme binds 8 mol of ATP per 440,000 g of protein.[81] Further support for an octamer came from the finding that eight free sulfhydryl groups could be titrated with Ellman's reagent [(5,5'-dithiobis) (2-nitrobenzoic acid)]. The amino acid composition of the enzyme indicated that nine half-cystine residues per subunit were present: in each subunit four cystines and one cysteine residue. The enzyme did not dissociate into subunits during chromatography or ultracentrifugation of the native enzyme. Interestingly, the ATP-sulfurylase isolated from corn root[84] had a molecular weight of 42,000 daltons. Is the native enzyme in this plant a monomer?

Burnell and Roy[63] purified the enzyme from rat liver and determined a molecular weight of 410,000 on Sepharose-4B. On a sucrose density gradient a $S_{20,w}$ of 4.8 was found, but ultracentrifugation showed a very complex Schlieren pattern, with $S_{20,w}$ values of 5.3 (corresponding to a molecular weight of 410,000), 8.6, 11, 18, and 20. The first two peaks were the major components, and the faster sedimenting material at 18 and 20 S was present only in trace amount. Since dilution of the protein did not change this sedimentation behavior, a rapidly equilibrating polymerizing system seems not very likely. Neither was the pattern due to denaturation because the enzyme activity was quantitatively recovered from the ultracentrifuge cell; this problem remains to be resolved. The mean value of the partial specific volume was 0.80 cm^3 / g. The authors discuss the possibility that this value indicates that the enzyme may be a lipoprotein. They found material with a high absorbance 410 nm associated with the enzyme, which might be a carotenoid-like substance, but has not yet been identified. Clearly, much work has still to be done in the complete physical characterization of the enzyme from various sources.

Purified ATP-sulfurylase from several sources proved to be stable for weeks at -18 to $-15°C$[59,66,76,79] or even at 5°C[60] unless it is in a Tris buffer.[78] However, it loses its activity on repeated freezing and thawing.[60,63,66,71] Tris strongly decreases the stability of the purified enzymer;[60,86] barbiturate less so, and in a phosphate buffer the enzyme is much more stable. ATP-sulfurylase from rat liver[63] was unstable in Tris, diethylbarbiturate, glycine, triethanolamine, and bicarbonate buffers of pH 7.8, but it was stable in a phosphate buffer, unless Tris was also present. The enzyme is rather heat labile: 1 min at 75°C, or 5 to 10 min at 60°C destroy most of the activity of the purified enzyme from various sources.[59,76,78,85] ATP seemed to protect the enzyme to a certain degree;[79] impure enzyme preparations may be more resistant against heat-inactivation than the purified enzyme.[84] Understandably, the ATP-sulfurylase from a thermophilic *Clostridium* species was stable at 60 to 65°C.[79] The detergent deoxycholate (1%) irreversibly destroyed activity of the rat-liver enzyme.[86]

The pH optimum of the reaction almost invariably is between 7.0 and 9.0. Variations within this range probably are due to the use of different buffers, assay methods (pH optima of interfering enzyme activities!) or, of course, differences in properties of the enzymes from different sources.

Analysis of the amino acid composition of the *Penicillium* enzyme revealed the presence of nine half-cystines per subunit of enzyme protein.[80] Together with the presence of only one titrable −SH group per subunit, this suggests that in each of the eight proposed subunits one free sulfhydryl group is available, which may or may not be involved in catalysis.[61] The reports on the effect of sulfhydryl-blocking agents are somewhat controversial. Levi and Wolf[86] report complete inhibition of the rat liver enzyme by 16 m*M* *p*–chloromercuribenzoate (PCMB); the effect of PCMB was prevented by the inclusion of reduced glutathione in the incubation medium, which could also reactivate the PCMB-inhibited enzyme. Burnell and Roy[63] similarly found strong inhibition of the purified rat-liver enzyme by PCMB and *N*-ethylmaleimide. The *Nitrobacter* enzyme was also inhibited by PCMB;[78] the untreated preparation was strongly activated by reduced glutathione and other −SH group-containing reagents, indicating that a reduced −SH group is essential to the optimally functioning ATP-sulfurylase. Interestingly, Shoyab and Marx[87] reported an activation of 40 to 90% of purified mouse mastocytoma enzyme by low concentrations of PCMB (0.05 to 0.1 m*M*), and inhibition at concentrations above 2 m*M* PCMB. *p*-Hydroxymercuri-benzoate had the same effect as PCMB, but iodoacetate, iodoacetamide, and mercuric chloride had no such effect. The enzymes from *Penicillium chrysogenum, Saccharomyces,* and spinach leaves were not inhibited by PCMB and several other sulfhydryl reagents.[59,76,88] Therefore, it seems that there may be a species difference in the role that sulfhydryl groups play in catalysis by ATP-sulfurylase. It is not yet clear whether this −SH group is involved in the binding of reaction intermediates, or may affect the conformation and activity of the enzyme through allosteric effects. Further, one has to consider the possibility that in impure preparations, PCMB (or any other compound under study) may affect any of the interfering enzymes, and thereby, indirectly, affect the measured enzyme activity. This might eventually be a very trivial explanation for the activation by PCMB, although it could equally well be a direct effect of PCMB on ATP-sulfurylase. When lysine was modified with pyridoxal, or tryptophan with 2-hydroxy-5-nitrobenzyl bromide, no inactivation of the *Penicillium* enzyme was observed.[88] However, modification of a single arginine residue (by 2,3-butanedione) or a single histidine (by light in the presence of methylene blue) residue per subunit caused complete inactivation. Modification of a tyrosine residue by tetranitromethane also caused inactivation. APS, ATP, and MgATP protected against some of these effects. Therefore, arginine, histidine, and tyrosine residues are essential for the functional integrity of the enzyme.

Many analogues of inorganic sulfate, ATP, and APS have been tested for their effects in the ATP-sulfurylase reaction: whether they could serve as substrate or whether they were (competitive) inhibitors. Dependent on the reaction measured (APS synthesis, reverse reaction, PP_i exchange), the effects may be different. The only sulfate analogue that seems to be activated by ATP-sulfurylase to an APS analogue is selenate, as was suggested by Bandurski et al. from rather indirect evidence.[8,71,89] They observed that selenate catalyzed the PP_i exchange with ATP (in the absence of sulfate) and that it is converted to a charcoal-absorbed form by ATP-sulfurylase in the presence of ATP (selenate itself is not absorbed to charcoal). Finally, they isolated from such incubations a selenium-containing compound (labeled with [^{75}Se]-selenate) with electrophoretic properties and acid lability similar to APS, which they suggested to be APSe. In a later publication Dilworth and Bandurski[90] further extended these studies by showing that a partly purified ATP-sulfurylase preparation from *Saccharomyces* catalyzed the formation of elemental selenium from selenate in the presence of ATP, inorganic pyrophosphatase, and reduced glutathione. The proposed APSe formed was reduced nonenzymatically by glutathione to elemental selenium, according to their reaction scheme. It proved impossible, however, to identify an APSe intermediate. On the other hand, 2 mol of P_i were released per mole of elemental selenium formed; furthermore, the reaction rate was decreased by omission of inorganic pyrophosphatase from the incubation medium, and even further by omission of Mg^{2+} (which strongly stimulates ATP-sulfurylase). They conclude that APSe must have been an intermediate in the formation of elemental selenium and that this mechanism may play a role in the ability of animals to utilize both selenite and selenate as a source of nutritionally required selenium. The fact that Shaw and Anderson[91] were not able to reproduce some of these findings was explained by Dilworth and Bandurski by the rather critical conditions required for the demonstrations of putative APSe by electrophoresis. Selenate catalyzes the $^{32}PP_i$-ATP exchange with a much lower K_m for selenate than that for sulfate, as shown for ATP-sulfurylase from *Penicillium*,[81] various *Astragalus* species,[91] spinach,[59] and rat liver.[63] Thus, it seems very likely that sulfate and selenate may bind to the same site of the enzyme; probably both are converted into an activated form. The latter remains, however, controversial so far,[91,92] the problem being that the presence of APSe has not been unequivocally identified by chemical means, but only inferred from indirect measurements.

It seems that sulfate "analogues" can not replace sulfate in the $^{32}PP_i$-ATP exchange reaction: CrO_4^{2-}, MoO_4^{2-}, ClO_3^-, or NO_3^- are either ineffective or even inhibitory towards the sulfate-dependent exchange.[59,63,81,93,94] The inhibition by both chlorate and nitrate was uncompetitive with respect to ATP and competitive with respect to sulfate with the spinach,[93] *Penicillium*,[94] and rat-liver[63] enzyme. Nitrate has been used in kinetic studies of ATP-sulfurylase as a dead-end inhibitor for sulfate;[94] the K_i values for the rat-liver enzyme were 2.2 mM (for nitrate) and 0.25 mM (for chlorate).[63] Some other anions that do not catalyze PP_i-ATP exchange are persulfate, thiosulfate, metabisulfate, dithionate, and selenite (40 mM each).[59] Farley et al.[81] have tested the inhibition of the forward reaction of ATP-sulfurylase from *Penicillium* by anions and found the following to be competitively inhibitory towards sulfate (in increasing order of potency): methylsulfate, NO_2^- n-hexylsulfate, HCO_3^-, SO_3^{2-}, phosphate, thiosulfate, formate, NO_3^- and ClO_3^- (Table 1). The *Nitrobacter* enzyme (forward reaction) was inhibited[78] by MoO_4^{2-}, CrO_4^{2-}, WO_4^{2-}, and SeO_4^{2-}. Sulfide, the end product of sulfate reduction in many bacterial strains, inhibited the molybdolysis by *Penicillium* ATP-sulfurylase, and behaved as an allosteric inhibitor of the K-type.[61] Interestingly, this feedback inhibition by sulfide is lacking in some wine yeasts that form sulfite, whereas in nonsulfite-producing yeast strains, there is a strong feedback by sulfide.[22]

It is important to realize that the "group VI anions" catalyze the ATP-sulfurylase-mediated hydrolysis of ATP to AMP and pyrophosphate,[71] which has led to the molybdolysis assay for ATP-sulfurylase. The rate of molybdolysis is about 100-fold faster than the rate of APS synthesis from sulfate, which may explain why sulfate inhibits molybdolysis.[61,76] It is interesting to note that several group VI anions that

Table 1
INHIBITORS OF THE FORWARD REACTION OF ATP-SULFURYLASE FROM
PENICILLIUM CHRYSOGENUM

Inhibitors competitive with ATP		Inhibitors competitive with SO_4^{2-}	
Compound[a]	Percentage inhibition	Compound[a]	Percentage inhibition
2'-AMP	1	Methylsulfate	21
3'-AMP	2	Nitrite	22
Ribose-5-Phosphate	9	*n*-Hexylsulfate	28
Adenosine	12	Bicarbonate	31
5'-AMS	13	Sulfite	34
5'-ADP	31	Phosphate	37
3',5'-ADP (PAP)	31	Thiosulfate	40
5'-AMP	32	Formate	46
NAD+	47	Nitrate	81
NADP+	51	Chlorate	91

[a]The concentration of the inhibitors was 3 mM.

From Farley, J. R., Nakayama, G., Cryns, D., and Segel, I. H., *Arch. Biochem. Biophys.*, 185, 376, 1978. Copyright, Academic Press, New York. With permission.

catalyze ATP hydrolysis by ATP-sulfurylase do not accelerate PP$_i$-ATP exchange.

Several analogues of ATP have been tested as to their effect on ATP-sulfurylase. The forward reaction of the enzyme is inhibited by free ATP, which inhibits competitive[61,94] in respect to the substrate form MgATP^{2-}. Table 1 shows a number of compounds listed in order of increasing potency, that inhibit the forward reaction competitive in respect to (Mg)ATP.[81] The inhibition by NAD and NADP is also competitive with respect to PP$_i$ and APS, as is to be expected for a rapid equilibrium ordered reaction sequence (see below). The fact that Spolter et al.[95] found an increase of $^{35}SO_4^{2-}$ incorporation into heparin by a mitochondria-free fraction of mouse mastocytoma in the presence of NAD remains to be explained; these authors, however, used a very impure enzyme preparation which complicates the analysis of their findings and makes clear-cut conclusions impossible.

The forward reaction of ATP-sulfurylase from the alga *Anabaena* was inhibited by ADP, AMP, and P$_i$ which could be overcome by increasing the ATP concentration, and, therefore, seemed competitive with respect to ATP.[96,97] GTP, UTP, TTP, ITP, and dATP also inhibited the forward reaction, of which GTP was shown to do so in a competitive fashion towards ATP.[96] APS also inhibited the partly purified ATP-sulfurylase from some wine yeast species;[27] some sulfite-producing strains possessed an ATP-sulfurylase that was much less sensitive to inhibition by APS than nonsulfite-producing strains.

In the reverse reaction, APS could not be replaced by GPS, IPS, ADP, or AMP as substrate,[60,75] but dAPS showed some activity; all of these substrates inhibited the reverse reaction with APS as substrate. The enzyme from rice roots was inhibited by ADP and adenosine, but was activated by AMP, especially at low ATP concentration.[98] The ^{32}PP$_i$-ATP exchange reaction by the rat-liver enzyme[63] was also inhibited by AMP and ADP. The inhibition was competitive with respect to ATP, and ADP had the higher affinity. dATP can serve as substrate for PP$_i$ exchange, but has a lower affinity and rate of exchange; in addition it inhibits the rate of exchange when ATP is used as substrate.[59]

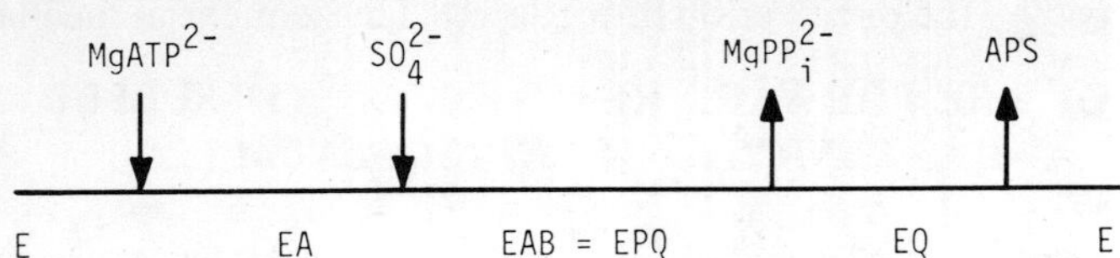

FIGURE 2. Sequential mechanism of the catalysis by ATP-sulfurylase.

GTP was not a substrate for PP$_i$ exchange.[59] In the molybdolysis assay CTP, GTP, UTP, ITP, and dTTP could not replace ATP.[71,75,76,79]

These results show that ATP-sulfurylase from various sources has a rather narrow substrate specificity, both as to the inorganic substrate and the nucleotide. Dead-end inhibitors are available for studies on the catalytic mechanism of the enzyme.

The activity of ATP-sulfurylase is very much dependent on the presence of sufficient Mg^{2+}, since the substrate for the enzyme is MgATP^{2-} (see below); therefore, EDTA is inhibitory. The effect of other, especially divalent cations depends on the assay method used. Very little has been done on the forward reaction. Farley et al.,[81] studying the purified enzyme from *Penicillium*, found that the forward reaction could not be sustained by Mn^{2+}, Co^{2+}, or Ca^{2+} instead of Mg^{2+}. They discuss the potential effects of these cations on inorganic pyrophosphatase, which indirectly affect the measured activity of ATP-sulfurylase. Further, the cation may interact with any of the components in the incubation: Mn^{2+} may form aggregates with PP$_i$. All these potential interactions should be kept in mind in the analysis of the results because they may be the reason for conflicting findings. Thus, Shoyab and Marx[99] reported that Mn^{2+} catalyzed the forward reaction by the mouse-mastocytoma enzyme.

In a thorough study, Farley et al.[81] compared the effectivity of Mg^{2+}, Mn^{2+}, Co^{2+}, and Ca^{2+} on the various reactions catalyzed by ATP sulfurylase. Mg^{2+} was effective in every reaction studied. Mn^{2+} and Co^{2+} could substitute for Mg^{2+} in the molybdolysis and the ^{32}PP$_i$-ATP exchange reaction, but Ca^{2+} was ineffective. They conclude that the enzyme from *Penicillium* possesses a divalent cation activator site that is involved in APS synthesis, and is distinct from the site for the metal ion-ATP complex. This activator site might accept all four cations, but functions only when occupied by Mg^{2+}. Other authors,[59,60,75,85] using enzyme preparations from various sources similarly found that ^{32}PP$_i$-ATP exchange and the reverse reaction could be supported by Co^{2+}, Mn^{2+}, and Zn^{2+}. The reports about Ni^{2+} are controversial.[59,60] Ba^{2+}, Ca^{2+}, Hg^{2+}, and Fe^{2+} were reported to be inhibitory towards the mouse-mastocytoma enzyme, measured in the reverse direction,[60] in decreasing order of potency.

Clearly, there is yet some confusion on the effect of the various cations, probably due to the use of so many different assay procedures and enzyme preparations. The main finding is, however, that Mg^{2+} seems physiologically involved in the catalytic action of the enzyme. Several authors[61,76,81,93,94] have put forward evidence that the real substrates for the ATP-sulfurylase are MgATP^{2-} and MgPP$_i^{2-}$. When the concentration of ATP is increased above that of Mg^{2+}, the enzyme activity is inhibited by the resulting free ATP. Excess of Mg^{2+} has no further effect on the rate of the reaction, but at very high Mg^{2+} concentrations complications may arise, such as precipitation of (insoluble) MgPP$_i$[93] which obviously decreases the ^{32}PP$_i$–ATP exchange.

D. Kinetic Mechanism

The kinetic mechanism of the ATP-sulfurylase reaction is an ordered Bi Bi sequential mechanism[63,81,93,94,99] (Figure 2). A suggestion by Levy and Wolf[86] that the reaction proceeded according to a Ping-Pong® mechanism has been disproved as most likely an artifact introduced by the purification procedure.[63] The sequential mechanism predicts that there are several partial reactions:[93,99]

$$E + MgATP^{2-} \rightleftharpoons E\text{--}MgATP^{2-} \tag{6}$$

$$E\text{--}MgATP^{2-} + SO_4^{2-} \rightleftharpoons E\begin{smallmatrix} \diagup MgATP^{2-} \\ \diagdown SO_4 \end{smallmatrix} \tag{7}$$

$$E\begin{smallmatrix} \diagup MgATP^{2-} \\ \diagdown SO_4 \end{smallmatrix} \rightleftharpoons E\begin{smallmatrix} \diagup MgPP_i^{2-} \\ \diagdown APS \end{smallmatrix} \tag{8}$$

$$E\begin{smallmatrix} \diagup MgPP_i^{2-} \\ \diagdown APS \end{smallmatrix} \rightleftharpoons E\text{--}APS + MgPP_i^{2-} \tag{9}$$

$$E\text{--}APS \rightleftharpoons E + APS \tag{10}$$

This reaction scheme has been thoroughly discussed by Farley et al.[81] (Figure 3). These authors showed binding of APS and $MgATP^{2-}$ to ATP-sulfurylase from *Penicillium* by (non) equilibrium dialysis; 8 mol of ATP bound to the enzyme (proposed to consist of eight subunits) with a K_s of 0.53 mM. This is in excellent agreement with the enzymatically determined K_i and K_m values for $MgATP^{2-}$ and free ATP, respectively (0.4 to 0.8 mM). Using column chromatography on Sephadex G-75, Shoyab and Marx[99] found similarly binding of ATP and APS to their mouse-mastocytoma enzyme. [^{35}S]-sulfate did not bind to the enzyme, not even in the presence of ATP (without Mg^{2+}) or ATP analogues; neither was $MgPP_i^{2-}$ bound.[81] An explanation for the somewhat unexpected lack of binding of sulfate is, that possibly $MgATP^{2-}$ is split before sulfate can be bound, with the hydrolysis products being bound in the active center (Equation 11):

$$E + MgATP^{2-} \rightleftharpoons E\text{--}MgATP^{2-} \rightleftharpoons E\begin{smallmatrix} \diagup AMP \\ \diagdown MgPP_i \end{smallmatrix} \tag{11}$$

Thermodynamic calculations about the equilibrium of reaction 11 suggest that most of the complex would be in the form of the nonhydrolyzed $E\text{--}MgATP^{2-}$ complex. However, the authors demonstrate that $MgATP^{2-}$ is indeed hydrolyzed by their very pure ATP-sulfurylase preparation to AMP and PP_i, which could not be due to contaminating enzyme activities. Similarly, there was a, be it very slow, $^{32}PP_i$-ATP exchange in the absence of sulfate as was to be expected from Equation 11. These interesting observations remain to be confirmed, although the authors have accumulated much (indirect) evidence that Equation 11 must exist. They found also hydrolysis of APS in the absence of PP_i, which may be related to the fact that for thermodynamic reasons the enzyme–APS complex is mainly in the form of

$$E\text{--}APS \rightleftharpoons E\begin{smallmatrix} \diagup AMP \\ \diagdown SO_4 \end{smallmatrix} \tag{12}$$

the "hydrolyzed" complex $E.AMP.SO_4$ (Equation 12). Since in the absence of $MgATP^{2-}$ the rate of resynthesis of APS from the latter complex is very slow, only an extremely slow rate of exchange of [^{35}S]-sulfate in the medium with the sulfate group in APS would be expected to take place, which is in agreement with the experimental findings: no such exchange was observed.[76,81,86,93]

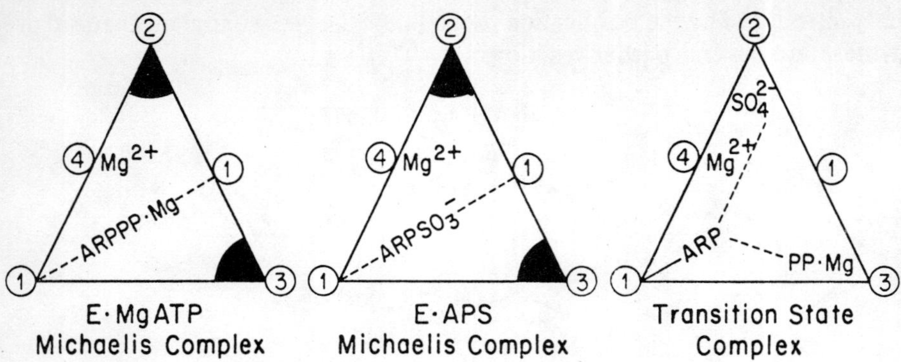

FIGURE 3.   Proposed schematic model of ATP-sulfurylase. The nucleotide substrate is bound initially at subsite 1 which recognizes the AMP moiety. Catalytic cleavage of the pyrophosphate or phosphosulfate anhydride bond results in the formation of E ~ AMP at part of subsite 1 and a conformational change in the enzyme that exposes subsites 2 and 3. Subsite 2 accepts SO_4^{2-} (or the sulfate portion of APS). Subsite 3 accepts $MgPP_1$ (or the $MgPP_1$ portion of MgATP). Water may be able to occupy subsites 2 and 3 or possibly, water has no actual site but occupancy of subsites 2 or 3 sterically hinders the attack of water on E ~ AMP. Subsite 4 is highly specific for Mg^{2+} (required for APS cleavage/synthesis). Ca^{2+} can bind to subsite 4, but with much less affinity than Mg^{2+}. (From Farley, J. R., Nakayama, G., Cryns, D., and Segel, I. H., *Arch. Biochem. Biophys.*, 185, 376, 1978. Copyright Academic Press, New York. With permission.)

The substrates and reaction products $MgATP^{2-}$, APS, sulfate, $MgPP_i$ are product inhibitors or substrate inhibitors in the various partial reactions in which they take part; usually, APS and $MgATP^{2-}$ were found to be competitive.[63,81,94] Several kinetic constants of the enzymes from *Penicillium* and mammalian sources are collected in Tables 2 and 3. Some data about properties of ATP-sulfurylase in rather impure preparations from soybean[100] and some higher plants[101] are available.

The intermediary formation of an enzyme.AMP.$MgPP_i$ complex from E–ATP (Equation 11) as suggested by Farley et al.[81] would seem to favor the mechanism proposed by Kosower[102] in which the sulfate ion reacts with the enzyme-bound AMP. Kossower argued that a nucleophilic attack on the α-phosphate group of ATP to release PP_i is highly unlikely because of the low nucleophilicity of the sulfate ion and the unfavorable interactions between the negatively charged sulfate and $MgATP^{2-}$ ions (although Mg^{2+} may facilitate the attack). The mechanism of molybdolysis might be a molybdate-catalyzed dissociation of the enzyme.AMP.$MgPPi_i$ complex, without a bond being formed between molybdate and AMP.

The ATP-sulfurylase equilibrium strongly favors the reverse reaction: the equilibrium constants as determined with the enzyme from several bacterial sources[71,75,79] are between 0.6 and 4×10^{-8}. In order to attain a high rate of the forward reaction, the products PP_i and APS must be rapidly removed by coupling reactions, for instance by inorganic pyrophosphatase or APS-kinase; both these reactions are strongly endergonic. Robbins and Lipmann[75] calculated a $\Delta F°$ of 46 kJ for the reaction, which indeed can be provided by the two subsequent reactions. The enzyme from the red alga *Rhodella* required an activation energy of 46 kJ.[83] The sulfate group-potential in APS must be about 80 kJ (as compared with a phosphate group-potential of about 34 kJ in ATP).

E. ADP-Sulfurylase

The properties of ADP-sulfurylase (ADP:sulfate adenylyltransferase; E.C. 2.7.7.5) will only briefly be discussed, since the activity so far has been studied only in bacteria

Table 2
KINETIC CONSTANTS OF ATP-SULFURYLASE FROM
PENICILLIUM CHRYSOGENUM

Kinetic constant	Value
K_m for $MgATP^{2-}$	0.38 mM
K_m for SO_4^{2-}	0.50 mM
K_m for $MgPP_i$	0.65 μM
K_i for APS	0.3—1.0 μM
K_i for APS as substrate inhibitor	0.3 mM
K_i for MgATP	0.6—0.7 mM
K_i for free ATP	0.5—0.8 mM
K_i for AMP	0.5—0.8 mM
K_i for MgADP	0.65 mM
K_i NO_3^-	0.18—0.24 mM
K_i ClO_3^-	0.13—0.21 mM
K_i $MgPO_4^-$	1.1—1.5 mM
V_{max} forward/V_{max} reverse	0.018
V_{max} forward (Mo_4)/V_{max} forward (SO_4)	20
K_{eq} (pH 8.0, 30°C experimental)	2.5×10^{-9}
K_{eq} (calculated from Haldane equation)	$6.0 \times 10^{-9} - 3.3 \times 10^{-8}$

From Farley, J. R., Cryns, D. F., Yang, Y. H. J., and Segel, I. H., *J. Biol. Chem.*, 251, 4389, 1976. With permission.

Table 3
KINETIC PARAMETERS OF ATP SULFURYLASE FROM MAMMALIAN SOURCES

Substrate or inhibitor	Source or enzyme	Reaction measured	K_m (mM)	K_i (mM)	Ref.
ATP	Rat liver	Molybdolysis	1.6		86
	Rat liver	Exchange	0.38		63
SO_4^{2-}	Rat liver	Exchange	2.5		63
	Rat liver	Forward	3.2		63
	Rat liver	PAPS synthesis	0.15		172
	Rat liver	PAPS synthesis by sulfation of 4-nitrophenol	0.10		86
	Rat liver	PAPS synthesis by sulfation of harmol	3.5		173
APS	Rat liver	Reverse	0.25		86
	Rat liver	Reverse	0.025		63
	Rat liver	Reverse	2.0		53
	Mouse mastocytoma	Reverse	0.1—0.05		85
	Sheep liver	Reverse	2.0		66
PP_i	Rat liver	Reverse	0.04		86
	Rat liver	Reverse	0.018		63
	Rat liver	Reverse	1.7		53
	Mouse mastocytoma	Reverse	0.2—0.15		85
	Sheep liver	Reverse	1.7		66
SeO_4^{2-}	Rat liver	Exchange	0.6	0.50	63
AMP	Rat liver	Exchange		0.6	63
ADP	Rat liver	Exchange		0.06	63
NO_3^-	Rat liver	Exchange		2.2	63
ClO_3^-	Rat liver	Exchange		0.25	63

and plants. This reaction seems to operate only in the reverse direction, and probably does not play a role in mammals. The forward reaction (Equation 13) would synthesize APS from ADP and inorganic sulfate.

$$ADP + SO_4^{2-} \rightleftharpoons APS + P_i \tag{13}$$

However, the forward reaction never has been shown to occur, and, in fact, is energetically even more unfavorable than the ATP-sulfurylase reaction: P_i is only removed by synthetic reactions, and is present in the cell at rather high concentrations. Therefore, most likely the reaction will operate in vivo in the reverse direction.

The enzyme was purified to some extent by Robbins and Lipmann[10] who measured the reverse reaction: production of ADP from APS. Since this reaction was not catalyzed by a purified ATP-sulfurylase preparation, it had to be due to another enzyme, which indeed could readily be separated from ATP-sulfurylase of yeast. Since both ATP-sulfurylase and inorganic pyrophosphatase require Mg^{2+}, whereas ADP-sulfurylase activity proceeds in the absence of Mg^{2+}, the observed production of P_i from APS in the absence of Mg^{2+} can not be due to a combination of ATP-sulfurylase and inorganic pyrophosphatase activities, yielding P_i (and ATP). Later work by Grunberg-Manago et al.[103] who purified the enzyme about 35-fold from yeast by a combination of protamine and ammonium sulfate fractionations and DEAE-cellulose, showed that it catalyzed an exchange reaction between $^{32}P_i$ and APS, ADP, and several other nucleoside diphosphates. No exchange occurred with the triphosphates, monophosphates, or PP_i, using this enzyme. The authors suggested that the mechanism of the enzymatic action is a displacement of phosphate from ADP (or sulfate from APS) through the formation of an intermediary enzyme-AMP complex. Inorganic sulfate had no effect on this exchange reaction.

ADP-sulfurylase was 300-fold purified from yeast by Adams and Nicholas[104] who confirmed the P_i-ADP exchange (presumably in the absence of sulfate) observed by Grunberg-Manago et al.[103] and reported on the kinetic properties of the enzyme. Some years later, Nicholls[105] proved that the $^{32}P_i$-ADP exchange, catalyzed by yeast ADP-sulfurylase, was independent of the presence of sulfate. The exchange could also be measured with APS as substrate (generating $AD^{32}P$ and SO_4^{2-}), and seemed to follow a Ping-Pong® reaction mechanism. Inorganic sulfate did not affect ADP-sulfurylase activity, unless concentrations of the order of 100 mM were used. Interestingly, related anions like arsenate, chromate, and vandate at 20 mM catalyzed the hydrolysis of ADP by yeast ADP-sulfurylase to AMP and P_i, whereas sulfate at this concentration catalyzed no such activity.[103]

The enzyme has also been purified from spinach-leaf tissue by Burnell and Anderson,[106] who devised a new $^{32}P_i$-ADP exchange method and have studied specificity and properties of the reaction. ADP-sulfurylase was found in the chloroplast fraction and was released by sonication. A serious complication in the analysis of this work is that the so-called "sulfate-independent" P_i-ADP exchange was consistently higher than the "sulfate-dependent" exchange, measured at 30 mM inorganic sulfate in the incubation medium. The authors have solved this problem by adding 3mM $BaCl_2$ to the assays which completely inhibited the sulfate-independent exchange, but activated the sulfate-dependent exchange to about twice the original activity of the untreated sulfate-independent exchange. It is hard to evaluate these findings; obviously, the presence of 30 mM sodium sulfate may reactivate the $BaCl_2$-inhibited enzyme, and therefore, the sulfate-dependent activity in the presence of $BaCl_2$ may include the previous sulfate-independent activity (because Ba^{2+} has been removed with the added sulfate). Why then the total activity should be twice that of the uninhibited sulfate-independent P_i-ADP exchange is not quite clear. It might be due to some activating effect of $BaCl_2$, although it is unlikely that such an activation would persist in the presence of sulfate (unless the activating effect were irreversible).

Although the enzyme has a wide distribution in bacteria and plants, more work is required to characterize the properties of the enzyme. It has been demonstrated in several microorganisms of which, for obvious reasons, the sulfur-metabolizing species have received most interest.[107-110] Peck has forwarded several possible roles of the enzyme in the intermediary metabolism of microorganisms.[109] It has not yet been demonstrated in mammalian tissues.

IV. APS-KINASE

Contrary to the relative wealth of data on ATP-sulfurylase, the knowledge on APS-kinase (ATP:Adenylylsulfate 3'-phosphotransferase; EC 2.7.7.4), the enzyme catalyzing the second step in sulfate activation, is very limited. The enzyme has been demonstrated in several tissues of many species.[22,111,112] Since the original purification and characterization,[10,71] only one further purification has been reported. The formation of PAPS has usually been measured by the production of a sulfate conjugate from a phenolic substance (e.g., naphthol) in a coupling reaction catalyzed by added phenolsulfotransferase.

Robbins and Lipmann[10] purified ATP-sulfurylase and APS-kinase from baker's yeast. By an acidification step (pH 5.8) they separated APS-kinase, which remained in solution, from ATP-sulfurylase, that was precipitated. After ethanol precipitation and ammonium sulfate fractionation, an enzyme preparation resulted that had a high affinity for APS; above 5 μM (the lowest measurable substrate concentration) APS showed substrate inhibition. IPS was not converted into the PAPS-analogue PIPS. The stoichiometry of PAPS synthesis was established and is shown in Equation 14. CTP, GTP, ITP, and UTP could replace

$$APS + ATP \rightleftharpoons PAPS + ADP \tag{14}$$

ATP in this reaction with equal effectivity. Mg^{2+}, Co^{2+}, and Mn^{2+} activitated the kinase, but Ca^{2+} had no effect; the pH optimum was between 8.5 and 9.0. The reaction was virtually irreversible and had a $\Delta F°$ of -25 kJ at pH 8.0 and 37°C.[75] In combination with the very high affinity for APS, this ensures an efficient synthesis of PAPS, even when the equilibrium of the first activating reaction (Equation 1) is very unfavorable. Since the enzyme preparations used in this early work[10,71] may still have been heavily contaminated, there is much need for confirmation of these findings with an APS-kinase preparation purified to homogeneity, using the more sophisticated techniques introduced in recent years. The only recent report available so far is by Burnell and Anderson,[113] who purified the enzyme from an extract of spinach-leaf tissue. The PAPS synthesis was measured by coupling it to sulfation of 2-naphthol, catalyzed by an added purified phenol sulfotransferase preparation from rabbit liver. A fluoride-insensitive 3'-nucleotidase, present in the extract, interfered with the assay since it hydrolyzed the 3'-phosphate group from PAPS. It could be effectively inhibited by the inclusion of 3'-AMP in the incubation medium, which competitively inhibited the hydrolysis of APS. When the spinach-leaf extract was subfractionated, the activity of APS-kinase was associated with the chloroplast fraction and was found mainly in the supernatant after sonication of this fraction (as was ATP-sulfurylase). The authors also studied the properties of APS-kinase *in situ* in isolated intact chloroplasts. Mercer and Thomas[114] had previously demonstrated this activity in chloroplasts of French-bean

(Phaseolus vulgaris) and maize *(Zea mays)* leaves. Burnell and Anderson[113] found that in the absence of 3'-AMP almost exclusively APS was formed. If, however, 3'-AMP was included, PAPS accumulated, and the amount of APS was very low. This may explain why, for example, Asahi[115] found only APS and no PAPS in his experiments with spinach-leaf chloroplasts; he did not use 3'-AMP in the incubation. Because no measurable 3'-nucleotidase was present in the chloroplasts, the effect of 3'-AMP may be due to some regulatory effect on overall PAPS synthesis in the chloroplasts; the site of regulation has, however, not been pinpointed by the authors.[113] Interestingly, the synthesis of PAPS in the isolated chloroplasts was increased by 50% when the chloroplasts were illuminated with a tungsten lamp.

In a later publication, Burnell and Whatley[92] have made use of the hydrolysis of PAPS by a 3'-nucleotidase for a rapid assay of APS-kinase. The production of ADP during the APS-kinase reaction (Equation 14) was measured by coupling it through pyruvate kinase and lactate dehydrogenase to the conversation of NADH into NAD. The 3'-nucleotidase regenerates APS from the PAPS formed and thereby keeps the substrate concentration constant. In impure enzyme preparations a quite high rate of "endogenous" NADH oxidation may be found, but when the enzyme is further purified, the assay becomes much more reliable, especially when fluoride is added to inhibit ATPase and ADP-sulfurylase activities. Cyanide inhibits a great part of the endogenous NADH oxidation. Thus, a convenient assay was devised which may facilitate the study of the kinetic properties of the purified enzyme. The authors observed substrate inhibition by APS of the spinach-leaf enzyme by concentrations above 20 μM; the K_m for APS was 5 μM, and that for ATP 1.3 mM. Selenate could not stimulate NADH oxidation in a purified APS-kinase preparation, and, therefore, probably did not form PAPSe. This coupled assay is easier to perform than the coupled assay with phenol sulfotransferase that has been used in most of the work on APS-kinase. Further work is much needed for a more complete characterization of the properties of the enzyme. No specific inhibitors or dead-end inhibitors are known, and the kinetic mechanism has not yet been studied. From rather indirect studies on the incorporation of [^{35}S] sulfate into chondroitin sulfate, Adams and Reinitz[116] concluded that galactosamine inhibits APS-kinase; this needs further confirmation.

V. ENZYMIC DEGRADATION OF APS AND PAPS

The three main points of attack of degrading enzymes in animal tissues on PAPS (Figure 4) are the 3'-phosphate group (3'-nucleotidase), the 5'-sulfatophosphate group (5'-nucleotidase), and the sulfatophosphate anhydride bond (sulfohydrolase). In bacteria, algae and plants in addition to these, the reduction of PAPS (and APS) plays an important role;[117-123] reductases and sulfotransferases are involved in this. Since the main interest of this book regards the situation in animals, and since these reductive reactions seem not to occur in animal tissues, they will not further be discussed, and the reader is referred to reviews on this subject.[22,25,26]

Of the three degrading pathways in animals, the sulfohydrolase pathway has been most extensively studied, and the nucleotidases have received relatively little attention. It is not yet clear to what extent the various pathways and enzymes contribute to the metabolism of APS and PAPS in the tissues. So far there has been no attempt to integrate all the knowledge from studies on the isolated enzymes, both of PAPS synthesis and PAPS breakdown, in order to get some insight into the in vivo regulation of PAPS metabolism. Similarly, no studies of the flux of [^{35}S]-sulfate through the sulfation pathway are available, though these are very much needed.

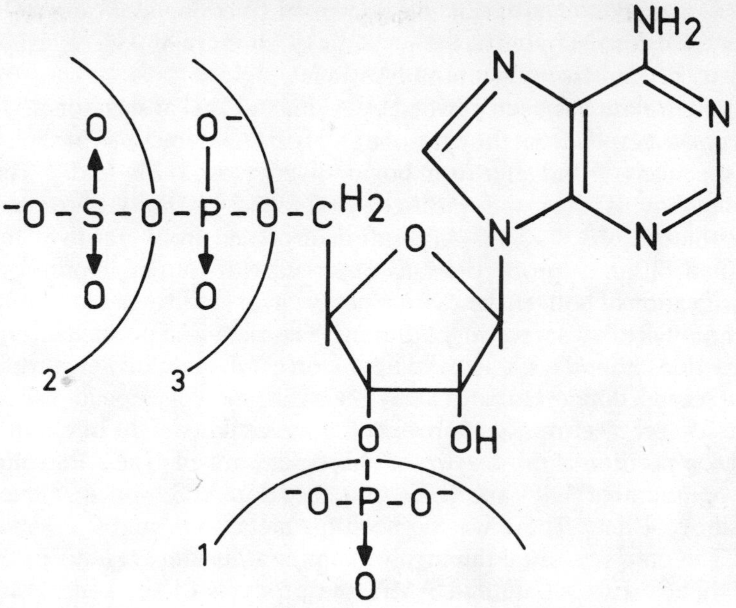

FIGURE 4. Hydrolytic breakdown of PAPS: 1. 3′-nucleotidase, 2. sulfohydrolase, and 3. 5′-nucleotidase.

3′-Nucleotidase activity converts PAPS into APS by hydrolysis of the 3′-phosphate bond.[34,36,124,125] This enzyme activity is ubiquitously present in nature, and it was used by Robbins and Lipmann[34] to establish the structure of active sulfate. APS can be hydrolyzed by 5′-nucleotidase activity with the ultimate formation of adenosine, phosphate, and sulfate.[34,67] Since this enzyme is also present in many tissues, it may play a role in vivo. Thus, when APS and PAPS were incubated with mitochondrial or microsomal fractions from rat liver, the activity of both 3′-nucleotidase and 5′-nucleotidase could be observed;[13,126] other enzymes further metabolize the products of the action of these nucleotidases and proposed sulfohydrolases. This in vitro breakdown could be partially inhibited by fluoride and EDTA.[126] Both the particulate and cystosolic fractions of rat liver contain degrading activity; whether the lysosomes play a physiological role is yet uncertain.[127-129]

Much more detailed knowledge is available on the sulfohydrolase(s). The existence of such enzymes was demonstrated in the early 1960s.[38,130-132] A crude enzyme preparation from sheep brain catalyzed the formation of PAP and inorganic sulfate from PAPS.[130] The pH optimum was 6.0 and several divalent cations, notably Co^{2+} and Mn^{2+}, seemed to activate the enzyme; EDTA had no effect, and Cu^{2+} was inhibitory. The enzyme had a high affinity for PAPS, the K_m being 45 μM. ADP was a powerful inhibitor: at 0.5 mM it inhibited over 60%. ITP, GTP, and UDP were only slightly inhibitory, and ATP and UTP even less.

The PAPS- and APS-sulfohydrolases were further investigated and purified from rat liver by the group of Dodgson and Rose.[129,133-135] PAPS-sulfohydrolysis is found in many species, from the flatworm to the chick.[129] In high-speed supernatants of various rat tissues the highest activities are present in spleen, liver, kidney, and gut; serum contains no such activity or only a very minor amount. When the liver was submitted to subcellular fractionation, APS-sulfohydrolase (measured by release of inorganic sulfate) was found both in the lysosomal and the cytosolic fraction. Since acid phosphatase, a marker enzyme of the lysosomal fraction, was (almost) completely absent from the cytosolic fraction, the cytosolic localization of APS-sulfohydrolase was not due to its release from disrupted lysosomes.[129,133]

APS-sulfohydrolase has been purified by Alumina-C gel adsorption and DEAE-Sephadex chromatography from the cytosolic and lysosomal fractions of rat liver 137- and 56-fold, respectively,[129] and later from bovine-liver cytosol 1200-fold.[133] The lysosomal enzyme from bovine liver was purified 8100-fold by affinity chromatography on 5'-AMP-Sepharose 4B.[135] The APS-sulfohydrolases from rat-liver cytosol and lysosomes had different properties[129] as observed with rather impure preparations. Further purification of both enzymes from bovine liver confirmed that the cytosolic and lysosomal sulfohydrolases were very different. The 1200-fold purified enzyme from the cytosolic fraction showed a single band upon polyacrylamide disc electrophoresis with and without sodium dodecyl sulfate (SDS).[133] Gel filtration on Sephadex G-100 and SDS polyacrylamide gel electrophoresis revealed a molecular weight of about 68,500; the amino acid composition of the enzyme has been determined. The APS-sulfohydrolases had a pH optimum of 5.4^{134} and a K_m of 1 mM for APS, which showed substrate inhibition above 4 mM. There was no need for metal ions, and Cu^{2+} and Hg^{2+} were inhibitory. The data suggested the involvement of a histidine residue in the catalysis. Inhibition studies with sulfate and AMP, the products of the hydrolysis, showed a pattern which is consistent with an ordered uni-bi reaction sequence; this was, however, not fully characterized. ATP and GTP inhibited competitively with APS (K_i of about 0.01 mM). Other nucleotides were also inhibitory, some competitive in respect to APS, some noncompetitive.

The lysosomal enzyme, purified 8100-fold also from bovine liver, behaved very differently.[135] The molecular weight of the single band on SDS-polyacrylamide gel electrophoresis was about 53,000. The enzyme turned out to be a relatively nonspecific hydrolase that split P_i from ATP, PP_i, and *bis*(4-nitrophenyl)phosphate, besides hydrolyzing the sulfate group from APS and PAPS. The authors argue that it is reasonable that APS and PAPS would not possess their own specific lysosomal sulfohydrolase, since these substrates would not be expected inside lysosomes. Even though this seems a reasonable assumption, the final purified preparation represents only 2% of the total activity in the starting material, the mitochondrial-lysosomal fraction, and a more specific (P)APS-sulfohydrolase may have been removed during purification.

PAPS-sulfohydrolase and APS-sulfohydrolase from bovine-liver cytosol can be separated by a simple ammonium sulfate fractionation from each other.[124] The pH optimum of the PAPS-sulfohydrolase was 9.5, that for PAPS-3'-nucleotidase between 5.5 and 6.0. Co^{2+} did not affect the sulfohydrolases, confirming findings with APS-sulfohydrolase from pig-kidney cortex[136] and from rat liver.[132] Co^{2+} (5 mM, however, activated PAPS-3'-nucleotidase about 5-fold.[124] The previous finding of activation of PAPS-sulfohydrolase by Co^{2+} (13 mM) in their opinion indicates that that PAPS-sulfohydrolase preparation[130] must have been contaminated with 3'-nucleotidase and APS-sulfohydrolase: Co^{2+} presumably had increased production of APS from PAPS by the contaminating 3'-nucleotidase, whereupon the contaminating APS-sulfohydrolase would increase the rate of sulfate release. However, Farooqui and Balasubramanian[125] who partially purified PAPS-3'-nucleotidase from sheep brain, found strong inhibition of PAPS-3'-nucleotidase by Co^{2+}. It is difficult to decide whether the differences in the effect of Co^{2+} are due to differences in the source of the enzyme, degree of purification, or methodology. Interestingly, the sheep brain 3'-nucleotidase preparation[125] was indeed activated about 3-fold by Co^{2+} when tested with 3'-AMP as substrate. Further work with pure, homogeneous enzyme preparations will solve these conflicting results.

PAPS degradation has also been studied in pig-kidney cortex.[128,136] PAPS-3'-nucleotidase was predominantly located in the smooth microsomal fraction, whereas PAPS-sulfohydrolase was present in several fractions. A complication in the analysis of the results of subfractionation studies is that many interfering enzyme activities may affect the outcome of specific assays to different extents in the various subcellular fractions, dependent on the subcellular distribution of these interfering enzymes. Unfortunately, most of the assays of the various PAPS-hydrolases are easily affected by interfering enzymes.

APS-sulfohydrolase from pig-kidney cortex has extensively been characterized.[136] It was concluded that there are two APS-sulfohydrolases, one with an acidic and one with a neutral pH optimum.

The findings on the low specificity of the lysosomal sulfohydrolase make it uncertain whether the lysosomes play a role in the physiological metabolism of APS and PAPS. Although the subcellular fractionation experiments in rat and bovine liver suggest a relatively high specific activity of the sulfohydrolases in the lysosomal fraction, the major amount of the hydrolase activity is in the other fractions.[124,127-129,133,136] Moreover, only an 80% increase in PAPS-degrading activity was observed when the lysosomal fraction from rat liver was treated with Triton® X-100,[127] whereas the activity of other lysosomal enzymes usually is enhanced severalfold by such a treatment.

The question remains whether there is much APS- or PAPS-breakdown under physiological conditions in vivo. Because of the unfavorable equilibrium of the ATP-sulfurylase reaction and the high affinity of APS-kinase for APS, one would expect a very low APS concentration. Under steady-state conditions the flux through the sulfate-activating pathway might be determined by physiological degradation of PAPS (slow?) and its consumption by sulfate conjugation of low-molecular weight substances or macromolecules.

VI. FACTORS AFFECTING SULFATE ACTIVATION IN VIVO

A. Vitamin A

From 1960 until about 1969 many papers have been published about the effect of vitamin A deficiency on sulfate metabolism. The data suggested that a deficiency of vitamin A caused a decrease in the rate of PAPS synthesis, owing to a decreased activity of ATP-sulfurylase. Since vitamin A deficiency causes serious illness in the animals, and since several investigators have not considered the effect of decreased food intake by the sick animals (which in itself already affects ATP-sulfurylase activity), the reported results are sometimes rather conflicting and confusing (see also Chapter 5, Section XI).

It had been known for some time that vitamin A deficiency influenced sulfate metabolism in vivo,[137,138] when Wolf and Varandani[139] found that the in vitro incorporation of [^{35}S]-labeled inorganic sulfate and [^{14}C]-glucose into glycosaminoglycans was decreased in colon segments and homogenates from vitamin A-deficient rats. The incorporation of [^{35}S]-sulfate could be restored by the addition of vitamin A (retinol) or its aldehyde (retinal) and acid (retinoid acid) derivatives to the incubation when inorganic [^{35}S]-sulfate was used as substrate. When however, preformed, [^{35}S]-labeled PAPS was used, vitamin A had no stimulatory effect on the incorporation of [^{35}S] into the glycosaminoglycans fraction.[140] The latter showed that not sulfation, but sulfate activation was affected by vitamin A deficiency and that vitamin A or its derivatives might enhance activity of the activating system. The stage for some controversy, however, was set by the report of Pasternak et al.[111] who could not find an effect of vitamin A deficiency in tissue preparations from the eye and colon of the rat and rabbit. Several other papers, on the other hand, confirmed the findings of Wolf and Varandani,[139] both the decrease of sulfate activation (ATP-sulfurylase) and the reactivation in vitro by retinol.[75,141-145] Subba Rao and Ganguly[146,147] further found that both sulfate activation and sulfate transfer in rat liver were decreased during vitamin A deficiency; in vitro sulfate activation could be completely restored to control levels by addition of retinol, whereas retinoic acid fully restored the sulfate transfer step in vitro. Retinol was only effective during the early stages of the vitamin A deficiency when the animals not yet had lost weight; once this occurred, the decrease of sulfate activation (measured in vitro) could no more be restored completely by addition of retinol in vitro, and in severely deficient rats it was completely without effect. Moreover, the pair-fed controls, that also lost weight, similarly showed decreased sulfate activation. The latter finding was confirmed by Geison et al.[148] who demonstrated that the specific activity of ATP-sulfurylase in rat liver and colon supernatants varied with the nutritional status of the rat. They came to the conclusion that the vitamin A effect in the rat might be completely due to the inadequate nutritional state of the deficient animals, and critically discuss the data on the effect of vitamin A deficiency available at that time. Indeed, other investigators[111,149] failed to observe a decrease of sulfate activation in several tissues of vitamin A-deficient rats, as compared to pair-fed controls; only in epiphysial cartilage a decrease was found. Levi et al.[150] confirmed the decrease of ATP-sulfurylase by starvation in rats, but concluded from nutritionally carefully controlled experiments that vitamin A deficiency caused an additional decrease of ATP-sulfurylase. Therefore, on balance, the decrease of sulfate activation (which is a decrease of ATP-sulfurylase activity) by vitamin A deficiency seems to occur; the experiments have to be carefully controlled in order to prevent confusion and misinterpretation due to the inadequate nutritional status of the vitamin A-deficient animals.

Interestingly, in fetal rat liver, PAPS synthesis and sulfation could be stimulated by approximately 25 to 50% when retinol or retinoic acid were added to liver preparations in vitro;[151] in the fetal liver a vitamin A-derived activating factor may be lacking. Sundaresan[142] indeed suggested that a lipid-soluble factor, derived from [^{14}C]-labeled retinol, was associated with the purified enzyme. Further, such a lipid-soluble factor isolated from ATP-sulfurylase of normal rats could restore the activity of ATP-sulfurylase from vitamin A-deficient rats to the normal level. However, Levi and Wolf[86] who obtained a much more purified enzyme, found no radioactivity of retinol associated with the enzyme. They suggest that the finding of Sundaresan[142] may have been due to contamination of his only partly purified enzyme and consider the possibility that vitamin A or a derivative may stabilize the rather labile ATP-sulfurylase in vitro. Perumal and Cama[143] reported stimulation of ATP-sulfurylase from rat liver, purified tenfold, by 5,6-monoepoxyretinoic acid when the enzyme was delipidated before; the delipidated enzyme from normal rats behaved similarly to the enzyme from vitamin A-deficient rats. However, in this work a very much contaminated enzyme preparation was used. The finding by Burnell and Roy[63] that a pigment with high absorption at 410 nm is present in their pure ATP-sulfurylase from rat liver, which may be carotenoid, is of interest. As yet, no definite conclusion can be reached whether a vitamin A-derived activator is associated with ATP-sulfurylase.

Since 1968 very few papers have been published on vitamin A and sulfate activation. Therefore, at present we are left with an unclear situation which requires much more in-depth work to solve this problem beyond doubt, and to elucidate the role of vitamin A or its derivatives in sulfate activation.

B. Hormones, Sex, and Age

Sulfation of glycosaminoglycans in rabbit and chick embryo cartilage is stimulated by thyroxine;[152,153] the exact site of action has not yet been determined, but synthesis of RNA is required for the effect. Similarly, somatomedine ("sulfation factor") stimulates the incorporation of sulfate into macromolecules.[12] No data on the effect of these hormones on sulfation of low-molecular weight substances are available, and the mechanism of action has not been clarified as yet.

Little is known about sex differences in sulfate activation. The activity of overall sulfation of 4-nitrophenol in female rats was reported to be about twice that in male rats. Fetal livers of both sexes contained almost the adult level of sulfate activation.[154,155] The development of sulfate activation in rat brain however, shows a different pattern: highest activity was found immediately after birth.[156,157] A second peak, 12 days after birth, which was observed by Balasubramanian and Bachhawat[156] could not be found by Jansen et al.,[157] which was ascribed by the latter authors to experimental artifacts in the earlier work. Gerlach[158] similarly found a gradual decrease in sulfate activation in rat heart muscle after birth. Indirect observations suggested that during development of the chick cornea, the degree of sulfation of cornea glycosaminoglycans may be regulated by the availability of PAPS.[149]

C. Food and Various Compounds

Starvation causes a pronounced decrease in ATP-sulfurylase activity and therefore of sulfate activation.[148,150] In rats on a 20% protein diet, the specific activity of the enzyme in the liver was about half of that in rats on an 80% protein diet.[150] The finding that low-protein feeding in rats caused low overall sulfation of phenols[160] is in agreement with these findings, although an effect on phenol sulfotransferase may also be involved.

The effect of feeding glucose, sucrose, or a polysaccharide from *Phaseolus mungo* (blackgram) on the sulfate-activating enzyme system of rats has been compared.[161] Sucrose feeding decreased the activity and the PAPS concentration in the liver, whereas the feeding of the polysaccharide increased these, both as compared to the glucose-fed controls.

D. Genetic Defeats in Sulfate Activation

One report so far has suggested that there may be genetic defects in sulfate activation. Schwartz et al.[162] investigated sulfate activation in epiphyseal cartilage from brachymorphic mice and found that [^{35}S]-incorporation into glycosaminoglycans was normal when [^{35}S]-labeled PAPS was the donor in vitro, but was defective when $^{35}SO_4^{2-}$ and ATP were used, both as compared to the activity in normal C57B1/6J mice. The exact nature of this difference still needs further clarification but seems to be due to a defective conversion of APS to PAPS.[163]

E. Regulation of Sulfate Activation in Bacteria and Plants

Although this subject is somewhat outside the scope of this book, some findings will be reported because regulation of the enzyme in animals may be along similar pathways. The dependence on food intake in animals shows that there certainly is regulation through (probably) repression and derepression of biosynthesis of the enzymes involved.

In both *Escherichia coli* and *Bacillus subtilis* sulfate-activating enzymes are repressed by cysteine and cystine.[22,25,164-166] In *Salmonella typhimurium* the genes for ATP-sulfurylase and APS-kinase could be located on the gene map, and mutants lacking the enzymes were isolated.[167] In *Desulphovibrio desulfuricans,* ATP-sulfurylase was not repressed by cysteine (or inorganic sulfite); in this species sulfate reduction is linked to the energy supply of the organism,[25] which may be the reason why ATP-sulfurylase is regulated differently from the situation in the other bacteria mentioned above, where APS may serve mainly a synthetic function.

In the filamentous fungus *Penicillium chrysogenum* ATP-sulfurylase is repressed by methionine and some of its metabolites.[61] There appeared to be a correlation between sulfate uptake, sulfate consumption and ATP-sulfurylase activity.[168] A *Neurospora* mutant that could not use sulfate for growth, but required sulfite or any more-reduced inorganic sulfur source, lacked ATP-sulfurylase, whereas the wild-type that uses also sulfate possesses this enzyme.[169]

Recently, repression and depression of ATP-sulfurylase have been studied in tobacco cells grown under different conditions.[170,171] ATP-sulfurylase appeared to be regulated by both a negative feedback and a positive mechanism. A negative feedback control mechanism in which an end product of the sulfate assimilatory pathway is the repressive factor is suggested because the enzyme is repressed when the sulfur supply is sufficient to support optimal growth (with sulfate, cysteine, or methionine as substrate) and is derepressed when sulfur becomes rate limiting (glutathione as substrate). The fact that low concentrations of selenate derepressed the enzyme in cells grown on sulfate, was explained by the proposed synthesis of a selenate analogue of the proposed repressor, which might relieve the end-product inhibition. The positive regulation was suggested by the fact that derepression of ATP-sulfurylase by sulfur limitation does not occur under conditions of starvation for nitrogen. The results suggest that also the decay of ATP-sulfurylase is regulated under derepressed conditions.

ACKNOWLEDGMENT

I am much indebted to Dr. A. B. Roy for reviewing the manuscript.

REFERENCES

1. **De Meio, R.H. and Tkacz, L.,** Conjugation of phenol by rat liver homogenate, *Arch. Biochem.,* 27, 242, 1950.
2. **De Meio, R.H. and Tkacz, L.,** Conjugation of phenol by rat liver slices and homogenates, *J. Biol. Chem.,* 195, 175, 1952.
3. **Bernstein, S. and MacGilvery, R.W.,** The enzymatic conjugation of *m*-aminophenol, *J. Biol. Chem.,* 198, 195, 1952.
4. **De Meio, R.H., Wizerkaniuk, M., and Fabiani, E.,** Role of adenosine triphosphate in the enzymatic synthesis of phenyl sulfate, *J. Biol. Chem.,* 203, 257, 1953.
5. **Bernstein, S. and MacGilvery, R.W.,** Substrate activation in the synthesis of phenyl sulfate, *J. Biol. Chem.,* 199, 745, 1952.
6. **Hilz, H. and Lipmann, F.,** The enzymatic activation of sulfate, *Proc. Nat. Acad. Sci. U.S.A.,* 41, 880, 1955.
7. **De Meio, R.H. and Wizerkaniuk, M.,** On the "active sulfate" intermediate, *Biochim. Biophys. Acta,* 20, 428, 1956.
8. **Bandurski, R.S., Wilson, L.G., and Squires, C.L.,** The mechanism of "active sulfate" formation, *J. Am. Chem. Soc.,* 78, 6408, 1956.
9. **Robbins, P.W. and Lipmann, F.,** The enzymatic sequence in the biosynthesis of active sulfate, *J. Am. Chem. Soc.,* 78, 6409, 1956.
10. **Robbins, P.W. and Lipmann, F.,** Separation of the two enzymatic phases in active sulfate synthesis, *J. Biol. Chem.,* 233, 681, 1958.
11. **Roy, A.B. and Trudinger, P.A.,** *The Biochemistry of Inorganic Compounds of Sulphur,* Cambridge University Press, London, 1970.
12. **De Meio, R.H.,** Sulfate activation and transfer, in *Metabolic Pathways,* Vol. 7, *Metabolism of Sulfur Compounds,* 3rd ed., Greenberg, D.M., Ed., Academic Press, New York, 1975, 287.
13. **Spencer, B.,** Endogenous sulphate acceptors in rat liver, *Biochem. J.,* 77, 294, 1960.
14. **Sasaki, S.,** The PAPS synthetic enzyme system in granulation tissue, *Clin. Chim. Acta,* 17, 215, 1967.

15. **Goldberg, I.H. and Delbrück, A.,** Transfer of sulfate from 3′-phosphoadenosine 5′-phosphosulfate to lipids, mucopolysaccharides and aminoalkylphenols, *Fed. Proc.,* 18, 235, 1959.
16. **Yoshida, H. and Egami, F.,** Formation of 3′phosphoadenosine 5′-phosphosulfate to charoninsulfuric acid, *J. Biochem. (Tokyo),* 57, 215, 1965.
17. **Kennedy, M.B.,** Products of biogenic amine metabolism in the lobster: sulfate conjugates, *J. Neurochem.,* 30, 315, 1978.
18. **Creange, J.S. and Szego, C.M.,** Sulphation as a metabolic pathway for oestradiol in the sea urchin *strongylocentrotus franciscanus, Biochem. J.,* 102, 898, 1967.
19. **Nozawa, A. and Kinoshita, S.,** Sulfate activating systems in developing sea urchin embryo, *J. Fac. Sci. Univ. Tokyo, Sect.,* 4, 14, 11, 1977, *Chem. Abstr.,* 89, 212344, 212345, 1978.
20. **Yang, R.S.H. and Wilkinson, C.F.,** Enzymic sulphation of *p*-nitrophenol and steroids by larval gut tissues of the southern armyworm *(Prodenia eridania,* Cramer), *Biochem. J.,* 130, 487, 1972.
21. **Yang, R.S.H. and Wilkinson, C.F.,** Sulphotransferases and phosphotransferases in insects, *Comp. Biochem. Physiol.,* 46B, 717, 1973.
22. **Schiff, J.A. and Hodson, R.C.,** The metabolism of sulfate, *Annu. Rev. Plant Physiol.,* 24, 381, 1973.
23. **Coughlan, S.,** Sulphate uptake in *Fucus serratus, J. Exp. Bot.,* 28, 1207, 1977.
24. **Skyring, G.W. and Trudinger, P.A.,** A comparison of the electrophoretic properties of the ATP-sulfurylases, APS-reductases and sulfite reductases from cultures of dissimilatory sulfate-reducing bacteria, *Can. J. Microbiol.,* 19, 375, 1973.
25. **Siegel, L.W.,** Biochemistry of the sulfur cycle, in *Metabolic Pathways,* Vol. 7, *Metabolism of Sulfur Compounds,* 3rd ed., Greenberg, D.M., Ed., Academic Press, New York, 1975, 217.
26. **Fitzgerald, J.W.,** Sulfate ester formation and hydrolysis: a potentially important yet often ignored aspect of the sulfur cycle of aerobic soils, *Bacteriol. Rev.,* 40, 698, 1976.
27. **Heinzel, M. and Trüper, H. G.,** Sulfite formation by wine yeast. 2. Properties of ATP-sulfurylase, *Arch. Microbiol.,* 107, 293, 1976.
28. **Bonish, G. W. and Eschenbruch, R.,** Sulphite reductase and ATP-sulfurylase in low- and high-sulphite forming wine yeasts. Relationship to sulphite accumulation during fermentation, *Arch. Microbiol.,* 109, 85, 1976.
29. **Skyring, G. W., Jones, H. I., and Goodchild, D.,** The taxonomy of some new isolates of dissimilatory sulfate-reducing bacteria, *Can. J. Microbiol.,* 23, 1415, 1977.
30. **Boström, H.,** Chemical and autoradiographic studies on the sulphate exchange in sulpho-mucopolysaccharides, *Ark. Kemi,* 6, 43, 1953.
31. **Dziewiatkowski, D. D.,** Autoradiographic studies with [^{35}S]-sulphate, *Int. Rev. Cytol.,* 7, 159, 1958.
32. **D'Abramo, F. and Lipmann, F.,** The formation of adenosine 3′-phosphate 5′-phosphosulfate in extracts of chick embryo cartilage and its conversion into chondroitin sulfate, *Biochem. Biophys. Acta,* 25, 211, 1957.
33. **Robbins, P. W. and Lipmann, F.,** Identification of enzymatically active sulfate as adenosine 3′-phosphate 5′-phosphosulfate, *J. Am. Chem. Soc.,* 78, 2652, 1956.
34. **Robbins, P. W. and Lipmann, F.,** Isolation and identification of active sulfate, *J. Biol. Chem.,* 229, 837, 1957.
35. **Baddiley, J., Buchanan, J. G., and Letters, R.,** Synthesis of "active sulphate," *Proc. Chem. Soc. (London),* p. 147, 1957.
36. **Baddiley, J., Buchanan, J. G., Letters, R., and Sanderson, A. R.,** Synthesis of "active sulfate" (adenosine 3′-phosphate 5′-sulphatophosphate), *J. Chem. Soc. (London),* p. 1731, 1959.
37. **Brunngraber, E. G.,** Nucleotides involved in the enzymatic conjugation of phenols with sulfate, *J. Biol.Chem.,* 233, 472, 1958.
38. **Suzuki, S. and Strominger, J. L.,** Enzymatic sulfation of mucopolysaccharides in the hen oviduct. 1. Transfer of sulfate from 3′-phosphoadenosine 5′-phosphosulfate to mucopolysaccharides, *J. Biol. Chem.,* 235, 257, 1960.
39. **Robbins, P. W.,** Preparation and properties of sulfuradenylates, in *Methods in Enzymology,* Vol. 6, Colowick, S. P. and Kaplan, N. O., Eds., Academic Press, New York, 1963, 766.
40. **Banerjee, R. K. and Roy, A. B.,** The sulfotransferase of guinea-pig liver, *Mol. Pharmacol.,* 2, 56, 1966.
41. **Balasubramanian, A. S., Spolter, L., Rice, L. I., Sharon, J. B., and Marx, W.,** Preparation of 3′-phosphoadenylyl sulfate in substrate quantities using mastocytoma enzymes, *Anal. Biochem.,* 21, 22, 1867.
42. **Hodson, R. C. and Schiff, J. A.,** Preparation of adenosine 3′-phosphate 5′-phosphosulfate (PAPS): an improved enzymatic method using *Chlorella pyrenoidosa, Arch. Biochem. Biophys.,* 132, 151, 1969.
43. **Sass, N. L. and Martin, W. G.,** Separation of sulfated nucleotides using polyacrylamide gel electrophoresis, *Anal. Biochem.,* 38, 559, 1970.
44. **Tsang, M. L., Lemieux, J., Schiff, J. A., and Bojarski, T. B.,** Preparation of adenosine 5′-phosphosulfate (APS) from adenosine 3′-phosphate 5′-phosphosulfate (PAPS) prepared by an improved procedure, *Anal. Biochem.,* 74, 623, 1976.

45. **Singer, S.,** Enzymatic sulfation of steroids. 6. A simple, rapid method for routine enzymatic preparation of 3′-phosphoadenosine-5′-phosphosulfate, *Anal. Biochem.,* 96, 34, 1979.

46. **Wilson, L. G. and Bierer, D.,** The formation of exchangable sulphite from adenosine 3′-phosphate 5′-sulphatophosphate in yeast, *Biochem., J.,* 158, 255, 1976.

47. **Cherniak, R. and Davidson, E. A.,** Synthesis of adenylylsulfate and adenylylsulfate 3′-phosphate, *J. Biol. Chem.,* 239, 2986, 1964.

48. **Melville, E. and Rutherford, F.,** A simple preparation of phosphoadenylyl sulphate labeled with [35]sulphur, *FEBS Lett.,* 37, 257, 1973.

49. **Horwitz, J. P., Neenan, J. P., Misra, R. S., Rozhin, J.,** Huo, A., and Philips, K. D., Studies on bovine adrenal estrogen sulfotransferase. 3. Facile synthesis of 3′-phospho- and 2′-phospho-adenosine 5′-phosphosulfate, *Biochim. Biophys. Acta,* 480, 376, 1977.

50. **Pennings, E. J. M. and Van Kempen, G. M. J.,** Analysis of 3′-phosphoadenylylsulphate and related compounds by paired-ion high performance liquid chromatography, *J. Chromatogr.,* 176, 478, 1979.

51. **Wong, K. P. and Yeo, T.,** Assay of adenosine 3′-phosphate 5′-sulphatophosphate in hepatic tissues, *Biochem. J.,* 181, 107, 1979.

52. **Van Kempen, G. M. J. and Jansen, G. S. I. M.,** Quantitative assay of 3′–phosphoadenosine-5′-phosphosulphate, "active sulphate," *Anal. Biochem.,* 51, 324, 1973.

53. **Stanley, P. E., Kelley, B. C., Tuovinen, O. H., and Nicholas, D. J. D.,** A bioluminicence method for determining adenosine 3′-phosphate 5′-phosphate (PAP) and adenosine 3′-phosphate 5′-sulfatophosphate (PAPS) in biological materials, *Anal. Biochem.,* 67, 540, 1975.

54. **Mulder, G. J. and Scholtens, E.,** The availability of inorganic sulphate in blood for sulphate conjugation of drugs in rat liver *in vivo.* [35S]-sulphate incorporation into harmol sulphate, *Biochem. J.,* 172, 247, 1978.

55. **Vijayakumar, S. T. and Kurup, P. A.,** Metabolism of glycosaminoglycans in atheromatous rats. Enzymes concerned with synthesis, degradation and sulphation of glycosaminoglycans, *Atherosclerosis,* 21, 245, 1975.

56. **Nambison, B. and Kurup, P. A.,** Ascorbic acid and glycosaminoglycans and lipid metabolism in guinea-pigs fed normal and atherogenic diets, *Atherosclerosis,* 22, 447, 1975.

57. **Vijayammal, P. L. and Kurup, P. A.,** Pyridoxine and atherosclerosis: role of pyridoxine in the metabolism of lipids and glycosaminoglycans in rates fed normal and high fat, high cholesterol diets containing 16% casein, *Aust. J. Biol. Sci.,* 31, 7, 1978.

58. **Sushama, D. C. S. and Kurup, P. A.,** Thyroid hormone and metabolism of glycosaminoglycans in rabbits, *Indian J. Biochem. & Biophys.,* 12, 43, 1975.

59. **Shaw, W. H. and Anderson, J. W.,** Purification, properties and substrate specificity of adenosine triphosphate sulphurylase from spinach leaf tissue, *Biochem. J.,* 127, 237, 1972.

60. **Shoyab, M., Su, L. Y., and Marx, W.,** Purification and properties of ATP-sulphurylase from Furth mouse mastocytoma, *Biochim. Biophys. Acta,* 258, 113, 1972.

61. **Tweedie, J. W. and Segel, I. H.,** Adenosine triphosphate sulfurylase from *Penicillium chrysogenum.* 2. Physical, kinetic, and regulatory properties, *J. Biol. Chem.,* 246, 2438, 1971.

62. **Reuveny, Z. and Filner, P.,** A new assay for ATP-sulfurylase based on differential solubility of the sodium salts of adenosine 5′-phosphosulfate and sulfate, *Anal. Biochem.,* 75, 410, 1976.

63. **Burnell, J. N. and Roy, A. B.,** Purification and properties of the ATP sulphurylase of rat liver, *Biochim. Biophys. Acta,* 527, 239, 1978.

64. **Balharry, G. J. E. and Nicholas, D. J. D.,** ATP-sulphurylase in spinach leaves, *Biochim. Biophys. Acta,* 220, 513, 1970.

65. **Balharry, G. J. and Nicholas, D. J. D.,** New assay for ATP-sulphurylase using the luciferin-luciferase method, *Anal. Biochem.,* 40, 1, 1971.

66. **Panikkar, K. R. and Bacchawat, B. K.,** Purification and properties of ATP-sulphate adenylyltransferase from liver, *Biochim. Biophy. Acta,* 151, 725, 1968.

67. **Baddiley, J., Buchanan, J. G., and Letters, R.,** Synthesis of adenosine 5′-sulphatophosphate. A degradation product of an intermediate in the enzymatic synthesis of sulphuric esters, *J. Chem. Soc. (London),* p.1067, 1957.

68. **Reichard, P. and Ringertz, N. R.,** Chemical synthesis of adenosine 5′-phosphosulfates, *J. Am. Chem. Soc.,* 81, 878, 1959.

69. **Shaw, W. H. and Anderson, J. W.,** Assay of adenosine 5′-triphosphate sulfurylase by pyrophosphate exchange, *Plant Physiol.,* 47, 114, 1971.

70. **Segal, H. L.,** Sulphate-dependent exchange of pyrophosphate with nucleotide phosphate, *Biochim. Biophys. Acta,* 21, 194, 1956.

71. **Wilson, L. G. and Bandurski, R. S.,** Enzymatic reactions involving sulfate, sulfite, selenate and molybdate, *J. Biol. Chem.,* 233, 975, 1958.

72. **Weil-Malherbe, H. and Green, R. H.,** The catalytic effect of molybdate on the hydrolysis of organic phosphate bonds, *Biochem. J.,* 49, 286, 1951.

73. **Wheldrake, J. F. and Pasternak, C. A.,** The control of sulphate activation in bacteria, *Biochem. J.,* 96, 276, 1965.
74. **Skyring, G. W., Trudinger, P. A., and Shaw, W. H.,** Electrophoretic characterization of ATP-sulfate adenylyltransferase (ATP-sulfurylase) using acrylamide gels, *Anal. Biochem.,* 48, 259, 1972.
75. **Robbins, P. W. and Lipmann, F.,** Enzymatic synthesis of adenosine 5'-phosphosulfate, *J. Biol. Chem.,* 233, 686, 1958.
76. **Hawes, C. S. and Nicholas, D. J. D.,** Adenosine 5'-triphosphate sulphurylase from *Saccharomyces cerevisiae, Biochem. J.,* 133, 541, 1973.
77. **Marx, W., Shoyab, M., and Su, L. Y.,** Yeast ATP-sulfurylase-ATP complex, *Int. J. Biochem.,* 5, 471, 1974.
78. **Varma, A. K. and Nicholas, D. J. D.,** Purification and properties of ATP-sulphurylase from *Nitrobacter agilis, Biochim. Biophys. Acta,* 227, 373, 1971.
79. **Akagi, J. M. and Campbell, L. L.,** Studies on thermophilic sulfate-reducing bacteria. 3. ATP-sulfurylase of *Clostridium nigrificans* and *Desulfovibrio desulfuricans, J. Bacteriol.,* 84, 1194, 1962.
80. **Tweedie, J. W. and Segel, I. H.,** ATP-sulfurylase from *Penicillium chrysogenum.* 1. Purification and characterization, *Prep. Biochem.,* 1, 90, 1971.
81. **Farley, J. R., Nakayama, G., Cryns, D., and Segel, I. H.,** Adenosine triphosphate sulfurylase from *Penicillium chrysogenum:* equilibrium binding, substrate hydrolysis and isotope exchange studies, *Arch. Biochem. Biophys.,* 185, 376, 1978.
82. **Menon, V. K. N. and Varma, A. K.,** Adenosine 5'-triphosphate sulphurylase from *Spirulina platensis, Experientia,* 35, 854, 1979.
83. **Møller, M. E. and Evans, L. V.,** Sulphate activation in the unicellular red alga *Rhodella, Phytochemistry,* 15, 1623, 1976.
84. **Onajobi, F. D., Cole, C. V., and Ross, C.,** Adenosine 5'-triphosphate-sulfurylase in corn roots and its partial purification, *Plant Physiol.,* 52, 580, 1973.
85. **Shoyab, M. and Marx, W.,** Two forms of ATP-sulfurylase in Furth mouse mastocytoma, *Life Sci.,* 9(II), 1151, 1970.
86. **Levi, A. S. and Wolf, G.,** Purification and properties of the enzyme ATP-sulfurylase and its relation to vitamin A, *Biochim. Biophys. Acta,* 178, 262, 1969.
87. **Shoyab, M. and Marx, W.,** Activation of mouse mastocytoma ATP-sulfurylase by *p*-hydroxymercuribenzoate, *Arch. Biochem. Biophys.,* 146, 368, 1971.
88. **Farley, J. R., Christie, E. A., Seubert, P. A., and Segel, I. H.,** Adenosine triphosphate sulfurylase from *Penicillium chrysogenum.* Evidence for essential arginine, histidine and tyrosine residues, *J. Biol. Chem.,* 254, 3537, 1979.
89. **Wilson, L. G. and Bandurski, R. S.,** An enzymatic reaction involving adenosine triphosphate and selenate, *Arch. Biochem. Biophys.,* 62, 503, 1956.
90. **Dilworth, G. L. and Bandurski, R. S.,** Activation of selenate by adenosine 5'-triphosphate sulfurylase from *Saccharomyces cerevisiae, Biochem. J.,* 163, 521, 1977.
91. **Shaw, W. H. and Anderson, J. W.,** Comparative enzymology of the adenosine triphosphate sulfurylase from leaf tissue of selenium-accumulator and non-accumulator plants, *Biochem. J.,* 139, 37, 1974.
92. **Burnell, J. N. and Whatley, F. R.,** A new, rapid and sensitive assay for adenosine 5'-phosphosulphate (APS) kinase, *Anal. Biochem.,* 68, 281, 1975.
93. **Shaw, W. H. and Anderson, J. W.,** The enzymology of adenosine triphosphate sulphurylase from spinach leaf tissue. Kinetic studies and a proposed reaction mechanism, *Biochem J.,* 139, 27, 1974.
94. **Farley, J. R., Cryns, D. F., Yang, Y. H. J., and Segel, I. H.,** Adenosine triphosphate sulfurylase from *Penicillium chrysogenum.* Steady state kinetics of the forward and reverse reaction, *J. Biol. Chem.,* 251, 4389, 1976.
95. **Spolter, L., Rice, L. I., Yamada, R., and Marx, W.,** Stimulation of sulfate activation by nicotinamide dinucleotide in presence of mastocytoma fraction free of mitochondria, *Biochem. Pharmacol.,* 16, 229, 1967.
96. **Sawhney, S. K. and Nicholas, D. J. D.,** Activation of sulphate in *Anabaena cylindrica, Planta,* 132, 189, 1976.
97. **Sawhney, S. K. and Nicholas, D. J. D.,** Effects of adenine nucleotides and phosphate on adenosine triphosphate sulphurylase from *Anabaena cylindrica, Biochem. J.,* 164, 161, 1977.
98. **Onajobi, F. D.,** Effects of adenine nucleotides on rice-root adenosine triphosphate sulphurylase activity *in vitro, Biochem. J.,* 149, 301, 1975.
99. **Shoyab, M. and Marx, W.,** Enzyme-substrate complexes of ATP-sulfurylase from mouse mastocytoma, *Biochim. Biophys. Acta,* 258, 125, 1972.
100. **Adams, C. A. and Johnson, R. E.,** ATP-sulfurylase activity in the soybean *(Glycine max (L)* Merr), *Plant Physiol.,* 43, 2041, 1968.

101. **Ellis, R. J.,** Sulphate activation in higher plants, *Planta,* 88, 34, 1969.
102. **Kosower, E. M.,** *Molecular Biochemistry,* McGraw-Hill, New York, 1962, 263.
103. **Grunberg-Manago, M.,** Del Campillo-Campbell, A., Dondon, L., and Michelson, A. M., ADP-sulfurylase de levure catalysant un échange entre l'orthophosphate et le phosphate terminal des nucleosides diphosphates, *Biochim. Biophys. Acta,* 123, 1, 1966.
104. **Adams, C. A. and Nicholas, D. J. D.,** Adenosine 5'-pyrophosphate sulfurylase in Baker's yeast, *Biochem. J.,* 128, 647, 1972.
105. **Nicholls, R. G.,** Purification and steady-state kinetics of adenosine 5'-pyrophosphate sulphurylase from Baker's yeast, *Biochem. J.,* 165, 149, 1977.
106. **Burnell, J. N. and Anderson, J. W.,** Adenosine diphosphate sulphurylase activity in spinach leaf tissue, *Biochem. J.,* 133, 417, 1973.
107. **Peck, H. D.,** Adenosine 5'-phosphosulfate as an intermediate in the oxidation of thiosulfate by *Thiobacillus thioparus, Proc. Natl. Acad. Sci. U.S.A.,* 46, 1053, 1960.
108. **Peck, H. D.,** The role of adenosine-5'-phosphosulfate in the reduction of sulfate to sulfite by *Desulfovibrio desulfuricans, J. Biol. Chem.,* 237, 198, 1962.
109. **Peck, H. D., and Stulberg, M. P.,** O^{18} studies on the mechanism of sulfate formation and phosphorylation in extracts of *Thiobacillus thioparus, J. Biol. Chem.,* 237, 1648, 1962.
110. **Thiele, H. H.,** Sulfur metabolism in *Thiorhodacea.* 5. Enzymes of sulfur metabolism in *Thiocapsa floridana* and *Chromatium* species, *Antonie van Leeuwenhoek J. Microbiol. Serol.,* 34, 350, 1968.
111. **Pasternak, C. A., Humphries, S. K., and Pirie, A.,** The activation of sulphate by extracts of cornea and colonic mucosa from normal and vitamin A-deficient animals, *Biochem. J.,* 86, 382, 1963.
112. **Mercer, E. I., Thomas, G., and Harrison, J. D.,** Occurrence of a 3'-phosphoadenosine 5'-phosphosulfate synthesizing system in two *Ochromonas* species, *Phytochemistry,* 13, 1297, 1974.
113. **Burnell, J. N. and Anderson, J. W.,** Adenosine 5'-sulphatophosphate kinase activity in spinach leaf tissue, *Biochem. J.,* 134, 565, 1973.
114. **Mercer, E. I. and Thomas, G.,** Occurrence of ATP-adenylsulfate 3'-phosphotransferase in the chloroplasts of higher plants, *Phytochemistry,* 8, 2281, 1969.
115. **Asahi, T.,** Sulfur metabolism in higher plants. 4. Mechanism of sulfate reduction in chloroplasts, *Biochim. Biophys. Acta,* 82, 58, 1964.
116. **Adams, J. B. and Reinitz, K. G.,** The biosynthesis of chondroitin sulphates. Influence of nucleotides and hexosamines on sulphate incorporation, *Biochim. Biophys. Acta,* 51, 567, 1961.
117. **Schmidt, A.,** A sulfotransferase from spinach leaves using adenosine-5'-phosphosulfate, *Planta,* 124, 267, 1975.
118. **Tsang, M. L. and Schiff, J. A.,** Sulfate-reducing pathway in *Escherichia coli* involving bound intermediates, *J. Bacteriol.,* 125, 923, 1976.
119. **Fankhauser, H. and Brunold, C.,** Localization of adenosine-5'-phosphosulfate sulfotransferase in spinach leaves, *Planta,* 143, 285, 1978.
120. **Schmidt, A. and Trüper, H. G.,** Reduction of adenylylsulfate and 3'-phosphoadenylylsulfate in phototrophic bacteria, *Experientia,* 33, 1008, 1977.
121. **Schmidt, A.,** Assimilatory sulfate reduction via 3'-phosphoadenosine 5'-phosphosulfate (PAPS) and adenosine 5'-phosphosulfate (APS) in blue-green algae, *FEMS Microbiol. Letters,* 1, 137, 1977.
122. **Sawhney, S. K. and Nicholas, D. J. D.,** Studies on degradation of adenosine-5'-sulphate (APS) and adenosine-3'-phosphate-5'-phosphosulphate (PAPS) in extracts of *Anabaena cylindrica, Plant Sci. Lett.,* 6, 103, 1976.
123. **Tsang, M. L. and Schiff, J. A.,** Properties of enzyme fraction A from *Chlorella* and copurification of 3'(2'), 5'-*bis*phosphonucleoside 3'(2')-phosphohydrolase, adenosine 5'-phosphosulfate sulfohydrolase and adenosine-5'-phosphosulfate cyclase activities, *Eur. J. Biochem.,* 65, 113, 1976.
124. **Denner, W. H. B., Stokes, A. M., Rose, F. A., and Dodgson, K. S.,** Separation and properties of the soluble 3'-phosphoadenosine 5'-phosphosulphate-degrading enzymes of bovine liver, *Biochim. Biophys. Acta,* 315, 394, 1973.
125. **Farooqui, A. A. and Balasubramanian, A. S.,** Enzymatic dephosphorylation of 3'-phosphoadenosine 5'-phosphosulfate to adenosine 5'-phosphosulfate in sheep brain, *Biochim. Biophys. Acta,* 198, 56, 1970.
126. **Lewis, M. H. R. and Spencer, B.,** The enzymatic degradation of nucleotide sulphatophosphate anhydrides, *Biochem. J.,* 85, 18P, 1962.
127. **Koizumi, T., Suematsu, T., Kawasaki, A., Hiramatsu, K., and Iwabori, N.,** Synthesis and degradation of active sulfate in liver, *Biochim. Biophys. Acta,* 184, 106, 1969.
128. **Austin, J., Armstrong, D., Stumpf, D., Luttenegger, T., and Dragoo, M.,** Subcellular distribution of two enzyme systems which degrade 3'-phosphoadenosine 5'-phosphosulfate ("active sulfate"), *Biochim. Biophys. Acta,* 192, 29, 1969.

129. **Bailey-Wood, R., Dodgson, K. S. and Rose, F. A.,** Purification and properties of two adenosine 5′-phosphosulfate sulphohydrolases from rat liver and their possible role in the degradation of 3′-phosphoadenosine 5′-phosphosulphate, *Biochim. Biophys. Acta,* 220, 284, 1970.

130. **Balasubramanian, A. S. and Bachhawat, B. K.,** Enzymic degradation of active sulphate, *Biochim. Biophys. Acta,* 59, 389, 1962.

131. **Adams, J. B.,** Acid mucopolysaccharide sulphokinases in human serum, *Biochim. Biophys. Acta,* 83, 127, 1964.

132. **Bailey-Wood, R., Dodgson, K. S., and Rose, F. A.,** A rat liver sulphohydrolase enzyme acting on adenylyl sulphate, *Biochem. J.,* 112, 257, 1969.

133. **Stokes, A. M., Denner, W. H. B., Rose, F. A., and Dodgson, K. S.,** Purification of a soluble adenosine 5′-phosphosulphate sulphohydrolase from bovine liver, *Biochim. Biophys. Acta,* 302, 64, 1973.

134. **Stokes, A. M., Denner, W. H. B., and Dodgson, K. S.,** Kinetic properties of the soluble adenosine 5′-phosphosulphate sulphohydrolase from bovine liver, *Biochim. Biophys. Acta,* 315, 402, 1973.

135. **Rogers, K. M., White, G. F., and Dodgson, K. S.,** Purification and properties of bovine lysosomal adenosine 5′-phosphosulphate sulphohydrolase. A non-specific enzyme with pyrophosphatase and phosphodiesterase activities, *Biochim. Biophys. Acta,* 527, 70, 1978.

136. **Armstrong, D., Austin, J., Luttenegger, T., Bachhawat, B., and Stumpf, D.,** Properties and sub-cellular distribution of two sulfatases which degrade adenosine 5′-phosphosulfate, *Biochim. Biophys. Acta,* 198, 523, 1970.

137. **Dziewiatkowski, D. D.,** Vitamin A and endochondral ossification in the rat as indicated by the use of sulfur-35 and phosphorous-32, *J. Exp. Med.,* 100, 11, 1954.

138. **Fell, H. B., Mellanby, E., and Pelc, S. R.,** Influence of excess vitamin A on the sulphate metabolism of bone rudiments grown *in vitro, J. Physiol.,* 134, 179, 1956.

139. **Wolf, G. and Varandani, P. T.,** Studies on the function of vitamin A in mucopolysaccharide biosynthesis, *Biochim. Biophys. Acta,* 43, 501, 1960.

140. **Varandani, P. T., Wolf, G., and Johnson, B. C.,** Function of vitamin A in the synthesis of 3′-phosphoadenosine-5′-phosphosulfate, *Biochem. Biophys. Res. Commun.,* 3, 97, 1960.

141. **Subba Rao, K., Sastry, P. S., and Ganguly, J.,** Studies on metabolism of vitamin A. 2. Enzymatic synthesis and hydrolysis of phenolic sulphates in vitamin A-deficient rats, *Biochem. J.,* 87, 312, 1963.

142. **Sundaresan, P. R.,** Vitamin A and the sulfate-activating enzymes, *Biochim. Biophys. Acta,* 113, 95, 1966.

143. **Perumal, A. S. and Cama, H. R.,** The role of 5,6-monoepoxyretinoic acid in the activation of ATP-sulfate adenylyltransferase, *Indian J. Biochem.,* 4, 152, 1967.

144. **Ponappa, B. C.,** Effect of vitamin A deficiency on lipids of rat intestines. *In vivo* incorporation of labelled sodium sulfate (^{35}S), *Environ. Physiol. Biochem.,* 2, 96, 1972.

145. **Sudhakaran, P. R. and Kurup, P. A.,** Vitamin A and glycosaminoglycan metabolism in rats, *J. Nutr.,* 104, 871, 1974.

146. **Subba Rao, K. and Ganguly, J.,** Studies on metabolism of vitamin A. 6. The effect of vitamin A deficiency on the activation of sulphate and its transfer to *p*-nitrophenol in rat liver, *Biochem. J.,* 90, 104, 1964.

147. **Subba Rao, K. and Ganguly, J.,** Studies on metabolism of vitamin A. The effect of the stage of vitamin A deficiency on sulphate activation in rat liver, *Biochem. J.,* 98, 693, 1966.

148. **Geison, R. L., Rogers., W. E., and Johnson, B. C.,** Comparative effects of vitamin A-deficiency and controlled food consumption on adenosine 5′-triphosphate: sulfate adenylyltransferase, *Biochem. Biophys. Acta,* 165, 448, 1968.

149. **Mukherji, B. and Bachhawat, B. K.,** Role of vitamin A in sulphate metabolism. Studies on the enzymatic activation of sulphate by various tissue extracts of normal and vitamin A-dificient rats, *Biochem. J.,* 104, 318, 1967.

150. **Levi, A. S., Geller, S., Roor, D. M., and Wolf, G.,** The effect of vitamin A and other dietary constituents on the activity of adenosine triphosphate sulfurylase, *Biochem. J.,* 109, 69, 1968.

151. **Carroll, J. and Spencer, B.,** Vitamin A and sulphotransferases in foetal rat liver, *Biochem. J.,* 96, 79P, 1965.

152. **Devi, C. S. S. and Kurup, P. A.,** Thyroid hormone and metabolism of glycosaminoglycans in rabbits, *Indian J. Biochem. & Biophys.,* 12, 43, 1975.

153. **Ben-Porath, E. and Gibson, K. D.,** Effect of RNA synthesis inhibitors on stimulation of sulfation by L-3,5,3′-triiodothyronine, *Biochem. Biophys. Res. Commun.,* 75, 311, 1977.

154. **Carroll, J. and Spencer, B.,** Sulphate activation and sulphotransferases in foetal and adult rats, *Biochem. J.,* 94, 20P, 1965.

155. **Wengle, B.,** Studies on ester sulphates. 17. Sulphate conjugation in extracts of foetal and juvenile rat liver, *Acta Soc. Med. Ups.,* 68, 154, 1963.

156. **Balasubramanian, A. S. and Bachhawat, B. K.,** Formation of active sulfate in rat brain, *J. Sci. Ind. Res.,* 20C, 202, 1961.

157. **Jansen, G. S. I. M., Van Elk, R., and Van Kempen, G. M. J.,** Developmental patterns of sulphate activation and phenolsulphotransferase in rat brain, *J. Neurochem.,* 20, 9, 1973.

158. **Gerlach, U.,** Über die Alternsabhängigkeit der Aktivität sulfataktivierender Enzyme im Herzen. (Ein Beitrag zur Biochemie des Alterns), *Klin. Wochenschr.,* 41, 873, 1963.

159. **Hart, G. W.,** Glycosaminoglycan sulfotransferases of the developing chick cornea, *J. Biol. Chem.,* 253, 347, 1978.

160. **Srinivas, L. and Rama, P. B. R.,** Studies on liver sulfurylase activity in rats. Vitamin A-deficient and low-protein diets, *Nutr. Metab.,* 19, 299, 1975.

161. **Menon, P. V. C. and Kurup, P. A.,** Nature of the dietary carbohydrate and metabolism of glycosaminoglycans and glycoproteins in rats., *J. Nutr.,* 106, 555, 1976.

162. **Schwartz, N. B., Ostrowski, V., Brown, K. S., and Pratt, R. M.,** Defective PAPS-synthesis in epiphysial cartilage from brachymorphic mice, *Biochem. Biophys. Res. Commun.,* 82, 173, 1978.

163. **Sugahara, H., and Schwartz, N. B.,** Defect in 3'-phosphoadenosine 5'-phosphosulfate formation in brachymorphic mice, *Proc. Natl. Acad. Sci. U.S.A.,* 76, 6615, 1979.

164. **Pasternak, C. A.,** Sulphate activation and its control in *Escherichia coli* and *Bacillus subtilis, Biochem. J.,* 85, 44, 1962.

165. **Wheldrake, J. F. and Pasternak, C. A.,** The control of sulphate activation in bacteria, *Biochem. J.,* 96, 276, 1965.

166. **Wheldrake, J. F.,** Intracellular concentration of cysteine in *Escherichia coli* and its relation to repression of the sulphate-activating enzymes, *Biochem. J.,* 105, 697, 1967.

167. **Collins, J. M. and Monty, K. J.,** Cysteine biosynthesis in *Salmonella typhimurium:* the presence of ATP-sulfurylase and APS-kinase in various cysteine requiring mutants, *Can. J. Biochem.,* 53, 1118, 1975.

168. **Farley, J. R., Mayer, S., Chandler, C. J., and Segel, I. H.,** ATP-sulfurylase from *Penicillium chrysogenum:* is the internal level of the enzyme sufficient to account for the rat of sulfate utilization?, *J. Bacteriol.,* 137, 350, 1979.

169. **Ragland, J. B.,** The role of ATP-sulfurylase in the biosynthesis of cysteine and methionine by *Neurospora, Arch. Biochem. Biophys.,* 84, 541, 1959.

170. **Reuveny, Z.,** Derepression of ATP-sulfurylase by the sulfate analogues molybdate and selenate in cultured tobacco cells, *Proc. Natl. Acad. Sci. U.S.A.,* 74, 619, 1977.

171. **Reuveny, Z. and Filber, P.,** Regulation of adenosine triphosphate sulfurylase in cultured tobacco cells. Effects of sulfur and nitrogen sources on the formation and decay of the enzyme, *J. Biol. Chem.,* 252, 1858, 1977.

172. **Hall, M. O. and Straatsma, B. R.,** The synthesis of 3'-phosphoadenosine 5'-phosphosulfate by retinae and livers of normal and vitamin A-deficient rats, *Biochim. Biophys. Acta,* 124, 246, 1966.

173. **Wong, K. P.,** Species differences in the conjugation of 4–hydroxy-3-methoxy-phenylethanol with glucuronic acid and sulphuric acid, *Biochem., J.,* 158, 33, 1976.

Chapter 5

SULFOTRANSFERASES

A. B. Roy

TABLE OF CONTENTS

I. INTRODUCTION

The sulfotransferases (EC 2.8.2.-, 3'-phosphoadenylylsulfate: X sulfotransferase) make up a group of enzymes of generally ill-defined specificity which catalyze the formation of sulfate esters, thiosulfates, or sulfamates from the appropriate acceptors with either adenosine 5'-sulfatophosphate (APS) or adenosine 3'-phosphate 5'-sulfatophosphate (PAPS) as the sulfate donor. These enzymes were called sulfokinases in the early literature.

In the case of the sulfotransferases responsible for the formation of sulfate esters and sulfamates, the sulfate donor is always PAPS so that the second reaction product is adenosine 3',5'-bisphosphate (PAP) and the reactions involved are therefore those represented in Equations 1 and 2.

$$R.OH + PAPS \longrightarrow R.OSO_3^- + PAP \tag{1}$$

$$R.NH_2 + PAPS \longrightarrow R.NHSO_3^- + PAP \tag{2}$$

These are irreversible except in a few special cases, for example, those in which R.OH is a nitrophenol, and Equation 1 is reversible because of the high sulfate potential of the nitrophenyl sulfate formed in the forward reaction.[1] Nothing is known of the chemistry of these reactions other than that the transfer of a sulfate group from PAPS to an acceptor occurs by a mechanism which does not lead to inversion of the configuration when the latter is asymmetric, as is, for example, a steroid. It seems likely that they must involve fission of the O–S bond in PAPS but this has not been shown.

Other sulfotransferases use more or less complex thiols as acceptors to form the corresponding thiosulfates, $R.SSO_3^-$. Different enzymes use either APS or PAPS as

Table 1
TYPES OF SULFOTRANSFERASE ACTIVITY WHICH WILL BE CONSIDERED IN THIS CHAPTER

Activity	Typical acceptors
Phenol sulfotransferase (EC 2.8.2.1)	4-Nitrophenol, tyrosine derivatives, biogenic amines
Steroid sulfotransferases	
Estrone sulfotransferase (EC 2.8.2.4)	Estrone
Androstenolone sulfotransferase	Dehydroepiandrosterone
Corticosteroid sulfotransferase	Cortisol
Bile-salt sulfotransferase (EC 2.8.2.14)	Lithocholate
Etiocholanolone sulfotransferase	3-Hydroxy-5β-steroids
Testosterone sulfotransferase	Testosterone
Cardenolide sulfotransferase	Digitoxigenin
Sterol sulfotransferase	Scymnol
Alcohol sulfotransferase	Aliphatic alcohols
Ascorbate sulfotransferase	Ascorbic acid
Calciferol sulfotransferase	Calciferol
Luciferin sulfotransferase (EC 2.8.2.10)	Luciferin
N-Hydroxyarylamine sulfotransferase	N-Hydroxyphenacetin
Arylamine sulfotransferase (EC 2.8.2.3)	2-Naphthylamine

Note: It is not certain how many of these activities are due to individual enzymes or, conversely, how many more specific enzymes are associated with each type of activity.

donor for these reactions which will not be considered here because they have not been shown to occur to any quantitatively significant extent in animals although they are very important in plants and microorganisms where they play a fundamental role[2] in the interconversions of SO_4^{2-} and SO_3^{2-}. As far as is known, the formation of thiosulfates plays no part in the metabolism of xenobiotics in animals and where simple thiosulfates, such as S-sulfocysteine and S-sulfoglutathione are formed, they may arise through the reaction of SO_3^{2-} with the corresponding disulfide rather than through a sulfotransferase-catalyzed reaction.[3]

Any discussion of the sulfotransferases is at present greatly hampered by the unfortunate fact that few, if any, of these enzymes have been obtained as homogeneous proteins. Claims of homogeneity have been made but, despite the evidence presented, it is difficult to accept them because the specific activities of the preparations are very low. The best available preparations have specific activities of the order of 1 $\mu mol.mg^{-1}.min^{-1}$: this should be compared with the specific activities of the phosphotransferases, which catalyze similar reactions, of about 100 to 1000 $\mu mol.mg^{-1}.min^{-1}$. Such a comparison may be unjustified, but it does give rise to doubts about the purity of the sulfotransferases so far prepared. This makes it impossible to decide how many sulfotransferases, as distinct from sulfotransferase activities, occur in animal tissues. Table 1 is an attempt to summarize the present position but it must be realized that the situation may finally prove to be quite different from that represented therein: there may be only a few relatively nonspecific sulfotransferases or there may be a much larger number of more highly specific enzymes.

The Enzyme Commission recognizes seven sulfotransferases of the type listed in Table 1: these are 3′-phosphoadenylylsulfate: phenol sulfotransferase (2.8.2.1); 3′-phosphoadenylylsulfate: 3β-hydroxysteroid sulfotransferase (2.8.2.2); 3′-phosphoadenylylsulfate: arylamine sulfotransferase (2.8.2.3); 3′-phosphoadenylylsulfate: estrone sulfotransferase (2.8.2.4); 3′-phosphoadenylsulfate: L-tyrosine-methyl-ester sulfotransferase (2.8.2.9); 3′-phosphoadenylylsulfate: luciferin sulfotransferase

(2.8.2.10) and 3'-phosphoadenylylsulfate: taurolithocholate sulfotransferase (2.8.2.14) with the trivial names aryl, 3β-hydroxysteroid, arylamine, estrone, tyrosine-ester, luciferin, and bile-salt sulfotransferase respectively. The trivial name aryl sulfotransferase is not satisfactory and the alternative, but not recommended, one of phenol sulfotransferase is preferable and will be used here because it more correctly describes the specificity of the enzyme. As will be considered later in section IVC, the name 3β-hydroxysteroid sulfotransferase is also not a satisfactory one because it implies that, for example, androsterone (a 3β-hydroxysteroid) could not be sulfated by the same enzyme as is dehydroepiandrosterone (a 3α-hydroxysteroid) whereas 3β-hydroxy-5β-androstan-17-one, with a very differently shaped carbon skeleton, could be: either of these implications may or may not be true and a less specific name must be used at this stage. The name used here, androstenolone sulfotransferase, is only marginally more satisfactory but at least it does not have any unwarranted authority. As will be considered below, the separate identities of phenol sulfotransferase (2.8.2.1) and tyrosine-ester sulfotransferase (2.8.2.9), although possible, are by no means proven (see Section IIID1) while the relation of bile-salt sulfotransferase (2.8.2.14) to other steroid sulfotransferases is quite obscure (see section IVE).

Finally it must be noted that Table 1 by no means lists all types of sulfotransferase found in animals. There also occur, for example, the many sulfotransferases known to be involved in the biosynthesis of sulfated glycosaminoglycans and of sulfolipids, while others must be presumed to be involved in the formation of tyrosine *O*-sulfate residues in fibrinopeptide B, gastrin II and other peptides. The latter reaction has not been studied: it presumably occurs at the post-translational stage but this has not been demonstrated. Bile pigment sulfates, of unknown structure, occur in mammalian bile[4] but nothing is known of their formation. In the lower animals still other sulfotransferases must exist for the synthesis of, for example, ommatin D, a wing and excretory pigment of the butterfly *Vanessa urticae*[5] or 11-hydroxysaxitoxin sulfate in the scallop *Pecten grandis* exposed to blooms of the dinoflagellate *Gonyaulax tamarensis* which contains 11-hydroxysaxitoxin itself.[6]

The sulfotransferases listed in Table 1, or at least those which occur in mammals, are all localized in the cytosol, as are the sulfate-activating enzymes (Chapter 4). However, their occurrence in the "soluble" fraction of a homogenate does not exclude the possibility of their being membrane-bound in the intact cell. They are, nevertheless, clearly distinguished from the sulfotransferases involved in the formation of sulfated glycosaminoglycans and sulfolipids because the latter are associated with the particulate fractions of the cell and are, at least in some cases, lipid-dependent.[7]

In this chapter we will be concerned primarily with the isolated sulfotransferases. The formation of sulfate esters in vivo will be considered only in special instances (see Chapter 6). Nevertheless, studies of this topic often provide the only, albeit indirect, information on the distribution of the various types of sulfotransferase in different species. A useful summary of comparative aspects of the metabolism of xenobiotics, from which most of the information comes, has been given by Smith.[8]

There has been much discussion of the nature of the "physiological" acceptors for the sulfotransferases listed in Table 1 and, with the exception of that for luciferin sulfotransferase (Section VIII), these are difficult to define. In the case of the steroid sulfotransferases there are many possible "physiological" acceptors, except for the unexpected cardenolide sulfotransferase activity in mammals (Section IVH), but no one steroid can be singled out as being "the" substrate for any one of them. Numerous aryl sulfates, presumably produced by phenol sulfotransferases, certainly occur in mammalian tissues but whether the parent phenols should be regarded as "physiological" substrates for these enzymes, in the sense that the enzymes have evolved to specifically handle them, is by no means clear. It may be that "physiological" acceptors in that sense do not exist for most of the sulfotransferases to be considered in this chapter and that these enzymes should be viewed in the same light as the microsomal mixed-function oxidases which often are regarded as having evolved to protect the organism from unwanted, but naturally occurring, compounds to which it might be exposed in its diet or its environment. The mixed-function oxidases produce many different types of hydroxyl-containing compounds which are in turn substrates for the relatively nonspecific sulfotransferases. If this is the correct view, then there are no "physiological" substrates, in the above strict sense, for the sulfotransferases which would be expected to be rather nonspecific enzymes. This low specificity may in turn explain the apparently low specific activities of the sulfotransferases which has already been mentioned and will be returned to in later sections. The situation is likely to be quite different with the sulfotransferases involved in the synthesis of sulfated glycosaminoglycans, sulfolipids, and sulfated polypeptides: there the products of the enzyme reactions do have specific roles to play and a corresponding specificity in the enzymes would be expected.

II. ASSAY OF THE SULFOTRANSFERASES

A. Introduction

The assay of sulfotransferases is by no means easy, if for no other reason than the difficulty of obtaining adequate amounts of PAPS. As has been pointed out in Chapter 2, Section V, a number of standard, but tedious, methods are available for the chemical synthesis of PAPS and [^{35}S]-PAPS. They can also be prepared biosynthetically by the reactions considered in Chapter 4, Section II. The method recently described by Singer[9] seems the most useful for this purpose, providing 100 to 150 μmol of PAPS in 2 days work, and having the capacity of being very easily scaled up if necessary. It is not immediately applicable for the preparation of [^{35}S]-PAPS.

Assuming the availability of PAPS, assays of sulfotransferase activity can be divided into two main groups: those using [^{35}S]-PAPS and those using unlabeled PAPS, with the latter further subdivided into those with more or less general applicability and those which have been devised for specific acceptors. Finally, there are methods which make use of the reversibility of the sulfotransferase reaction in the case of the nitrophenol-nitrophenyl sulfate system and so do not require PAPS.

Several of the methods are rather complex and not readily adaptable for detailed kinetic studies of the sulfotransferases, although they are useful for preliminary experiments. Methods in which PAPS is not provided as such but is generated by a sulfate-activating system from ATP and SO_4^{2-} either simultaneously with the sulfotransferase reaction or prior to the sulfotransferase reaction, can give no precise information. The concentration of PAPS is not known and it is not generally possible to have both the activating system and the sulfotransferase functioning under their respective optimum conditions in a single reaction mixture. Nevertheless, these methods are undoubtedly valuable for preliminary work provided that their limitations are kept in mind.

Complications are likely to arise when only crude preparations of the sulfotransferases are available, as is unfortunately very frequently the case. Such preparations are likely to contain sulfatases and other enzymes, such as 3'-nucleotidases, which attack PAPS (see Chapter 4, Section V). Once again accurate kinetic data cannot be obtained with such preparations, not only because of the decreasing concentration of PAPS but also because of the accumulation of adenosine 3', 5'-bisphosphate which is a powerful inhibitor of most, if not all, sulfotransferases. The possible presence of enzymes destroying PAPS must also be kept in mind when investigating the effect of metal ions on sulfotransferase activities in crude preparations: any observed effect need not necessarily arise only from changes in the sulfotransferase activity because many PAPS-degrading enzymes are themselves influenced by metal ions.[10] Only when purified enzyme preparations are available can kinetic studies be carried out with any confidence.

Crude tissue extracts,[11] and even partially purified sulfotransferases,[12] contain endogenous sulfate acceptors, and this is likely to be a general phenomenon so that care is required in interpreting the results of experiments in which [^{35}S]-PAPS of high specific activity is the sulfate donor.

Further complications have been introduced by the important observations[13] that Triton® X-100, and the oligomers separated from it, can be sulfated by crude sulfotransferase preparations from bovine adrenal cortex or rat liver. As this detergent, a polyoxyethylene diisobutylphenol, is widely used in biochemistry to solubilize both enzymes and substrates, the possibility of its causing spurious results must be kept in mind.

It should also be noted that many types of sulfotransferase are very susceptible to substrate inhibition by their acceptors so that care must be taken in developing methods for their assay, especially in crude preparations (see Section IVD2).

B. Methods Using [^{35}S]-PAPS

These are of widespread applicability and can, in principle, be used with almost any type of acceptor although the detailed procedure must vary with the chemistry of the latter.

Many of the methods are based on that of Wengle[14] which makes use of the fact that PAPS and SO_4^{2-} give insoluble barium salts while the barium salts of sulfate esters are, in general, soluble. [^{35}S]-sulfate esters can therefore be determined as the amount of ^{35}S remaining in solution after the removal of insoluble barium salts. Such methods, using $Ba(OH)_2$ and H_2SO_4, have been used for the assay of steroid sulfotransferases[15] and of phenol sulfotransferases[16] while others using $Ba(OH)_2$ and $ZnSO_4$ have been used to follow the synthesis of 4-nitrophenyl sulfate[17,18] or of the sulfates of catecholamines.[19] On the other hand, it has been shown that this type of method cannot be used when the acceptor is acidic as are, for example, phenolic carboxylic acids[19] or bile salts[20] because the barium salts of their sulfate esters are themselves insoluble.

Another fairly general, and very sensitive, method for the assay of phenol, steroid, and alcohol sulfotransferases has recently been described:[21] this depends upon the separation of the sulfate esters from the reactants and from other products by thin-layer chromatography on cellulose.

Other less generally applicable methods separate the [^{35}S]-sulfate esters from other labeled compounds by paper[16,22] or thin-layer[23] chromatography, or by electrophoresis.[16] Less widely applicable is the separation of PAPS and SO_4^{2-} from serotonin O-[^{3}S]-sulfate by the removal of the former on a column of Biorex-4 under acidic conditions.[24] The sulfate esters of estrogens[25] or of bile salts[26] can be separated from [^{35}S]-PAPS and $^{35}SO_4^{2-}$ by extraction with suitable solvents.

An interesting method has been developed for use with N-hydroxypurines (purine N-oxides) as acceptors: these give very reactive sulfate esters which easily undergo nonenzymic reactions to reform, in part, the acceptor and to quantitatively liberate SO_4^{2-}. After correcting for the hydrolysis of the [^{35}S]-PAPS (see Chapter 4), the amount of $^{35}SO_4^{2-}$ produced is a measure of the sulfotransferase activity.[27]

Obviously, with such a multiplicity of methods, details cannot be given here but must be sought in the original papers. For kinetic work, methods based on that of Wengle[14] have been most used and seem the most suitable, provided that the barium salt of the sulfate ester is soluble, although an ever-present danger must be the adsorption of the sulfate ester by precipitates of $BaSO_4$ or denatured protein. Surprisingly, only Wengle[14] and Foldes and Meek[19] appear to have measured the recovery of sulfate esters from reaction mixtures. The former showed that the recovery of C_{19} steroid sulfates was 80 to 90%, that of C_{21} steroid sulfates was 66 to 77%, while that of ethyl and phenyl sulfates was about 90%. The latter workers obtained recoveries of 82 to 90% for the sulfate esters of a number of neutral and basic phenols. These losses are by no means negligible, especially with the rather nonpolar steroids. They might be decreased by using purer sulfotransferase preparations, and therefore smaller amounts of protein, but this has not been established. Further, as the recoveries seemed[14] to depend to some extent upon the polarity of the steroid, care would have to be taken in interpreting small differences in the apparent rates of sulfation of different acceptors. The chromatographic method recently devised by Sekura et al.[21] would appear to obviate some of the problems encountered with the Wengle method, but it has not yet been widely used.

C. Methods Using Unlabeled PAPS

Of these, the only one of fairly general applicability is based on the solubility of the methylene blue salts of certain sulfate esters in chloroform (see Chapter 2, Section IIB). This method can be used with any acceptor which is sufficiently nonpolar: it has, for example, been used to follow the synthesis of aryl and steroid sulfates[28-30] and of some aryl sulfamates.[28] It cannot be used to follow the sulfation of the lower alcohols, carbohydrates, tyrosine, or biogenic amines because these do not give methylene blue salts of sufficient solubility in chloroform. Again the method must be used with care to ensure that the recovery of the sulfate ester is adequate. This is particularly important with relatively nonpolar steroids such as cholesterol because cholesteryl sulfate is rather firmly bound to protein which must be precipitated with ethanol to allow a good recovery of the ester.[31] In fact, with crude enzyme preparations, precipitation of the protein with ethanol is recommended, whatever the acceptor. Unfortunately this step complicates the procedure because the ethanol must be completely removed before the methylene blue method can be applied.

Many methods, some now of only historic interest, are available for the determination of sulfotransferase activity with specific acceptors such as 3-aminophenol,[32] 4-nitrophenol,[33,34] serotonin,[35] 4-methylumbelliferone,[36] and harmol.[37] The first two of these methods are simple spectrophotometric ones, but the others require the separation of the sulfate ester from the unreacted acceptor by suitable chromatographic techniques.

Of particular interest are methods for detecting the formation of the very unstable sulfate esters of N-hydroxyarylamines: these cannot be isolated and are determined by their reaction with methionine to give, after suitable treatment, methylmercapto derivatives of the arylamine. Methods have been described for the determination of the sulfotransferase involved in the sulfation of N-acetyl-N-hydroxy-2-aminofluorene by determining the amount of N-acetyl-1-methylmercapto-2-aminofluorene produced, either by gas chromatography[38] or by using [*methyl*-³H]methionine as a reactant.[39] Similar methods have been described for other N-hydroxyarylamines[40] (see Chapter 8, Section I).

When the acceptor is readily available in a labeled form, then the methods using unlabeled PAPS become considerably more sensitive. Techniques of this type have been particularly valuable with the steroid sulfotransferases where extensive use has been made of [4-¹⁴C]dehydroepiandrosterone[41] and of [6,7-³H]estrone,[42] in both cases the free steroid being separated from the steroid sulfate by extraction with the appropriate solvents. More recently,[21] steroid sulfates have been separated from the parent steroids by adsorption of the former on silica-gel impregnated glass fiber sheets followed by extensive washing with suitable solvents. Again this method seems likely to be a valuable one, but it has not yet been widely used.

D. Other Methods

All of the above methods use PAPS as a sulfate donor and, in view of the difficulty in preparing large amounts of this nucleotide, methods in which it was not required would be useful. Such methods are available, and are based on the fact that 4-nitrophenyl sulfate, and nitroaryl sulfates in general, have a high sulfate potential[1] so that the reaction between, say, 4-nitrophenol and PAPS is reversible. This reversibility can be used in two ways for the assay of sulfotransferases.

The first is restricted to the phenol sulfotransferases and simply requires the spectrophotometric determination of the nitrophenol formed by the reaction between the nitrophenyl sulfate and adenosine 3′,5′-bisphosphate,[29] that is, by the reverse of Equation 1. Obviously, adenosine 3′,5′-bisphosphate is required in substrate amounts in this type of assay.

In the second type of assay only catalytic amounts of adenosine 3′,5′-bisphosphate are required, and the sulfate is transferred from the nitroaryl sulfate, usually 4-nitrophenyl sulfate, to an acceptor which will form a sulfate ester of a sulfate potential low relative to that of 4-nitrophenyl sulfate, as represented in Scheme 3. Again the activity can be

$$\text{4-nitrophenyl sulfate} \rightleftharpoons \text{PAPS} \rightleftharpoons \text{acceptor sulfate} \qquad (3)$$
$$\text{4-nitrophenol} \qquad \text{PAPS} \qquad \text{acceptor}$$

followed by the spectrophotometric determination of the liberated 4-nitrophenol.[1] Among the first to use this method were Segal and Mologne[43] in their investigation of the sulfation of tyrosine derivatives by rat-liver cytosol, but it has since been used to follow the sulfation of biogenic amines,[44] *N*-hydroxyphenacetin,[45] and even of glycosaminoglycans[46] so that it is apparently not restricted to the assay of phenol sulfotransferases, although Gregory and Lipmann[1] could not, in their rabbit system, detect any transfer of sulfate from 4-nitrophenyl sulfate to steroids. Also, for reasons not understood, Banerjee and Roy[29] could not detect any significant transfer of sulfate from 4-nitrophenyl sulfate to either phenol or 2-naphthol by a purified phenol sulfotransferase which could, nevertheless, catalyze the simple reverse reaction between 4-nitrophenyl sulfate and adenosine 3′,5′-bisphosphate. In view of this observation negative results with this type of assay should be viewed with caution. It should also be noted that this method is not suitable for detailed kinetic studies of a sulfotransferase reaction, especially if more than one sulfotransferase is involved, as is likely to be the case in the transfer of sulfate from 4-nitrophenyl sulfate to an acceptor which is not a phenol, for example, *N*-hydroxphenacetin or a glycosaminoglycan. Adenosine 3′,5′-bisphosphate cannot be replaced by inosine 3′,5′-bisphosphate, and adenosine 2′,5′-bisphosphate gives only about 1.4% of the activity achieved with the 3′,5′-bisphosphate.[1]

III. PHENOL SULFOTRANSFERASE

A. Introduction

That animals can form aryl sulfates has been known since the classical work of Baumann over 100 years ago, and it was through the study of this process that Bernstein and McGilvery[47] were led to the discovery of "active sulfate," subsequently identified as adenosine 3′-phosphate 5′-sulfatophosphate. Nevertheless, despite this long history, the nature of the phenol sulfotransferase(s) of animal tissues still remains obscure because it is now clear that phenol sulfotransferase activities can be shown by several enzymes, but whether all of these should be regarded as distinct phenol sulfotransferases is by no means certain.

Banerjee and Roy[28] were the first to separate, by chromatography on DEAE-Sephadex, three phenol sulfotransferase activities, each capable of using 4-nitrophenol as an acceptor, from guinea-pig liver. Two of these were associated with steroid sulfotransferase activities, whereas the third, which was more clearly resolved, showed only phenol sulfotransferase activity. The latter activity appeared to be due to a true phenol sulfotransferase. Barford and Jones[48] made a similar observation in rat liver: they separated two phenol sulfotransferase activities, one of which again was associated with a steroid sulfotransferase activity. More recently Sekura and Jakoby[49] have separated two apparently specific phenol sulfotransferases from rat liver by chromatography on DEAE-cellulose. It seems likely that animal tissues in general will show this pattern of having several phenol sulfotransferase activities, some of which will be associated with other types of sulfotransferase activity.

Other problems are caused by the multiplicity of acceptors. From studies in intact animals[50] it would have been expected that most phenols would be capable of being sulfated, and this has been, in general, born out by studies of sulfotransferase activities in tissue extracts. The acceptors fall into three groups: first, more or less simple phenols, of which 4-nitrophenol and 4-methylumbelliferone have been most studied; second, derivatives of tyrosine, such as tyrosine methyl ester; and third, biogenic amines such as dopamine and their metabolites such as 4-hydroxy-3-methoxyphenylethylene glycol. At one stage it was thought that at least the first two of these groups of acceptors were sulfated by different enzymes because it seemed possible to partially separate the two activities;[16] however, subsequent work, to be described below, appeared to show that the separation was only apparent and simply reflected changes in specificity associated with changes in the oxidation state of a single enzyme. The situation with the third group of acceptors is perhaps less clear, but it is now generally considered[19,44,51-53] that they are substrates for the same phenol sulfotransferases as are the other two groups of acceptors. Unfortunately the recent studies of Sekura and Jakoby[49] do not support the above generalizations. Neither of the two phenol sulfotransferases, sulfotransferases I and II, which they have isolated from rat liver, will sulfate tyrosine methyl ester or dopamine, so that the possibility of there being several relatively specific phenol sulfotransferases must be considered anew. Further evidence for this is given by the demonstration that rat liver contains a second pair of phenol sulfotransferases, distinct from sulfotransferases I and II, which can use tyrosine methyl ester or, most interestingly, hydroxylamine derivatives (see Section IX) as acceptors.[81a]

In this section a phenol sulfotransferase will be defined as an enzyme which can use simple phenols, tyrosine derivatives, and biogenic amines, or their derivatives, as sulfate acceptors but which show no steroid or other sulfotransferase activities.

B. Purification and General Properties

The preparation of phenol sulfotransferases is not easy: they are generally rather unstable, for example, to organic solvents, although their stability is improved by EDTA and by thiols. Nevertheless, as will be considered below (Section IIIC), the uncontrolled use of the latter can cause problems. They are also stabilized by polyols such as sucrose or glycerol. They have generally been obtained by ammonium sulfate precipitation, gel filtration or ion-exchange chromatography and only recently have affinity techniques been developed for their purification.

The most useful preparation of the phenol sulfotransferases is undoubtedly that of Sekura and Jakoby[49] from rat liver. A crude sulfotransferase fraction was obtained by chromatography of the liver extract on an agarose-Cibacron Blue column, and this was separated into the fractions containing sulfotransferases I and II by chromatography on DEAE-cellulose. These two enzymes were purified by further chromatography, finally on a column of agarose-ATP from which they were eluted with a liner gradient of PAPS, from 0 to 45 μM in phosphate buffer, pH 6.5. The purified enzymes were stored in the presence of 0.25 M sucrose and 3 mM 2-mercaptoethanol, in the absence of which they lost their activity within a few days: glycerol gave a much lesser degree of protection than did sucrose. Sulfotransferases I and II were apparently specific phenol sulfotransferases with no detectable steroid, alcohol, N-hydroxyarylamine or, arylamine sulfotransferase activities.[49] Both of them have, to judge by electrophoresis, been obtained as homogeneous proteins of molecular weight 65,000 and are made up of two apparently identical subunits. Phenol sulfotransferase I had an isoelectric point of 8.05 and both had rather high extinction coefficients, $A^{1\%}_{280\ nm}$ being 19 and 20 for phenol sulfotransferases I and II, respectively. These values were based on protein determinations by the Lowry method. Phenol sulfotransferases I and II are obviously very similar enzymes, both physically and kinetically, and apart from their separation on DEAE-cellulose and different isoelectric points, they differ significantly only in their amino acid compositions, especially in their contents of lysine, alanine, and isoleucine. The relationship between these two enzymes remains to be established.

Borchardt and Schasteen[177] have used affinity chromatography to prepare a single phenol sulfotransferase from rat liver. The adsorbent was agarose-4-hydroxyphenyl-acetic acid, and the enzyme was eluted with a linear gradient, from 5 to 200 mM, of phosphate buffer, pH 7.4. The length of the spacer arm between the ligand and the matrix was critical, and one approximately 25 Å long gave the best results, a purification of 45- to 65-fold from an ammonium sulfate fraction of rat-liver cytosol. This phenol sulfotransferase, which was not obtained as a homogeneous protein, also had a molecular weight of 65,000 but, unlike phenol sulfotransferases I and II,[49] was stable in buffers containing 10% glycerol.

All of the other phenol sulfotransferases so far prepared also have molecular weights in the region of 60,000 to 70,000[29,55] to judge by their behavior in gel chromatography, but there are indications that aggregation can occur.[48,56]

The phenol sulfotransferases have surprisingly low specific activities. The best preparation from guinea-pig liver[29] (and unpublished observations) had a specific activity of only 0.04 μmol.mg^{-1}.min^{-1} with 4-nitrophenol as acceptor, while two different preparations from rat liver gave values of 0.6 and 0.1 μmol.mg^{-1}.min^{-1} with 4-nitrophenol[54] and tyrosine methyl ester,[16] respectively, as acceptors. The two phenol sulfotransferases recently prepared[49] from rat liver, apparently as homogeneous proteins, had specific activities of 0.25 and 0.28 μmol.mg^{-1}.min^{-1} with 2-naphthol as acceptor. Unfortunately, most of the preparations used for kinetic work have been considerably less purified, and in many cases it is not possible to give the specific activities in absolute terms.

With regard to the enzymic activity of the phenol sulfotransferases there is general agreement on one point. Their activity is, unlike that of most other types of sulfotransferase, not increased by Mg^{2+} or other divalent cations, nor decreased by EDTA.

C. Effects of Thiols and Thiol Reagents

There were early reports of rat-liver phenol sulfotransferase being inhibited both by thiols[54] and by thiol reagents.[16,48,54] Some protection against the latter was given by PAPS

Table 2
**VALUES OF K_m FOR SOME PARTLY PURIFIED PHENOL
SULFOTRANSFERASES**

| | | | K_m (μM) | | |
Tissue	pH	Acceptor (A)	A	PAPS	Ref.
Guinea-pig liver	5.6	4-Nitrophenol	70	36	29
Rat liver	8.0	4-Nitrophenol	51	14	54
	7.5	4-Nitrophenol	1.5	30	48
		4-Nitrophenol[a]	340	30	48
		Tyrosine methyl ester	2900	—	48
	6.5	2-Naphthol[b]	60	6.5	49
		2-Naphthol[c]	90	12	49
Ox kidney	5.5	4-Nitrophenol	1100	14	55
Rat brain	7.4	4-Methylumbelliferone	11	10	63
		4-Hydroxy-3-methoxy-phenylethylene glycol	32	11	63
	6.4	Phenol	40	0.3	19
		4-Hydroxy-3-methoxy-phenylethylene glycol	18	0.3	19

[a] Aged (oxidized) enzyme.
[b] Sulfotransferase I.
[c] Sulfotransferase II.

but not by tyrosine methyl ester.[57] The effects of thiols were complex and differed with different acceptors: the sulfation of 4-nitrophenol was inhibited while that of tyrosine methyl ester was activated.[6]

More detailed investigations have clarified some of these findings.[48,54] The properties of the phenol sulfotransferase of rat liver change on keeping, presumably through oxidation, because they are restored to those of the freshly prepared enzyme by treatment with dithiothreitol. Oxidation is accompanied by a large increase in the K_m for 4-nitrophenol, from 1.5 to 340 μM, along with a fourfold increase in V. There is no change in the K_m for PAPS which is 30 μM with both the oxidized and reduced enzymes (Table 2). More striking, however, is the fact that the oxidized enzyme is unable to use tyrosine methyl ester as an acceptor. The picture which therefore emerged from these studies was that the apparent specificity of at least some phenol sulfotransferases was a function of the oxidation state of the enzyme, and presumably of the oxidation state of the thiol groups in it.

However, not all preparations of phenol sulfotransferases show these effects. The enzyme from guinea-pig liver was activated by 2-mercaptoethanol[29] and that of ox kidney was unaffected by a number of thiols,[55] in both cases the acceptor being 4-nitrophenol, while the two highly purified sulfotransferases from rat liver were both activated by 2-mercaptoethanol,[49] with 2-naphthol as acceptor.

It should be obvious that the action of thiols on phenol sulfotransferases is still by no means clearly understood and that in future much greater care should be taken in their use, for example during the preparation of the enzymes, than has been done in the past.

D. Kinetics
1. Specificity
As has already been pointed out, it is difficult to give much reliable information on the specificity of the phenol sulfotransferases, not only because of their multiplicity, but

also because their specificity may appear to vary with changes in the oxidation state of the enzyme. However, most simple phenols, except estrone, are acceptors, as are derivatives of tyrosine which do not contain a free carboxyl group and also many biogenic amines and their metabolites. Indications of the general specificities of a number of phenol sulfotransferases can be gained from References 19, 29, 44, and 55 to 59.

The inability to sulfate estrone, at least at a detectable rate, is surprising because it is a typical phenol, and the closely related compounds equilin (3-hydroxyestra-1,3,5, (10), 7-tetraen-17-one) and equilenin (3-hydroxyestra-1, 3, 5(10), 6, 8-pentaen-17-one) are substrates, at least for the phenol sulfotransferase of guinea-pig liver.[29]

In some early studies[43] it was stated that for a tyrosine derivative to be an acceptor for phenol sulfotransferase, the amino group had to be free and unprotonated and the carboxyl group blocked because, for example, *N*-acetyltyrosine ethyl ester was not a substrate. More recently, however, it has been shown[57] that a partially purified phenol sulfotransferase from rat liver will sulfate *N*-acetyltyrosine ethyl ester with a V of about 40% of that of tyrosine ethyl ester. There is no obvious reason for this difference in results, but in the early experiments the sulfate donor was 4-nitrophenyl sulfate whereas PAPS was the donor in more recent studies.

Tables 2 and 3 give some values for the kinetic constants of a number of phenol sulfotransferases. There are some surprising differences in the values for different enzymes: for example, the values of K_m for 4-nitrophenol range from 1.5 μM to 2.5 mM. Further values are available for other substrates: biogenic amines and similar compounds,[19] tyrosine derivatives,[57] and benzo[*a*]pyrene derivatives.[59] The values of v in the latter reference are only relative because known concentrations of PAPS were not used in their determination.

As can be seen from Table 3, there are big changes in the kinetic constants, and hence the apparent specificity, of rat-liver phenol sulfotransferase depending upon whether it is in the oxidized or reduced state.[58] In the oxidized state there is a reasonable correlation between the Hammett substitution constant, σ, and V, 4-nitrophenol being sulfated much more rapidly than 4-(2'-aminoethyl)-phenol. With the reduced enzyme there is no such correlation, but V is greater when nucleophilic substituents are present in the phenol. In this case 4-(2'-aminoethyl)-phenol is sulfated more rapidly than 4-nitrophenol. It has been argued, therefore, that in the cell, where the sulfotransferase is likely to be in the reduced form, biogenic amines will be the preferred acceptors.[58]

The most detailed specificity studies are those of Sekura and Jakoby[49] with the two purified phenol sulfotransferases, transferases I and II, of rat liver. Their results are summarized in Table 3 from which it can be seen that there are only slight differences between the values for the two enzymes. In contrast to the earlier preparations of phenol sulfotransferases from rat liver,[54,57] but like that from ox kidney,[55] neither sulfotransferase I nor sulfotransferase II could use L-adrenaline, dopamine, or tyrosine methyl ester as acceptor despite the enzymes being stored, and assayed, in 5 mM 2-mercaptoethanol so that they presumably are in the reduced form. Unfortunately there is too little overlap between the data for sulfotransferases I and II and reduced rat-liver phenol sulfotransferase to allow detailed comparison, but where this can be made, there are few similarities except that neither set of data could be fitted to any Hammett relationship.[49,58]

It should be clear that although most phenols can be sulfated by sulfotransferases in vitro, as they are in vivo, there is no certainty about the number of sulfotransferases which are involved. Until recently it seemed fairly certain that phenols, tyrosine derivatives, and biogenic amines were sulfated by one type of enzyme, a phenol

Table 3
VALUES OF KINETIC CONSTANTS FOR THE SYNTHESIS OF ARYL SULFATES BY PARTLY PURIFIED PHENOL SULFOTRANSFERASES

| | K_m (μM) | | | | | | V_{rel} (4-Nitrophenol = 1.0) | | | |
| | | | | | | | Rat liver[58] | | Rat liver[49] | |
Acceptor	Guinea-pig liver[29]	Ox kidney[55]	Rat liver I[49]	Rat liver II[49]	Guinea-pig liver[49]	Ox kidney[35]	Oxidized	Reduced	I	II
Phenol	2500	—	1800	2600	0.30	0.07	0.47	2.1	0.22	0.14
4-Acetamido	—	—	2100	1600	—	—	—	—	0.18	0.08
3-Aldehydo	—	—	—	—	—	0.21	—	—	—	—
4-Aldehydo	—	—	—	—	—	0.76	—	—	—	—
4-(2'-Aminoethyl)	—	—	—	—	—	—	0.12	1.8	—	—
3-Amino	—	—	—	—	—	—	0.24	1.8	—	—
2-Chloro	—	—	150	190	—	—	—	—	1.5	1.2
3-Chloro	—	—	120	160	—	—	0.74	1.1	0.85	0.57
4-Chloro	—	—	1500	1200	—	0.80	0.65	0.66	1.6	0.79
4-Methoxy	—	—	4200	6500	—	—	0.35	2.1	3.0	2.30
2-Methyl	—	—	—	—	—	0.22	—	—	—	—
3-Methyl	—	—	1000	1400	—	0.08	—	—	0.63	0.32
4-Methyl	—	—	2900	2200	—	—	—	—	—	—
3-Nitro	—	—	600	440	—	0.50	—	—	2.0	0.9
4-Nitro	70	1100	1600	2500	1.0	1.0	1.0	1.0	1.0	1.0
4-Phenyl	—	—	180	250	—	—	—	—	0.54	0.3
1-Naphthol	25	—	—	—	1.0	0.33	—	—	—	—
4-Nitro	18	—	—	—	0.39	—	—	—	—	—
2-Naphthol	25	—	—	—	0.95	—	—	—	1.6	1.1
5,6,7,8-Tetrahydro	56	—	—	—	0.63	—	—	—	—	—
2-Phenanthrol	17	—	—	—	0.51	—	—	—	—	—
15,16-Dihydro-3-hydroxy-17-oxocyclopentena[a]phenanthrene	15	—	—	—	0.13	—	—	—	—	—
Equilin	20	—	—	—	0.21	—	—	—	—	—
Equilenin	15	—	—	—	0.10	—	—	—	—	—
Estrone	—	—	—	—	0.0	0.0	—	—	0.0	0.0
3-Hydroxyindole	—	—	80	70	—	—	—	—	1.5	0.76
4-Hydroxyindole	—	—	290	300	—	—	—	—	1.3	0.73
5-Hydroxytryptamine	—	—	1600	530	—	—	—	—	0.05	0.01
L-Tyrosine methyl ester	5000	—	—	—	—	0.0	0.0	0.60	0.0	0.0

sulfotransferase, but more recent studies[49,55] cast some doubt on this interpretation. More highly purified samples of the enzymes sulfating tyrosine derivatives and biogenic amines will have to be prepared before the specificity of phenol sulfotransferase can be understood.

Other problems also require investigation. For example, tyrosine O-sulfate residues occur in proteins and peptides,[60] but there is no information on their incorporation. In some preliminary studies, Barford and Jones showed[61] that a crude phenol sulfotransferase preparation from rat liver could neither sulfate L-tyrosyl t-RNA nor catalyze an exchange between [^{35}S]-PAPS and tyrosyl O-sulfate residues in fibrinogen, although it could catalyze such a transfer with 4-nitrophenyl sulfate or tyramine O-sulfate. They therefore concluded[61] that there was nothing to implicate phenol sulfotransferase in the formation of the tyrosyl O-sulfate residues of fibrinogen.

Another interesting problem which has not been investigated is the formation of the disulfates of di- and trihydroxy phenols.[62] Presumably these must be formed by a hydroxyphenyl sulfate acting as an acceptor for the transfer of a further sulfate group; it would be interesting to know if phenol sulfotransferase, as normally understood, can carry out such a reaction.

2. pH Effects

The optimum pH of the phenol sulfotransferase reaction varies with the nature of the acceptor. With simple phenols it has been variously reported between pH 5.5[29] and 7.5,[54] while with amines it seems to be nearer pH 9.[19,44] With 2-naphthol as acceptor there were two pH optima, at pH 6.5 and pH 9.5; only the former was found with 4-nitrophenol as acceptor.[49] More detailed studies have led to the suggestion[57] that for a phenol to be an acceptor for the phenol sulfotransferase of rat liver, the hydroxyl group must not be ionized, and that any amino group which is present must be in the unprotonated form. Some further evidence for this view is given by the observation [52] that the sulfation of 4-methylumbelliferone or 4-hydroxy-3-methoxyphenylethylene glycol at pH 7.4 is not inhibited by dopamine and related amines which are protonated at this pH, but that it is inhibited by their deaminated metabolites.

It has also been suggested that the phenol sulfotransferase of rat liver contains an ionizing group with a pK of about 9.5, perhaps a thiol, which is involved in the binding of PAPS.[57] As has been mentioned in Section IIIC, PAPS can protect this enzyme from inactivation by thiol reagents.[57]

3. Reaction Mechanism

Only two detailed kinetic studies have been carried out. Banerjee and Roy[29] investigated the kinetics of the phenol sulfotransferase of guinea-pig liver (specific activity 0.01 μmol.mg^{-1}.min^{-1}, with 4-nitrophenol as acceptor at the optimum pH of 5.6. From initial velocity studies of both the forward and reverse reactions, and from product inhibition studies, it was shown that the kinetics were consistent with the reaction being rapid-equilibrium random bi-bi with one dead-end complex containing 4-nitrophenol and adenosine 3′,5′-bisphosphate. This can be represented as in Scheme 4 where A is 4-nitrophenol and AS is 4-nitrophenyl sulfate. The values of K_m were 70 μM, 36 μM, 110 μM, and 14 μM for 4-nitrophenol, PAPS, 4-nitrophenyl sulfate, and adenosine 3′, 5′-bisphosphate, respectively.

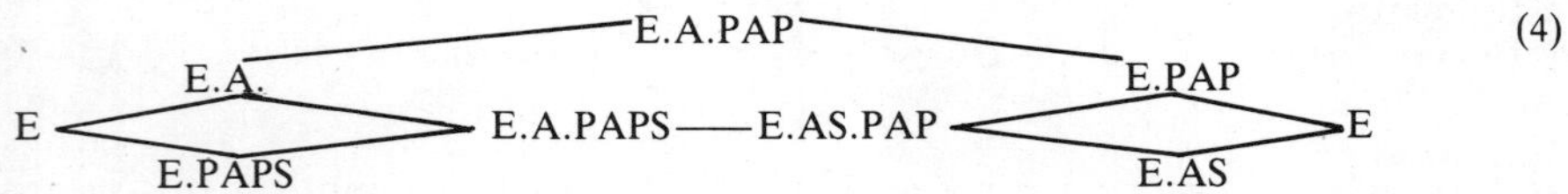

(4)

A similar conclusion was reached from less detailed studies of the forward reaction of the phenol sulfotransferase of rat liver[57] at pH 7.5 with tyrosine methyl ester as acceptor.

On the other hand, with the corresponding enzyme from rat brain (specific activity 0.4×10^{-3} μmol.mg^{-1}.min^{-1}) a different picture has emerged,[63] although in this case only the forward reaction could be studied because of the irreversibility of the phenol sulfotransferase reaction with the substrates used, 4-methylumbelliferone and 4-hydroxy-3-methoxyphenylethylene glycol, at their respective pH optima of 7.4 and 7.8. In this case the reaction was sequential ordered bi-bi, again with a dead-end complex containing acceptor and adenosine 3′,5′-bisphosphate. The kinetics were consistent with PAPS being the first substrate bound and PAP being the last product released. Again the K_m for the latter is low, about 10 μM. Values of the several kinetic constants for the other reactants are also given.[63] This mechanism can be represented as in Scheme 5 with A and AS being 4-methylumbelliferone or 4-hydroxy-3-methoxy-phenylethylene glycol and their sulfates, respectively. At pH 7.4, the pH optimum, substrate inhibition by either of these acceptors was pronounced but it did not occur at pH 6.2 or 9.0.

$$E\text{---}E.PAPS\text{---}E.A.PAPS\text{---}E.AS.PAP\text{---}E.PAP\text{---}E \tag{5}$$
$$|$$
$$E.A.PAP$$

The two mechanisms shown in Schemes 4 and 5 are rather different, and only further work will resolve the discrepancy which may, however, be more apparent than real and arise from the different pH values at which the reactions were carried out. At pH 5.6 the guinea-pig enzyme did not show any substrate inhibition at high concentrations of the acceptor, 4-nitrophenol, but at pH values greater than about 6.2 substrate inhibition became more and more pronounced as the pH was raised.[29] This certainly suggests that the reaction mechanism might be different at higher pH values and, as pointed out by Pennings et al.,[63] the occurrence of such a substrate inhibition is incompatible with a rapid-equilibrium random mechanism. More detailed studies over a wide pH range are required to resolve this situation.

There have been no studies of the kinetics or detailed mechanism of the transfer of sulfate from 4-nitrophenyl sulfate to an acceptor with adenosine 3',5'-bisphosphate as a cofactor[1] (Scheme 3). This reaction has been used by several groups studying sulfation reactions (see Section IID), although Banerjee and Roy[29] could not detect it with the purified phenol sulfotransferase of guinea-pig liver. The latter finding is not entirely unexpected if the reaction is a random one (Scheme 4), whereas the sequential mechanism (Scheme 5) shown by the rat enzyme at higher pH values could favor such a transfer. Again, more detailed kinetic studies are required.

4. Inhibition

Adenosine 3',5'-bisphosphate, a product of the forward reaction, is generally a powerful inhibitor of phenol sulfotransferases, competitive with PAPS and noncompetitive with the acceptor, and with its K_i being considerably less than the K_m of the former.[29,49,63] Likewise, ADP is a rather powerful inhibitor competitive with respect to PAPS, noncompetitive with respect to acceptor.[63] Oxidation of carbon atoms 2 and 3 of the ribose of ADP by periodate gives ADP-dialdehyde. This is an active-site directed irreversible inhibitor of phenol sulfotransferase which first forms a dissociable complex with the enzyme and then reacts with it to form a covalent bond, presumably at the PAPS-binding site because PAPS gives essentially complete protection against the inhibitor.[64] Although this has not so far been tested, it appears likely that ADP-dialdehyde will be a general inhibitor of sulfotransferases and not specific for phenol sulfortransferase. Reduction of ADP-dialdehyde gives 2',3'-acyclic-ADP which is not an inhibitor.[64]

Mulder and Scholtens[65] have shown that some phenols are powerful inhibitors of phenol sulfotransferase, not only in vitro but apparently also in vivo. Pentachlorophenol and 2,6-dichloro-4-nitrophenol are particularly effective, concentrations of 10 μM giving complete inhibition of phenol sulfotransferase activity with 0.15 mM harmol or 1 mM phenol as acceptors. There is no obvious explanation of this unexpected effect which cannot simply be due to a competition for PAPS.

The effects of probenecid [4-(dipropylsulfamoyl)-benzoic acid] on the phenol sulfotransferase activity of a homogenate of rat brain are interesting.[66] It may either inhibit or activate, depending upon the ratio of the modifier to acceptor (4-methylumbelliferone or 4-hydroxy-3-methoxyphenylethylene glycol) and not upon the concentration of the former alone. In view of the influence of probenecid on brain metabolism this effect might be worth reinvestigating with purer preparations of the sulfotransferase from rat brain. Probenecid is a simple inhibitor of the phenol sulfotransferase of rat liver.[66]

As has already been stated, there is no information on the chemistry of the phenol sulfotransferase reaction. It is, therefore, interesting that there is evidence for the participation of arginyl residues in the binding of PAPS. This is suggested by the inactivation of phenol sulfotransferase by butane-2,3-dione or by phenylglyoxal[17] under conditions in which these are believed to react specifically with arginyl residues.

E. Distribution and Control

It is hardly surprising that little information is available on these aspects of the phenol sulfotransferases considering that there is little certainty about the number of such enzymes which exist, even in such a well-investigated organ as the liver. Bearing this in mind, it can be said that most tissues in most mammals, and probably in most vertebrates, can synthesize aryl sulfates and so presumably contain phenol sulfotransferases. Somewhat unexpected is the recent finding of phenol sulfotransferase activity in human blood platelets:[67] if this holds for other species, it could pose problems in the interpretation of the results of investigations of the formation of sulfate esters by perfused organs. Phenol sulfotransferase also occurs in invertebrates,[8] particularly in insect gut tissues[30,68] and in the lobster *Homarus americanus* where phenol sulfotransferase has been found in the hepatopancreas[69] and in nervous tissue.[70] Strangely enough, phenol sulfotransferase has not been found in molluscs,[8] although it presumably must occur in at least those species containing the substituted indoxyl sulfates[71] which are the precursors of Tyrian Purple and probably in others.[6]

Quantitative values for different organs and different species are difficult to provide because in many cases PAPS has not been used as the sulfate donor, and only the overall synthesis of aryl sulfates from SO_4^{2-} and ATP has been measured; obviously this can do little other than show the presence, in indeterminate amounts, of a phenol sulfotransferase. Values of the phenol sulfotransferase activity of different tissues have been given for the rat,[72] man,[73] and the human fetus:[74] liver is generally the richest source. Some values for the brains of different species, and for different regions in the brain, are available.[72]

In mammalian liver and kidney it is clear that phenol sulfotransferase occurs in the cytosol, but the distribution of the activity in brain is less certain. There have been reports that in rat brain the phenol sulfotransferase activity, with either 4-methylumbelliferone or 4-hydroxy-3-methoxyphenylethylene glycol as acceptor, is associated with a subclass of synaptosomes,[51,75] probably those containing catecholamines.

There is the same lack of clear information about possible changes in the level of phenol sulfotransferase during development, but fetal tissues generally seem to have a low activity. At birth rat liver[56,76-78] and brain[79] have only about 10% of the adult level of activity: this rises to the adult level within about a week in the case of the liver[76] and within several weeks for the brain.[79] In the mouse the situation is more complicated. At birth the phenol sulfotransferase activity in the liver is about twice that of the adult; this increases to about five times the adult level at about 20 days and then falls to the adult level which is attained at about 40 days.[80,81]

Some observations by Powell and Jones (quoted in Reference 58) deserve greater attention than they seem to have received. These authors showed that in the fetal rat there was a sudden and complete loss of phenol sulfotransferase activity in homogenates of the gut one day before birth. This was due to the appearance in the gut of an unidentified inhibitor of rather high molecular weight. The inhibitor was not specific for the phenol sulfotransferase of gut but also influenced that of liver. It was not suggested that this inhibitor had a physiological role to play but rather that homogenization allowed it to come in contact with the phenol sulfotransferase. Obviously, should this phenomenon be a general one, then great care would have to be taken in the interpretation of any studies using unfractionated tissue preparations.

Sex differences in the levels of phenol sulfotransferase activity are not as striking as those found with many of the steroid sulfotransferases (see Section IV). In the rat, the activity in male liver is about 1.5 to 2 times that in female,[77,78] but no such sex difference is found in mouse[80] or guinea-pig liver.

In conclusion it must be emphasized that the statements made in this section should be accepted with caution. As has already been said, many tissues show several different sulfotransferase activities, not all of which may be due to a true phenol sulfotransferase, yet most of the information on the distribution and control of the phenol sulfotransferases has of necessity been obtained with unfractionated tissue preparations. When specific determinations of the different sulfotransferases become possible, the picture may become quite different.

IV. STEROID SULFOTRANSFERASES

A. Introduction

Several types of steroid sulfotransferase are found in mammalian tissues, but their detailed study is complicated by the fact that most of them have not been obtained free from other types of sulfotransferase activity. The steroid sulfotransferases of guinea-pig liver,[28] for example, were consistently associated not only with phenol sulfotransferase activity but also with arylamine sulfotransferase activity, both of which appeared to be intrinsic to at least two different steroid sulfotransferases. This has not been proven, and the association of these activities could have been due to strong interactions between a number of specific sulfotransferases, an interpretation which is perhaps suggested by the preparation from other sources of steroid sulfotransferases apparently free from phenol and arylamine sulfotransferase activities. The partially purified adrostenolone sulfotransferase of rat liver[22] can use butan-1-ol as an acceptor, but it has usually been thought that this represented the activity of a contaminating alcohol sulfotransferase. This may not be the case, because the three homogeneous hydroxysteroid sulfotransferases of Jakoby et al.[176] all show alcohol sulfotransferase activity (see below and Section V). It is, therefore, very likely that present ideas on the specificity of the steroid sulfotransferases in particular, and of the sulfotransferases in general, are considerably in error.

The steroids, being fairly complex but rigid molecules, lend themselves to detailed specificity studies. Up to the present the interpretation of these has been difficult because homogeneous steroid sulfotransferases have not been available. Figure 1 shows the numbering of those carbon atoms in the steroid nucleus which are of interest in this particular connection and also the conformations of the two commonly occurring series of steroids, the 5α-steroids (e.g., cholestanol, androsterone) and the 5β-steroids (e.g., coprostanol, cholic acid, etiocholanolone). The Δ5-steroids (e.g., dehydroepiandrosterone) have a conformation similar to that of the 5α-steroids, while in the estrogens the A ring is aromatic and hence planar. In a few steroids, such as the cardenolides and the bufadienolides (see Section IVH), rings C and D are *cis*-linked so that these compounds have a nonplanar conformation in this region of the molecule.

Most types of steroid seem to be able to form sulfate esters in vivo. Phenolic hydroxyl groups in position 3, primary alcoholic hydroxyl groups in positions 21 and 27, and secondary alcoholic hydroxyl groups at positions 3, 7, 12, 20, and 24 are sulfated so that

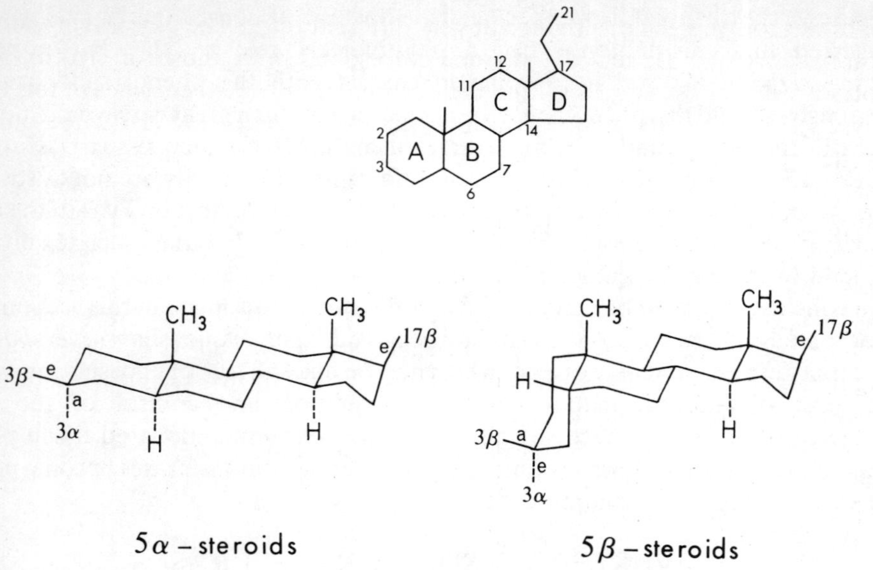

FIGURE 1.   Conformation of the two commonly occurring series of steroids.

several different steroid sulfotransferases might be expected to exist. These have apparently been found, although not necessarily separated, and in general their apparent specificity in vitro parallels that which would have been predicted from the types of steroid sulfate formed in vivo.

Complications which have not yet been investigated include the formation of steroid disulfates, for example, of the 3β,17β-, and 3β,20β-dihydroxy steroids.[82] The latter type of compound is important because it seems to be the only evidence that steroid 20-sulfates can be formed in vitro although one, 20β-sulfooxy-5β-pregan-3β-ol, has been isolated from pregnant mare's urine.[83] Mixed conjugates such as estriol 3-sulfate 16-glucuronide and pregnanediol 3-sulfate 20-glucuronide also occur naturally, and the former is obtained when estriol 16-glucuronide is incubated[84] with extracts of guinea-pig liver in the presence of ATP and SO_4^{2-}. Whether or not this reaction is catalyzed by the same sulfotransferase as normal sulfates, the phenolic hydroxyl group of estriol is unknown.

Of the sulfotransferase activities considered in this section, five—estrone, androstenolone, cortiocosteroid, bile salt, and sterol sulfotransferase activities have generally been considered to be due to specific enzymes which have been appropriately named, although, with the exception of estrone sulfotransferase, all preparations show a considerable lack of specificity with respect to the types of steroid which they can use as acceptors. The separate existence of the other three sulfotransferase activities—etiocholanolone, testosterone and cardenolide sulfotransferase activities—is more doubtful and supported only by circumstantial evidence. However, such a subdivision of the steroid sulfotransferase activities may be quite unjustified. One of the first suggestions of this came from the work of Singer et al. (see Section IVD) who isolated, from rat liver, sulfotransferases I, II, and III: the purification of these was followed by their ability to sulfate cortiocosteroids, but they could also use many other types of steroid as acceptors and sulfotransferase II seemed, in fact, to be identical to the so-called androstenolone sulfotransferase of rat liver. More recently, Jakoby et al.[81a] have isolated, also from rat liver, hydroxysteroid sulfotransferases I, II, and III as homogeneous proteins. Each of these can sulfate hydroxyl groups at positions 3, 17, and

21 of the steroid molecule, although at very different rates. The physical properties of sulfotransferases I, II, and III do not correspond with those of hydroxysteroid sulfotransferases I, II, and III so that the number of individual enzymes of this type in rat liver seems to be rather large. Much further work is needed to clarify the situation.

In general, the steroid sulfotransferases differ from the phenol sulfotransferases considered in Section III by being activated by Mg^{2+}, and some other divalent cations, although there is nothing to indicate an absolute requirement for these ions. It is therefore interesting that the phenol sulfotransferase activities associated with the steroid sulfotransferases of guinea-pig liver[28] are, unlike the specific phenol sulfotransferase, activated by Mg^{2+} which could be taken as further evidence for the view that both the former activities are functions of the steroid sulfotransferases.

Again in general, most steroid sulfotransferases are activated by thiols, but the nature of the activation is not understood.

Several steroid sulfotransferases have been shown to exhibit non-Michaelis kinetics in that the initial velocities of their reactions do not show a hyperbolic relationship with the substrate concentration. These enzymes show "wavy" substrate curves of the general type shown in Figure 2. As will be considered in subsequent sections, a number of possible explanations for these curves has been proposed, but their origin has still not been established. Whatever it be, it effectively prevents the determination of K_m and V for these enzymes.

B. Estrone Sulfotransferase
1. Introduction
Many of the general comments which have been made about phenol sulfotransferase apply with equal force to estrone sulfotransferase because its relationship to other sulfotransferases is by no means clear. Nose and Lipmann[85] were the first to show the existence of several steroid sulfotransferases by separating, from extracts of rabbit liver, an enzyme sulfating dehydroepiandrosterone from another sulfating estrone. The latter also sulfated 4-nitrophenol, but there were indications that two distinct sulfotransferases were involved. Banerjee and Roy[28] obtained similar results with guinea-pig liver, separating a sulfotransferase using dehydroepiandrosterone as an acceptor from an estrone sulfotransferase; the separation was not complete, and both steroid sulfotransferases showed phenol and arylamine sulfotransferase activities with 4-nitrophenol and 2-naphthylamine, respectively, as acceptors. More recent work has provided evidence for the existence of an estrone sulfotransferase which will use many derivatives of 3-hydroxyestra-1,3,5(10)-triene as acceptors; to this extent it is obviously a phenol sulfotransferase, but it differs from the phenol sulfotransferase discussed in Section III in that it cannot sulfate simple phenols. It can, however, use more complex phenols as acceptors (see Section IVB4). As phenol sulfotransferase can sulfate polycyclic phenols such as 2-phenanthrol, equilin, and equilenin[29] (Table 3), the distinction between phenol sulfotransferase and estrone sulfotransferase is by no means as clear-cut as is implied by their names.

In what follows, a purely operational approach will be used and an estrone sulfotransferase will be taken to be a sulfotransferase which can use estrone and related compounds as acceptors but which has little or no activity towards simple phenols.

2. Purification and General Properties
Estrone sulfotransferase has been purified only from bovine adrenal gland[86] and placenta,[87] but the specific activities of the final preparations are very low, 0.005 and 0.01 $\mu mol.mg^{-1}.min^{-1}$, respectively. Despite this, it has been claimed that these preparations of estrone sulfotransferase are essentially homogeneous.[86,87] They show a

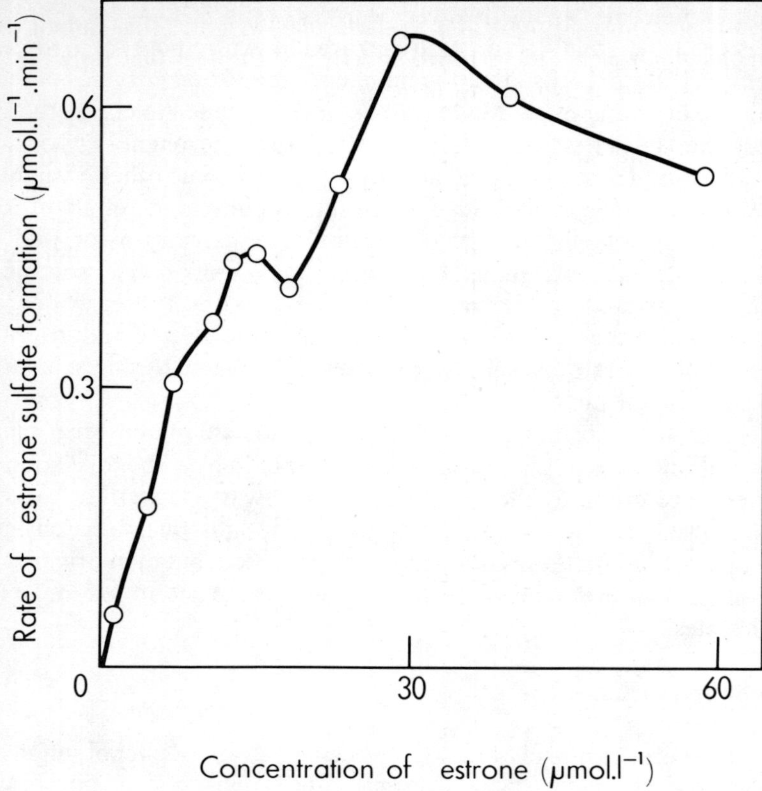

FIGURE 2. Typical "wavy" substrate curve shown by many estrone and androstenolone sulfotransferases. The figure shows the response of the former enzyme from ox adrenal.[86]

characteristic four-banded pattern on electrophoresis in acrylamide gel, and the corresponding four isoenzymes of estrone sulfotransferase can be separated by repeated chromatography on DEAE-cellulose. These isoenzymes differ in specific activity and charge but not in molecular weight,[86] and they can be isolated from organs of individual animals.[86,87] The aminoacid compositions of the isoenzymes differ only slightly from one another, probably only in the values for lysine and aspartic acid. These differences could be correlated with the different electrophoretic mobilities of the isoenzymes, but more information is required. The mixture of isoenzymes sedimented as a single boundary in the ultracentrifuge with an $s^0_{20,w}$ of 4.9 S. There was no indication of any concentration dependence of s. Molecular weight determination by equilibrium ultracentrifugation gave a value of 78,000, consistent with that obtained by density gradient centrifugation.[86] The sedimentation behavior was not altered by the presence of PAPS or of estrone, and no evidence was found for the existence of subunits.

Unfortunately it is difficult to reconcile these observations with earlier ones which described two forms, A and B, of the estrone sulfotransferase of bovine adrenal.[15,88] Form A, the more stable, was produced from form B on standing, and only form B was obtained when the entire isolation procedure was carried out in the presence of 3 mM mercaptoethanol. Further, it was shown by gel chromatography that form B was a trimer or tetramer of form A, and that the latter had a molecular weight of 67,000. More recently[86] it has been stated that forms A and B of estrone sulfotransferase were artifacts arising through an incomplete separation of isoenzymes of different specific activities, but as these isoenzymes do not differ in molecular weight,[86] this cannot explain the different molecular weights of forms A and B, nor the fact that only the latter was isolated when mercaptoethanol was present.[15,88]

An interesting feature of the estrone sulfotransferases is that, as isolated, they contain estrone.[12,87] The amount is small, 0.3 mol/mol protein (assuming homogeneity), but it is a constant feature of the preparations.

Only one other general property requires comment. Estrone sulfotransferase has apparently no requirement for exogenous metal ions because it is not inhibited by EDTA.[15,28] On the other hand, its activity is increased by Mg^{2+}, although high concentrations inhibit.[15] Similar effects are given by other divalent cations.

3. Effects of Thiols and Thiol Reagents

The effects of thiols on estrone sulfotransferase are complex. In early studies it was found that the enzyme was activated, to an extent varying from preparation to preparation, by cysteine and inhibited by chloromercuribenzoate and other SH reagents.[15] The effect of any given concentration of chloromercuribenzoate varied with the concentration of estrone used as acceptor.[15] Quantitative determination of the thiol content of native estrone sulfotransferase gave a value of 0.18 mol SH per mole enzyme, compared with a total of 23 half-cystine residues per mole of enzyme.[86] The presence of substrate did not increase the apparent thiol content of the enzyme, but denaturation by sodium dodecyl sulfate increased it to 0.9 mol SH per mole enzyme.[86] It is therefore interesting that the substrate analogue 4-mercuri-17β-estradiol can react with the native enzyme to the extent of 1 mol SH per mole enzyme.[89] This thiol group is presumably close to the active center of the enzyme, but as no protection is offered by estradiol, it cannot be in the steroid-binding site. Surprisingly, some protection was afforded by 11-deoxycorticosterone or by testosterone, neither of which is a substrate for the enzyme.

Therefore, although thiol groups are clearly implicated in the activity of estrone sulfotransferase, it is by no means clear in what way they are implicated.

4. Kinetics

In general terms the estrone sulfotransferase of bovine adrenal cannot use simple phenols,[15,25] 2-naphthylamine,[15] nor *N*-acetyl-*N*-hydroxy-2-aminofluorene[25] as acceptors although the synthetic estrogens stilbestrol and hexestrol are sulfated at rather a low rate.[15] As will be discussed below, more complex phenols are sulfated.[25] The pH optimum of the bovine adrenal enzyme is about 8.[15,25,86] The crude estrone sulfotransferase from guinea-pig liver had rather a broad optimum at about pH 6, but the activity trailed well into the alkaline with about 25% of it remaining at pH 8.[28]

The first investigations of the kinetics of estrone sulfotransferase were those of Adams[15,88] with the A and B forms of the enzyme from bovine adrenal gland (see Section IVB3). The A form was reported as showing the normal Michaelis kinetics of a sequential reaction, with K_m values of 14 μM estradiol and 70 μM PAPS. In striking contrast to this, the B form gave "wavy" substrate curves, similar to that in Figure 2 with varying concentrations of estradiol.[88] Further, in the presence of cysteine the A form also gave "wavy" substrate curves with estradiol. More recently it has been stated[86] that the earlier[15] reports of Michaelis kinetics with the A form of estrone sulfotransferase were incorrect and had arisen because an insufficient number of experimental points had been used, and that the A form, like all four of the isoenzymes presently recognized[86] gave "wavy" substrate curves with varying concentrations of estradiol. In contrast, all the isoenzymes gave normal Michaelis kinetics with PAPS which had a K_m of 35 μM. Similar findings have been made with the estrone sulfotransferase of bovine placenta.[87] An explanation of these "wavy" substrate curves has been proposed in terms of the existence of a number of different conformers of estrone sulfotransferase, and so presumably of each of the four isoenzymes, because they individually gave the typical "wavy" curves with varying concentrations of acceptor.

The interpretation of these results is made much more difficult when those of Rozhin et al.[25] are taken into account. These authors have prepared the A form estrone sulfotransferase from bovine adrenal glands by the method of Adams and Poulos[15] and have used this for detailed kinetic studies. As originally reported by Adams and Poulos,[15] Rozhin et al.[25] find this preparation of estrone sulfotransferase to give normal Michaelis kinetics with varying concentrations of acceptor, a finding which is, of course, at variance with the more recent observations of Adams et al.[86] No explanation of this discrepancy can be given, and it is unfortunate that insufficient data are available for any other estrone sulfotransferase. Banerjee and Roy[28] found no evidence of any anomalies with the estrone sulfotransferase of guinea-pig liver, but their preliminary observations were not made in sufficient detail to be certain that they did not occur.

a. Acceptor Specificity

The detailed observations of Rozhin et al.[25] have shown that while bovine estrone sulfotransferase can use many derivatives of 3-hydroxyestra-1,3,5(10)-triene as acceptors, it cannot sulfate derivatives of estra-1,3,5(10)-triene with the phenolic hydroxyl group in positions 2 or 4, nor can it sulfate simple phenols. It can, however, use more complex phenols as acceptors. From detailed investigations of over 60 compounds it was concluded that to be an acceptor the phenol required a lipophilic substitutent, about 7 Å long and *para* to the hydroxyl group, and, in the steroid acceptors, an oxygen function in the D ring which was available for hydrogen bonding to an area in the enzyme which lay about 3.7 Å above the plane of the ring.

No kinetic studies have been made in sufficient detail to allow any deductions to be made about the mechanism of the reaction. It is, however, sequential,[15,25] and the fact that the enzyme very firmly binds endogenous estrone[12,87] suggests either that the reaction must be a random one or that estrone is the first substrate in an ordered reaction. The latter possibility seems less likely because it would be very different from the situation with phenol sulfotransferase (see Section IIID3).

Not many values of K_m have been reported, but those of estrone (3.8 μM) and estradiol (6.7 μM) are probably typical.[25] Much information on the relative rates of sulfation of different estrogens, at an arbitrary substrate concentration, is tabulated in Reference 25. There are no very striking effects, but in view of the existence of mixed conjugates (see Section IVA) it is interesting that estradiol 17β-glucuronide is sulfated at only about 10% of the rate of estrone.

Further information on the specificity for steroids has been obtained from inhibition studies. Neither estra-1,3,5(10)-triene nor androst-5-ene are inhibitors, but the introduction of one or more oxygen functions at positions 3, 16, or 17 gives rather powerful inhibitors of estrone sulfotransferase.[42] In a series of such estratriene derivatives, K_i ranged from 3.5 to 90 μM while in a series of androstane derivatives it ranged from 35 to 302 μM, with the planar 5α-androstane derivatives binding more strongly than the nonplanar 5β-androstane derivatives. In the estratriene series a hydroxyl group at position 3 was not required for binding, and the introduction of suitable substituents in the A ring could greatly decrease K_i so that 2,4-dibromoestradiol and 4-nitroestradiol both had K_i values of about 0.1 μM. These observations led to the synthesis of 3-methoxy-4-nitroestra-1,3,5(10)-trien-17-one as a powerful inhibitor of estrone sulfotransferase with a K_i of 4.3 μM. As it itself cannot be sulfated and does not compete with estradiol for the estrogen receptor,[42] it should be of considerable use in investigations of the role of sulfation in the biochemistry of the estrogens. Inhibition studies have also led to the suggestion[42] that in the transition state of the estrone sulfotransferase reaction there is stacking between the A ring of the acceptor and the adenine of PAPS.

b. Donor Specificity

The specificity of estrone sulfotransferase towards PAPS is not absolute: adenosine 2′-phosphate 5′-sulfatophosphate can be used by the enzyme as a sulfate donor and gives about 30% of the rate obtained with an equal concentration of PAPS.[90] This relatively high activity with the 2′-phospho derivatives is interesting when it is recalled that adenosine 2′,5′-bisphosphate cannot replace the 3′,5′-bisphosphate as cofactor for the transfer of sulfate from 4-nitrophenyl sulfate to an acceptor.[1] Changes in the adenine moiety of PAPS also influence its ability to act as a sulfate donor:[178] 7-deazaadenosine 3′-phosphate 5′-sulfatophosphate and 8-bromoadenosine 3′-phosphate 5′-sulfato-phosphate give values of V about 50% of that obtained with PAPS as donor. These analogues bind quite strongly to estrone sulfotransferase and are competitive inhibitors with respect to PAPS. Removal of the 6-amino group of the adenine, to give purine 3′-phosphate 5′-sulfatophosphate, or its replacement by a hydroxyl group, to give inosine 3′-phosphate 5′-sulfatophosphate, causes a loss of 90% and 100%, respectively, of the ability to act as a sulfate donor.

c. Inhibition

As seems to be generally the case with the sulfotransferases, adenosine 3′,5′-bisphosphate is a powerful inhibitor of estrone sulfotransferase, competitive with PAPS. Values of 56 μM and 7 μM have been reported for K_i at pH 7.1[86] and 7.5,[91] respectively. A number of analogues of adenosine 3′,5′-bisphosphate have been prepared,[91] and it has been shown that both the 3′-phosphate and the 6-amino group are important for binding to the enzyme. Alterations in the pyrimidine part of the adenosine generally increased the K_i while alterations in the imidazole portion could give a greatly increased inhibitory power. For example, 7-deazaadenosine 3′,5′-bis-phosphate had a K_i of 0.6 μM. These analogues of adenosine 3′,5′-bisphosphate will presumably be inhibitors of sulfotransferases in general and not only of estrone sulfotransferase.

Other inhibitors are less interesting. Again like other sulfotransferases, estrone sulfotransferase is rather weakly inhibited by ADP but surprisingly this is noncompetitive with respect to PAPS: the K_i is 2.8 mM.[86] Estrone sulfotransferase is inhibited by some fatty acids, but not by their methyl esters. In the saturated series the inhibition is only significant from the C_{11} to the C_{16} acids, with the maximum effect shown by tetradecanoic acid, but the C_{18} unsaturated acids are powerful inhibitors. The extent of the inhibition is related to the ratio of the concentrations of fatty acid and enzyme, not to the former itself, and seems generally to be related to detergent effects.[92]

Although a considerable amount of information is obviously available on the kinetics of the estrone sulfotransferase reaction, much remains to be explained, particularly why some preparations show Michaelis kinetics with varying concentrations of acceptor while others, prepared by similar methods from the same organ, do not. Perhaps pertinent is the fact, already noted, that the specific activities of the available preparations of estrone sulfotransferase are low, at the best 0.01 μmol.mg^{-1}.min^{-1}, which is less than those of preparations of phenol sulfotransferase (0.6 μmol.mg^{-1} .min^{-1}) or N-hydroxyarylamine sulfotransferase (2 μmol.mg^{-1}.min^{-1}) which are not homogeneous. This suggests either that estrone sulfotransferase is only a minor component of the preparations at present available or, if the preparations are indeed homogeneous, that estrogens are not the physiological acceptors for this enzyme, despite their high affinity for it. The former possiblity seems the more likely.

5. Distribution and Control

If the formation of estrogen sulfates is accepted as evidence for the occurrence of estrone sulfotransferase, then this enzyme must be widely distributed. Its occurrence in bovine tissues has been measured only by using the endogenous sulfate-activating system to produce PAPS from ATP and SO_4^{2-}: under these conditions by far the greatest activity was found in the placenta and adrenal (50% of the placental activity) with that in the liver being much less (about 10% of the placental level).[93] Other organs, including the ovary and testis, contained only low levels of activity. More direct determinations, using PAPS as sulfate donor, have shown that human liver has about double the activity of the adrenals while again other organs have only a low activity.[73] Estrone sulfotransferase activity has been found in chick embryo cartilage,[94] in adult hen liver, oviduct and vagina,[95] the gut of the larval Southern Armyworm, *Prodenia eridania*,[68] and the gut of the sea urchin *Strongylocentrotus franciscanus*.[96]

In the human fetus the estrone sulfotransferase activity in the liver is only about 25% of that in the adult,[97] while the fetal adrenal has a very high activity, about five times that of the adult gland.[73,74,97,98]

Sulfate esters are believed to play an important role in the metabolism of estrogens, although direct evidence for this has yet to be provided, so it is not surprising that much interest has been shown in the estrone sulfotransferase activity of endocrine tissue. Pack and Brooks[99] have shown indirectly by measuring the production of sulfated metabolites of estradiol, that there are cyclic changes in the level of estrone sulfotransferase in the pig uterus. The activity is very low at estrus and reaches a peak at day nine of the cycle, about the middle of diestrus. Much interest has also been shown in paraendocrine tissue, such as mammary carcinoma. This, unlike normal breast tissue, shows estrone sulfotransferase activity,[100,101] and there are suggestions[102] that the sulfotransferase pattern of mammary tumor may be a guide to the prognosis of the condition.

Finally, it is worth noting the suggestion[89] of a possible genetic relationship between bovine estrone sulfotransferase and bovine serum albumin—both contain many half-cystine residues but only one free thiol group, and both bind one molecule of estrone. The evidence for such a relationship remains scanty, but is certainly worth further investigation.

C. Androstenolone Sulfotransferase

1. Introduction

Once again the early work of Nose and Lipmann[85] had shown the existence of a sulfotransferase utilizing dehydroepiandrosterone as an acceptor, and this was extended by the work of Banerjee and Roy[28] who partially separated such an enzyme from guinea-pig liver. As in the case of the corresponding estrone sulfotransferase, from which it was incompletely separated, this steroid sulfotransferase also showed phenol sulfotransferase and arylamine sulfotransferase activities. The specificity of the sulfotransferase which uses dehydroepiandrosterone as an acceptor is still not known, and a suitable name for the enzyme is difficult to find (see Section I). The names steroid sulfotransferase or steroid alcohol sulfotransferase are frequently used but, having regard to the other types of steroid sulfotransferase known, they are too general. A name which has been suggested previously[103] will be used here: this is androstenolone sulfotransferase, androstenolone being an alternative trivial name for its typical acceptor, dehydroepiandrosterone (androst-5-en-3β-ol-17-one or 3β-hydroxyandrost-5-en-17-one), but this name is undoubtedly too specific.

2. Purification and General Properties

The first important study of androstenolone sulfotransferase was that of Adams and Edwards[104] who used the unfractionated cytosol of human adrenal gland as a source of the enzyme. Gel filtration showed a number of peaks of androstenolone sulfotransferase activity, all of which appeared to be polymers of a unit of molecular weight 65,000. The polymeric species, which were in an equilibrium only slowly attained over several days, could be separated by density gradient centrifugation, and the position of the equilibrium was shown to be influenced by the substrates and modifiers of the enzyme. Dissociation to the monomer was favored by PAPS, a concentration of 0.15 mM causing complete dissociation, while dehydroepiandrosterone favored association, as did Mg^{2+} and cysteine, both of which activate the enzyme. More recently Adams and McDonald[105] have developed an affinity procedure for the separation of this androstenolone sulfotransferase, using the ligand dehydroepiandrosterone-17-(O-carboxymethyl) oxime linked to Sepharose-4B. The enzyme was adsorbed and eluted batch-wise, 0.1 mM dehydroepiandrosterone in phosphate buffer, pH 7.5, containing 2% propylene glycol being used as eluant. The resulting enzyme was stated to be 95% pure, as judged by electrophoresis on acrylamide gel, and it gave a single zone of activity, corresponding to a molecular weight of 68,000, on sucrose density gradient centrifugation. Electrophoresis in sodium dodecyl sulfate showed that the enzyme was made up of two subunits of molecular weight 35,000 which were, to judge by peptide maps, identical. No mention was made[105] of any tendency of this enzyme to polymerize; yet the density gradient centrifugation was carried out in the same way as it had been previously[104] when extensive polymerization did occur. This suggests that in the latter case there was in fact interaction between the androstenolone sulfotransferase and other proteins in the cytosol rather than simple polymerization. The specific activity of the preparation was only 0.007 μmol.mg^{-1}.min^{-1} which again seems remarkably low for a pure enzyme, especially as Ryan and Carroll[22] have prepared an androstenolone sulfotransferase from rat liver which has a specific activity of 0.017 μmol.mg^{-1}.min^{-1} and which is not homogeneous.

Two other preparations of androstenolone sulfotransferase have been briefly examined but neither were highly purified. Both had specific activities of about 0.003 μmol.mg^{-1}.min^{-1} and were obtained from rat[41] and guinea-pig[105] liver, respectively. Their respective molecular weights were about 50,000 and 67,000.

3. Kinetics

The results of kinetic studies with this enzyme are confusing. The pH optimum has been variously reported as about 5.0[22] and about 7.5.[28,41,104] Some preparations are activated by Mg^{2+} or other divalent cations,[28,41,104] while others[22] are not. It is of interest that Ryan and Carroll[22] showed that whereas the activity of their purified preparations of androstenolone sulfotransferase was not increased by Mg^{2+}, the activity in crude preparations was so increased: as mentioned in Section IIA, it is important to consider the influence of divalent ions on PAPS-degrading enzymes when only crude preparations are available.

With the liver enzymes[22,41,106] the kinetics are Michaelis in type and are consistent with a sequential reaction: K_m values for PAPS range from 4 to 45 μM, and for dehydroepiandrosterone from 6 to 20 μM. The apparent K_m of 45 μM PAPS for the guinea-pig enzyme[106] is likely to be too high because the preparation contained PAPS-degrading enzymes. The picture with the enzyme from human adrenal is quite different:[104,105] here the kinetics are non-Michaelis and the substrate curves, either with PAPS or dehydroepiandrosterone as variable substrate, are "wavy" and quite similar to the curve in Figure 2. It is, therefore, impossible to give values for the kinetic constants for this enzyme. These anomalous kinetics are not a function of the method of preparing the enzyme because it has been reported[105] that androstenolone sulfotransferase prepared from bovine liver by the affinity technique used for the adrenal enzyme gives Michaelis kinetics.

Little can be said of the specificity of androstenolone sulfotransferase except that it is obvious that the available preparations do not use only 3β-hydroxy-Δ^5 steroids and the similarly planar 3β-hydroxy-5α steroids as acceptors. Not only can 3α-hydroxy-5α steroids be sulfated but also the highly nonplanar 3-hydroxy-5β steroids. Even hydroxyl groups in other positions in the steroid molecule can be sulfated. Some data, extracted from the quite large amount available[22,41,105] are given in Table 4. It is certainly of interest that the preparation having the highest specific activity, that of Ryan and Carroll,[22] has the least ability to use hydroxyl groups other than those at position 3 as acceptors, and it seems highly probable that the available preparations of androstenolone sulfotransferase contain other steroid sulfotransferases (Sections IVF and IVG).

A potential acceptor of particular interest is cholesterol because of the possible role of cholesteryl sulfate as a precursor of other steroid sulfates, such as dehydroepiandrosterone sulfate[107] and thence other steroids.[108] Cholesterol can be sulfated by some,[22,105,106] but not all[22,41] preparations of androstenolone sulfotransferase and again not by the most highly purified preparation,[22] thus some doubt must remain as to whether or not the synthesis of cholesteryl sulfate is a function of androstenolone sulfotransferase itself. One possible source of error which must be noted is the rather firm binding of cholesteryl sulfate to protein: if not recognized, poor recoveries of the ester could easily be obtained.[106] Other aspects of the synthesis of cholesteryl sulfate require investigation. For example, it is readily formed in slices of guinea-pig liver, kidney, skin, or lung, yet it is hardly, if at all, produced in slices of adrenal gland, ovary or testis, an observation[109] which must raise doubts as to the source of cholesteryl sulfate in the adrenal gland.

4. Distribution and Control

Androstenolone sulfotransferase activity seems to be fairly widely distributed, but in bovine[93] and adult human[73] tissues only the liver and adrenal are quantitatively important. Bovine placenta is also a rich source. Although other organs seem to contain only small amounts of androstenolone sulfotransferase, this is not to say that these are unimportant: they may have highly specific functions. The human fetal adrenal gland contains large amounts of androstenolone sulfotransferase,[74] about ten times as much as does adult liver or adrenal, but other fetal organs generally have very low activities of this, as of most other, sulfotransferases. Androstenolone sulfotransferase activity has also been found in chick embryo[110] and in insects.[30]

Androstenolone sulfotransferase differs from the other sulfotransferases so far mentioned in that there is a striking sex difference in the activities in the liver of the adult rat, female liver having at least twice the activity of male liver. This was first noted by Roy[111] and has since been confirmed by others, both in the rat[77,112] and in the mouse.[81,112] This sex difference does not occur in the fetal livers, and in the mouse the activity in the liver rises rapidly after birth to a peak at 20 days, when there is still no sex difference, after which it falls to the adult levels.[81] In the rat, androstenolone sulfotransferase activity in the liver rises steadily from birth to give the adult levels at about 7 weeks.[77] There is apparently no sex difference in the levels of androstenolone sulfotransferase in adult human tissues.[73]

As will be considered in the next section, it appears that one of the corticosteroid sulfotransferases of rat liver, STII, is identical with androstenolone sulfotransferase: information on the control of this enzyme is given in Section IVD3.

Table 4
**RELATIVE RATES OF SULFATION OF SOME STEROIDS
(DEHYDROEPIANDROSTERONE = 1.0) BY PARTIALLY PURIFIED
PREPARATIONS OF ANDROSTENOLONE SULFOTRANSFERASE**

	Relative velocity with enzyme from		
Acceptor	Human liver[41]	Human adrenal[105]	Rat liver[22]
3α-Hydroxy-5α-androstan-17-one (androsterone)	—	0.44	0.53
3β-Hydroxy-5α-androstan-17-one (epiandrosterone)	—	1.6	1.4
3α-Hydroxy-5β-androstan-17-one (etiocholanolone)	0.45	0.89	0.05
3β-Hydroxy-5β-androstan-17-one	—	—	0.45
3β-Hydroxyandrost-5-en-17-one (dehydroepiandrosterone)	1.0	1.0	1.0
17β-Hydroxyandrost-4-en-3-one (testosterone)	0.0	0.15	0.02
3β-Hydroxypregn-5-en-20-one (pregnenolone)	—	1.0	0.61
11β,20-Dihydroxypregn-4-ene-3,20-dione (corticosterone)	—	—	0.06
21-Hydroxypregn-4-ene-3,20-dione (deoxycorticosterone)	—	0.10	0.10
11β,17α,21-Trihydroxypregn-4-ene-3,20-dione (cortisol)	0.0	—	0.0
3β-Hydroxycholest-5-ene (cholesterol)	0.0	—	0.0
3-Hydroxyestra-1,3,5 (10)-trien-17-one (estrone)	0.08	—	0.0

Note: The measurements were made at arbitrary concentrations of steroids, and the enzymes were not necessarily free from other types of steroid sulfotransferase activities.

D. Corticosteroid Sulfotransferase

1. Introduction

It has long been known that corticosteroid sulfates can be formed in vivo, and the early work of Roy and Banerjee[113] showed that guinea-pig liver contained a corticosteroid sulfotransferase which could use deoxycorticosterone as an acceptor and which was distinct, but inseparable, from estrone and androstenolone sulfotransferases. Its activity was apparently much lower than those of the latter two enzymes. Although a homogeneous corticosteroid sulfotransferase still has not been obtained, a number of partially purified preparations are available, as is also a considerable amount of information on its control.

2. Purification and General Properties

Singer et al.[114] separated, by chromatography on DEAE-Sephadex, approximately equal amounts of three corticosteroid sulfotransferases (STI, STII, STIII) from the cytosol of female rat liver. The livers of male rats yielded mainly STIII with small amounts, about 10 to 20% of the total, of STII. Cortisol (11β,17α,21-trihydroxy-pregn-4-en-3,20-dione) was routinely used as the acceptor in these studies, but other steroids could be sulfated and there were differences in the specificities of the different fractions, as shown in Table 5. The same three sulfotransferases were obtained from female rat liver when corticosterone (11β,21-dihydroxypregn-4-ene-3, 20-dione) was used as acceptor.[115] Fractions STI and STII showed a greater activity with cortisol than with corticosterone, whereas the reverse was true with fraction STIII. With both acceptors sulfation was shown to occur at position 21.[114,115]

Sulfotransferase STI with a specific activity of 0.012 μmol.mg^{-1}.min^{-1} has been prepared from female rat liver,[116] the final step being affinity chromatography on agarose-adenosine 3′,5′-bisphosphate with ADP as eluant. It is much less stable than

Table 5
THE RELATIVE ACTIVITIES, UNDER ARBITRARY CONDITIONS, OF CORTI-COSTEROID SULFOTRANSFERASES STI, STII, AND STIII OF RAT LIVER

	Activity relative to cortisol (= 1.0) with					
Enzyme	Dehydroepiandrosterone		Testosterone		Estradiol	
fraction	Male	Female	Male	Female	Male	Female
STI	—	1.6	—	0.24	—	0.60
-purified	—	1.7	—	0.33	—	0.47
STII	2.5	7.0	0.56	0.80	1.1	0.89
STIII	1.0	3.8	0.27	0.34	1.2	0.91
-purified	0.30	—	0.09	—	0.31	—

Note: Data, from References 114, 116, and 117, are given for both the fractions as originally obtained and after purification.

most other sulfotransferases, and during chromatography, at pH 7.5, on Sephadex G-150 or G-200 it lost 90 to 95% of its activity, although it was stable on G-100 under the same conditions. It lost about 50% of its activity when stored at $-20°C$ for 2 days: on the other hand, little activity was lost on storage at 0°C for 2 weeks. Its molecular weight, from sedimentation velocity measurements, was 156,000, double that of most other steroid sulfotransferases but similar to that of the bile salt sulfotransferase of rat liver.[23] In contrast, the small amounts of activity remaining after chromatography of STI on Sephadex G-200 eluted as two peaks with molecular weights of 50,000 and 70,000. The pH optimum of STI is 6.0, and at pH 6.8 the values of K_m are 7.1 μM cortisol and 11 μM PAPS. It is inhibited by 4-mercuribenzoate and is activated by Mg^{2+} and some other divalent cations, Cr^{2+} being particularly effective, 5 mM giving a 2.5-fold activation: Zn^{2+} and Ca^{2+}, on the other hand, inhibited. Like other corticosteroid sulfotransferases, STI showed other types of steroid sulfotransferase activity (Table 5): the ratios of these activities remained fairly constant during the final stages of the preparations, and Singer[116] has suggested that they all are associated with a single enzyme. Many steroids inhibit STI with cortisol as substrate:[116] some of these, such as dehydroepiandrosterone, testosterone, and estradiol, could be functioning as alternative substrates (Table 5) but others, such as progesterone (pregn-4-ene-3, 20-dione), could not.

Sulfotransferase STIII has been partially purified from male rat liver, in which it is the major corticosteroid sulfotransferase,[117] to give a preparation with a specific activity of 0.001 $\mu mol.mg^{-1}.min^{-1}$. More highly purified, and apparently homogeneous, preparations have been obtained from female rat liver.[179] The molecular weight of STIII is 61,500. Its activity is modified, similarly but not identically to that of STI, by divalent cations, some activating and some inhibiting, and it is inhibited by 4-mercuribenzoate. The optimum pH is 6.0 and at pH 6.8, where it is more stable, the kinetics are consistent with those of a sequential reaction with K_m values of 6.8 μM cortisol and 6.3 μM PAPS. As shown in Table 5, the preparation still shows other types of sulfotransferase activity: the changes in the relative activities during purification[117] suggest that the sulfation of testosterone is due to a contaminating enzyme but that of estradiol and dehydroepiandrosterone is due to STIII. The kinetics with corticosterone are more complex because there is pronounced substrate inhibition with this steroid:[115] the maximum activity is attained at about 15 μM corticosterone and by 40 μM the activity has dropped by about 50%. Singer[115] has discussed the problems arising from this phenomenon, which are compounded by the biological and seasonal variations in the enzyme levels, and he has developed a "mosaic" assay using three different concentrations of substrate, each at several different enzyme concentrations. Many types of steroid inhibit STIII, the inhibition being competitive in those cases which have been examined in sufficient detail, a finding which is perhaps surprising in the case of progesterone.[117] Neither AMP, ADP, nor ATP inhibited STIII at concentrations of 8 mM, 33 times that of the PAPS.

Much further work is needed to elucidate the relationships of the various corticosteroid sulfotransferases not only with each other but also with the other steroid sulforansferases. For example, Singer[116] has suggested, on the basis of their chromatographic behavior, that STII is the androstenolone sulfotransferase of Ryan and Carroll:[22] this, however, seems unlikely because the latter enzyme cannot[22] sulfate cortisol.

Although conclusive information is not available, it seems that at least one other corticosteroid sulfotransferase, a mineralocorticoid sulfotransferase, must exist in rat liver.[116,117]

3. Control

This particular group of sulfotransferases has been much studied from the standpoint of their control, and it should be remembered that the findings may have implications for other steroid sulfotransferases because of the possible identity of one of the "corticosteroid" sulfotransferases (STII) with androstenolone sulfotransferase.[117,118] Elucidation of the control of steroid sulfotransferases will not be easy when the different enzymes have overlapping specificities.

The first investigations were made with deoxycorticosterone:[119] with this acceptor the corticosteroid sulfotransferase activity in the liver of newborn rats was high, about 6 nmol/mg protein: this fell to about 2 nmol/mg by 1 week, kept this level for 4 weeks, after which it began to rise in females and fall in males to the adult levels of 6 nmol/mg and 1.5 nmol/mg, respectively, which were attained at an age of about 8 weeks. The adult female level was not altered by ovariectomy, either neonatally or postpubertally, while neonatal orchidectomy caused the level of corticosteroid sulfotransferase in adult male liver to rise to the female level. Postpubertal orchidectomy gave some increase in the liver corticosteroid sulfotransferase activity, but not to the female level. From these results, and from the effects of administered estrogens and androgens, it was concluded[119] that the level of corticosteroid sulfotransferase activity in female liver was maintained by nongonadal factors, while that in the male was suppressed by testicular androgens in two ways — by an irreversible imprinting in the neonatal period and by a reversible suppression postpubertally. Further evidence for these views were obtained from studies on male pseudohermaphroditic rats.[120]

With the demonstration[114] that rat liver contained three types of corticosteroid sulfotransferase activity, with either cortisol or corticosterone as acceptors, the situation became much more complex. Briefly, Singer et al.[114] showed that the total corticosteroid sulfotransferase activity in female rat liver was about five times that in male rat liver, and that while the activity in the female rose steadily from birth, that in the male dropped after puberty (about 4 weeks). In both sexes the adult levels were reached at about 7 or 8 weeks of age. The levels of the different sulfotransferases changed during development. In newborn females STII (androstenolone sulfotransferase?) was the major enzyme, by puberty STI had become dominant, and subsequently all three activities increased to their adult levels. In the male, on the other hand, STIII had begun to appear by puberty, and the adult pattern, in which it is the dominant enzyme, developed within 7 or 8 weeks. From these results, and later studies on gonadectomized[121] and adrenalectomized[122] rats, the following picture emerged. In females, the adrenals are the main determinant of the corticosteroid sulfotransferase activity of the liver, while in males the adrenals are important but their effects are modified by suppressive effects of the testes and by an unidentified factor which predominantly increases the level of STII. Singer[122] has suggested that the presence of the latter factor can explain the irreversible imprinting of corticosteroid sulfotransferase activity which was postulated by Carlstedt-Duke and Gustafsson.[119] If the factor is present in neonatal males, as is suggested by the high level of STII in these animals, then neonatal orchidectomy could allow it to continue to exert its effect in the absence of the testes and during a period of submaximal adrenal activity. This could give a greatly increased activity of STII (androstenolone sulfotransferase?) in neonatally orchidectomized males and account for the apparent feminization of the hepatic corticosteroid sulfotransferase activity.[119]

More recent studies[123] have shown that the pituitary plays an important role in the regulation of hepatic corticosteroid sulfotransferase activity. This is particularly clear in the female rat where hypophysectomy causes a fall in the activities of all three corticosteroid sulfotransferases, although at different rates. In the male rat the situation is more complex and still not fully understood.

In male rats there are striking changes in the levels of the corticosteroid sulfotransferases with age.[118] Although there is little difference in the total activities in the livers of young (9 to 19 weeks) and old (20 to 27 months) rats—66 and 81 nmol/hr/100g body weight, respectively—there were big differences in the levels of the different enzymes. In young male rats STIII accounts for 80 to 90% of the total hepactic corticosteroid sulfotransferase activity and STII accounts for the remainder. In old rats the proportions are altered so that STII (androstenolone sulfotransferase?) is a major fraction of the whole and, further, STI is not unimportant. This gives a change in the relative rates of sulfation of different steroids in young and old rats: in particular, a greater ability to sulfate dehydroepiandrosterone in the latter. These differences may explain the different effects of glucocorticoids in young and old rats.[118]

Finally, it is worth noting the suggestions that the corticosteroid sulfotransferases, alone among the steroid sulfotransferases, may have specific roles in a number of metabolic processes. These include the induction of tyrosine transaminase,[118'] an involvement in several types of hypertension in male rats[124] and in some types of cancer.[125]

E. Bile-Salt Sulfotransferase

It has been known since the work of Palmer[126] that lithocholic acid 3-sulfate is formed in vivo, but it is only recently that the appropriate sulfotransferase has been examined. Once again it must be noted that the relationship of this enzyme to the other steroid sulfotransferases is unknown, except for the observation[23] that the bile-salt sulfotransferase of rat liver can be separated from estrone sulfotransferase by isoelectric focusing.

A bile-salt sulfotransferase has been obtained from the cytosol of rat liver[23] but its specific activity is very low, only 0.7×10^{-3} μmol. mg^{-1}.min^{-1} with taurolithocholate as acceptor. The apparent molecular weight, by gel filtration, is 130,000; the isoelectric point, by isoelectric focusing, is 5.3; and the pH optimum is 6.5. Detailed kinetic studies have not been made, but the apparent K_m values are 8 μM PAPS and 50 μM taurolithocholate. A very similar bile-salt sulfotransferase has been prepared from rat kidney[20] with the higher specific activity of 0.005 μmol.mg^{-1}.min^{-1}. Its molecular weight is 80,000 and its isoelectric point 5.8. The K_m values are 2 μM PAPS and 40 μM taurolithocholate. Both of these bile-salt sulfotransferases are inhibited by SH reagents and by EDTA, although there is no evidence of an absolute requirement for metal ions.

There have been few comments on the specificities of these sulfotransferases. Both the free bile acids and their glyco- or tauro- conjugates (i.e., compounds in which the carboxyl group of the bile acid is linked through a peptide bond with glycine or taurine, respectively) are acceptors, although the rates, at an arbitrary substrate concentration, are greater with the latter. Dihydroxy and trihydroxy bile acids are acceptors, but the products differ with the different enzymes: the liver sulfotransferase[23] gave two and three products, presumably the $3\alpha,7\alpha$-di and the $3\alpha,7\alpha,12\alpha$-trisulfates with taurochenodeoxycholate and taurocholate, respectively, while the kidney preparation[20] gave only the 7α-sulfate with chenodeoxycholate. It is of interest that the perfusion of rat kidney with chenodeoxycholate likewise gave only 7α-sulfate.[127] Whether different sulfotransferases are involved in sulfation at the 3, 7, and 12 positions has not been established, but such a situation seems not unlikely although Chen et al.[20] reported no success in attempts to separate activities towards the 3α- and 7α-hydroxyl groups. It is of interest that some years ago it was shown[128] that 7α-hydroxyandrostenolone (3β, 7α-dihydroxyandrost-5-en-17-one) gave the 7α-sulfate when incubated with rat-liver cytosol, SO_4^{2-} and ATP: whether this reaction would require yet another sulfotransferase is not known.

Some values for the relative rates of sulfation of the different acceptors are given in Table 6.

Isolithocholate (3β-hydroxy-5β-cholanic acid) is not an acceptor, at least with the kidney enzyme,[20] and is in fact an inhibitor of the sulfation of glycolithocholate.

Recently, the bile-salt sulfotransferase activity in the unfractionated cytosol of human liver has been examined.[26] The specificity appears to be different from that of the rat-liver enzyme because lithocholate and glycolithochlate are sulfated at approximately equal rates (Table 6), but the difference may not be real because the rates given are V for the human enzyme and v under arbitrary conditions, for the rat enzymes. The values of V were 0.28×10^{-3} and 0.23×10^{-3} μmol.mg^{-1}.min^{-1}, respectively, while the corresponding values of K_m were 2 μM and 3.3 μM, respectively. The latter values are much less than those for the rat enzyme.

Bile-salt sulfotransferases have been found in the rat,[20,23] guinea pig,[129] and man,[26] and they probably occur generally in mammals. So far the enzyme has been found only in the liver and kidney, although there is some disagreement about its occurrence in the latter organ of the human: Imperato et al.[130] reported that bile-salt sulfotransferase did occur in human kidney while Lööf and Wengle[26] could not detect it therein. Like many other sulfotransferases, the activity of bile-salt sulfotransferase in human and guinea-pig fetal liver is low, only about 10% of the adult value.[129] In the rat, bile-salt sulfotransferase activity in female liver is about three times that in male liver: postpubertal ovariectomy causes the level to drop to close to that of the male, and this fall is prevented by the administration of estradiol which has no effect on the activity in male liver.[131] These results seem to distinguish rather clearly bile-salt sulfotransferase from corticosteroid sulfotransferase: as considered above (Section IVD3), the high level of the latter in female rat liver is not lowered by postpubertal ovariectomy, and the low level in male liver is increased by the administration of estradiol, both contrary to the behavior of bile-salt sulfotransferase. Finally, it should be noted that these findings in vitro correlate well with the sex differences in the formation of the sulfate ester of taurolithocholate in vivo.[131]

It has been suggested[132] that the high susceptibility of the rhesus monkey, compared with man, to the hepatotoxic effects of lithocholate can be correlated with the lower ability of the former species to sulfate the bile acid.

Table 6
RELATIVE RATES OF SULFATION OF BILE SALTS BY SOME PARTIALLY PURIFIED BILE SALT SULFOTRANSFERASES

Acceptor	Relative rate (lithocholate = 1.0) with enzyme from		
	Rat liver	Rat kidney	Human liver
Taurolithocholate	3.7	1.6	—
Glycolithocholate	4.4	1.6	0.82
Lithocholate	1.0	1.0	1.0
Taurochenodeoxycholate	—	0.72	—
Glycochenodeoxycholate	—	0.62	—
Chenodeoxycholate	—	0.42[a]	—
Taurocholate	—	0.36	—
Glycocholate	—	0.29	—

Note: The values for the rat tissues were obtained under arbitrary conditions (References 20 and 23) while those for human liver are relative values of V (Reference 26).

[a]Rate of formation of the 7α-sulfate.

F. Etiocholanolone Sulfotransferase

Preparations of androstenolone sulfotransferase from rat liver,[22] human liver,[41] and ox adrenal[105] can sulfate the etiocholanolones, 3α- and 3β-hydroxy-5β-androstan-17-one, but, as can be seen from the data in Table 4, the rates of sulfation of these compounds relative to that for dehydroepiandrosterone are very different in the different species. In the rat, the etiocholanolones are sulfated more slowly than dehydroepiandrosterone, while in the ox and the human the rates with the two different types of acceptor are quite comparable. Similar differences had been noted, many years ago, between crude preparations of the cytosol of rat liver[111] on the one hand and human liver[133] or adrenal[98] on the other. Although obviously inconclusive, these observations do suggest the separate existence of an etiocholanolone sulfotransferase which preferentially utilizes the 3-hydroxy-5β-androstan-17-ones, and perhaps other 3-hydroxy-5β steroids, as acceptors.[111] This conclusion might have been predicted from the very different conformations of the 5α and 5β steroids: the former are essentially planar while the latter are not. It is also interesting that, whatever their rates of sulfation relative to that of dehydroepiandrosterone, 3β-hydroxy-5β-androstan-17-one is sulfated more rapidly than 3α-hydroxy-5β-androstan-17-one.[22,111,133] This is somewhat surprising because the 3β-hydroxyl group is an axial one and therefore might have been expected to be less reactive.

As the bile salts are 5β steroids, it seems not impossible that the postulated etiocholanolone sulfotransferase might be identical to bile-salt sulfotransferase, although the latter (see Section IVE) will not sulfate 3β-hydroxy-5β-cholanic acid, while the former can sulfate both 3α- and 3β-hydroxy-5β-androstan-17-one. Only further work can resolve this problem.

It should be noted that ecdysone (2β,3β,14α,22β,25-pentahydroxy-5β-cholest-7-en-6-one) is a 5β steroid, and so the sulfotransferase involved in the formation of ecdysone sulfate in insects[30,68] could perhaps be regarded as an etiocholanolone sulfotransferase.

G. Testosterone Sulfotransferase

Testosterone (17β-hydroxyandrost-4-en-3-one) can be used as an acceptor by several sulfotransferase preparations, for example, the androstenolone sulfotransferase preparations from rat liver[22] and guinea-pig liver,[28] but it is clear[113] that testosterone is sulfated by an enzyme distinct from androstenolone sulfotransferase and from estrone sulfotransferase. On the other hand, testosterone sulfotransferase activity could not be resolved from the corticosteroid sulfotransferase (with deoxycorticosterone as acceptor) of guinea-pig liver.[113] It is therefore interesting that the purification of the latter enzyme from rat liver seemed also to concentrate a testosterone sulfotransferase activity (Table 3 of Reference 117). However, structural considerations would seem to make it unlikely that the same enzyme could utilize as an acceptor both the primary 21-hydroxyl of a corticosteroid and the secondary 17β-hydroxyl of testosterone, so that the existence of a testosterone sulfotransferase is likely. If it does exist, it will probably not be specific for testosterone but will also sulfate the 17β-hydroxyl groups in androstanediols and androstenediols[82] and in estradiol.[82,114]

Wengle and Boström[82] considered the effects of various substituents on the sulfation of a 17β-hydroxyl group and suggested that it was inhibited by a 17α-methyl or a 17α-ethyl group, but not by a 17α-ethinyl group. However, as actual rates of sulfation were not measured, the interpretation of the results must remain in some doubt.

It has long been known[82,111] that crude extracts of rat liver can sulfate epitestosterone (17α-hydroxyandrost-4-en-3-one). Whether this reaction is brought about by the same enzyme as sulfates testosterone is not known.

H. Cardenolide Sulfotransferase

Herrmann and Repke[134] showed that the cytosols of guinea-pig, human-, and fetal-human livers could sulfate a number of cardioactive genins of both the 5α and 5β series. These cardenolides have a *cis* junction of the C and D rings compared with the *trans* junction of the more typical animal steroids, a change which completely alters the shape of the steroid molecule in this region. The constant presence of a 14β hydroxyl group is a further difference from the hormonal steroids. Of the eight cardenolides tested, seven were sulfated by the cytosol of guinea-pig liver: these were digitoxigenin (3β,14-dihydroxy-5β,14β-card-20(22)-enolide), epidigitoxigenin (3α,14-dihydroxy-5β,14β-card-20(22)-enolide), uzarigenin (3β,14-dihydroxy-5α,14β-card-20(22)-enolide), epiuzarigenin (3α,14-dihydroxy-5α,14β-card-20(22)-enolide), sarmentogenin (3β,11α,14-trihydroxy-5β,14β-card-20(22)-enolide), digoxigenin (3β,12β,14-trihydroxy-5β,14β-card-20(22)-enolide), and gitozigenin (3β,14,16β-trihydroxy-5β, 14β-card-20(22)-enolide). In these, the only common hydroxyl groups were in the 3α or 3β and 14β positions. As the latter is a tertiary hydroxyl which would be expected to be rather unreactive, it seems probable that sulfation was occurring at position 3. On the other hand, strophanthidin (3β,5,14-trihydroxy-19-oxo-5β,14β-card-20(22)-enolide) was not sulfated, but this could reflect the rather different structure in the region of rings A and B, particularly the aldehyde function at position 10.

Once again structural considerations suggest that these cardenolides must be sulfated by a sulfotransferase distinct from those already considered. If this is so, it is difficult to visualize its physiological acceptor because cardenolides do not occur in mammals, although the conformationally similar bufadienolides are constituents of toad venoms. It is of interest that at least one of these, bufalin (3β,14-dihydroxy-5β, 14β-bufa-20,22-dienolide), exists as the 3-sulfate, and this has been isolated from the skin of *Bufo vulgaris formosus*.[135] It is possible that androstenolone sulfotransferase and etiocholanolone sulfotransferase might be the enzymes responsible for the sulfation of the corresponding cardenolides, but, if so, then the structural requirements of these enzymes with respect to rings C and D must be small indeed.

I. Sterol Sulfotransferase

The biles of lower vertebrates contain sterol sulfates[136] in which the sulfate group occurs in the side chain rather than in the nucleus of the steroid. Bridgewater and Ryan[137] showed that homogenates of the liver from the frog *Rana temporaria* could form such esters when incubated with the steroid, ATP, and SO_4^{2-}. The compounds shown to be acceptors were ranol ($3\alpha,7\alpha,12\alpha,24\xi,26$-pentahydroxy-$5\alpha$-27-norcholestane), scymnol ($3\alpha,7\alpha,12\alpha,24\xi,26,27$-hexahydroxy-$5\beta$-cholestane), $3\alpha,7\alpha,12\alpha,24$-tetrahydroxy-$5\beta$-cholane, and 24-hydroxy-5β-cholane, and so again both 5α and 5β steroids could be sulfated. With ranol, sulfation was shown to occur at position 24.

Enzyme preparations from the toad *Xenopus laevis* will catalyze similar reactions with PAPS as the sulfate donor.[138] The appropriate sulfotransferase, which could be separated from the accompanying alcohol sulfotransferase (see Section V), was activated by Mg^{2+} but unaffected by thiols. The two acceptors used were ranol and β-cyprinol ($3\alpha,7\alpha,12\alpha,26,27$-pentahydroxy-$5\beta$-cholestane): presumably, sulfation occurred at positions 24 and 26 or 27, respectively, but this was not shown. Again it seems possible that sterol sulfotransferase is a complex of enzymes because at last two types of hydroxyl group can be sulfated: the secondary hydroxyl group at position 24 in ranol and the primary hydroxyl group at position 27 in scymnol, cyprinol, and related compounds.[136]

Sterol sulfotransferase activity could not be detected in rat or chick liver.[138]

V. ALCOHOL SULFOTRANSFERASE

It has been known since the work of Vestermark and Boström[139] that the primary alcohols from methanol to pentan-1-ol (the latter being the highest member of the series tested) can be sulfated when incubated with the cytosol of rat liver together with ATP and SO_4^{2-}. The same reaction must occur in vivo because Boström and Vestermark[140] showed that these alkyl sulfates could be formed in rats dosed with the appropriate alcohols, but there is little to show that such a pathway is important in the metabolism of xenobiotics, at least in mammals. Known examples are the formation of small amounts of the sulfate ester of 1,2-propanediol 3-(4'-chlorophenoxy)-1-carbamate (chlorophenesin carbamate: a muscle relaxant) by rats[141] and of 2-sulfooxymethyl-1-methyl-5-nitroimidazole as a major metabolite of 1,2-dimethyl-5-nitroimidazole (dimetridazole: used in control of histomoniasis) in turkeys.[142] The formation of alkyl sulfates may be of greater importance in birds than in mammals because it has long been known that chick embryos contain propan-2-yl sulfate and other sulfate esters.[143]

The presumption is that a specific sulfotransferase, alcohol sulfotransferase, must be involved in the formation of alkyl sulfates from monohydric[139] or polyhydric[144] alcohols. Some of the latter can give disulfates. However, no attempts to purify the alcohol sulfotransferase of mammalian liver have been reported, and the possibility of its being identical with one or more of the steroid sulfotransferases, which also use alcoholic hydroxyl groups as acceptors, cannot be discounted. Indeed, as already pointed out (Section IVA), the three hydroxysteroid sulfotransferases of rat liver[176] can use a number of simple alcohols as acceptors. In general, the more hydrophobic the alcohol, the greater is its ability to act as an acceptor. With hydroxysteroid sulfotransferase I the values of K_m for dehydroepiandrosterone, ethanol, butan-1-ol and pentan-1-ol are 0.012, 42, 3, and 1.7 mM, respectively, while the corresponding values of V are 0.67, 0.049, 0.092, and 0.15 μmol.mg^{-1}.min^{-1}, respectively.[81a] The values for hydroxysteroid sulfotransferases II and III are similar. It may well be, therefore, that a specific alcohol sulfotransferase does not exist in mammalian tissues and that the activity assigned to it is simply a reflection of the activity of the steroid sulfotransferases.

There have been preliminary reports[138] of the purification of alcohol sulfotransferase from the liver of the toad *Xenopus laevis*, but these have done little other than clearly distinguish this enzyme from the sterol sulfotransferase which also occurs in this organ (see Section IVI). The alcohol sulfotransferase activity, with PAPS as sulfate donor, did not require added Mg^{2+} and was activated by thiols, a quite different pattern of behavior from sterol sulfotransferase. Again, the primary aliphatic alcohols up to pentan-1-ol were sulfated, and the latter was apparently the most efficient acceptor. No other information was given about its specificity.

Alcohol sulfotransferase activity, like that of most sulfotransferases, is low in extracts of rat and guinea-pig fetal livers: it is present in the livers of chick embryos and reaches a peak of about five to ten times the adult values just before hatching, after which the adult level is reached within 3 days.[110]

The ability of liver extracts to sulfate compounds such as ethanol and propane-1,2-diol[11] must be kept in mind when these are used as solvents for the addition of, say, steroids to reaction mixtures. Circumstances could arise where these might compete with the added acceptor for the available PAPS and so cause erroneous results. Although in some cases it has been shown[106] that these solvents have no effect on the activity of partially purified steroid sulfotransferases, there are reports of unexplained effects on the conjugation of progesterone metabolites by unfractionated liver preparations.[145]

The sulfation of the oligomers of Triton® X-100 by crude sulfotransferases from a number of mammalian organs[13] must also be recalled here because it is possible that it is an alcohol sulfotransferase which is involved in this reaction (see also Section IIA).

VI. ASCORBATE SULFOTRANSFERASE

Ascorbate 2-sulfate is known to be of widespread occurrence, but there is little information on its biosynthesis. It has been shown to be formed by the transfer of sulfate from PAPS to ascorbate in a reaction catalyzed by a sulfotransferase in rat liver and colon.[146] No information is available on the enzyme or on its relation to other sulfotransferases. It should be noted that the pK values of ascorbic acid are 4.1 and 11.8, and it has a certain phenolic character, therefore it could conceivably be an acceptor for phenol sulfotransferase. Perhaps pertinent is the fact that ascorbate 2-sulfate is rapidly hydrolyzed by sulfatase A, an arylsulfatase.[147]

VII. CALCIFEROL SULFOTRANSFERASE

There have been sporadic reports of the occurrence of vitamin D sulfate in milk[148] and urine,[149] although the characterization of the compound was not convincing. Higaki et al.[150] have claimed that homogenates of rat liver formed calciferyl sulfate when incubated with calciferol, ATP, and SO_4^{2-}, but again the evidence was not convincing. Traces of activity were claimed to occur in other rat tissues.[151] Very little information was given so that speculation on the nature of the presumed sulfotransferase is pointless, but it should be noted that the partially purified androstenolone sulfotransferase of rat liver[22] cannot use calciferol as an acceptor.

VIII. LUCIFERIN SULFOTRANSFERASE

This enzyme has been most studied in the Sea Pansy, *Renilla reniformis* (an anthazoon), but it occurs in those other coelenterates in which luciferin is the substrate for the bioluminescence reaction.[152] Partially purified extracts of *Renilla* could bring about the formation of luciferin sulfate from luciferin and PAPS,[153] but they could not use 4-nitrophenol as an acceptor.

The role of luciferin sulfotransferase in vivo, unlike that of all the other sulfotransferases so far known, appears to be the catalysis of what would normally be considered the reverse reaction, that between luciferin sulfate and adenosine 3′, 5′-bisphosphate to give luciferin and presumably PAPS, although the latter has not been detected in the reaction mixtures.[153] The K_m for adenosine 3′,5′-bisphosphate is very low, about 70 pM. Luciferin sulfate is the sulfate ester of the enolic form of an oxoimidazopyrazine[154] which would be expected to have a rather high sulfate potential, and it in fact has a lability to acid very similar to that of PAPS.[153] The ease with which the reverse of the usual sulfotransferase reaction occurs is therefore not surprising.

It appears that luciferin sulfate is the storage form of the relatively unstable luciferin[152] and, if this is the case, then the question of the way in which luciferin sulfate is synthesized is a most interesting one. It is unusual for a single enzyme to be involved in both the synthesis and breakdown of a metabolite which suggests that a second luciferin sulfotransferase may exist. The details of the control of the luciferin — luciferin sulfate equilibrium — will be most interesting.

Luciferin sulfotransferase also differs from the other sulfotransferases considered in this chapter because it, and the associated light-producing system, are localized not in the cytosol but in specific intracellular structures, the lumisomes.[155]

The great ease with which luciferin sulfotransferase catalyzes the reaction between luciferin sulfate and adenosine 3′,5′-bisphosphate to give luciferin, which can readily be determined through its reaction with the luciferase system to produce light, has provided a useful means of determining adenosine 3′,5′-bisphosphate and, less directly, PAPS.[156] As little as 10 pmol of adenosine 3′,5′-bisphosphate can easily be measured.

IX. *N*-HYDROXYARYLAMINE SULFOTRANSFERASE

This sulfotransferase is of great interest because it catalyzes the formation of hydroxylamine derivatives containing the grouping $>$N.OSO$_3^-$. These are highly reactive compounds[157] which in many cases cannot be isolated but detected only by their reactions with other compounds (see Chapter 2, Section IIB2; this chapter, Section IIC; and Chapter 8) Much of the interest in these hydroxylamine derivatives stems from their role in carcinogenesis, first clearly shown for the sulfate of *N*-acetyl-*N*-hydroxy-2-aminofluorene.[158,159]

DeBaun et al.[38] showed that the cytosol of rat liver contained a sulfotransferase which could utilize PAPS for the synthesis of the sulfate ester of *N*-acetyl-*N*-hydroxy-2-amino-fluorene. This sulfotransferase was stimulated somewhat by Mg^{2+} or Mn^{2+}, had an optimum pH of 6.5 to 6.7, and could use any of several *N*-acetyl-*N*-hydroxyarylamines as acceptors.[38,40] Other acceptors which have been investigated in detail are *N*-hydroxy-*N*-methyl-4-aminoazobenzene,[38] *N*-hydroxyphenacetin,[45] and 3-hydroxyxanthine.[78] It has not been established that the one enzyme sulfates all these compounds, and it is possible that a number of more specific enzymes is involved, although this seems improbable. For example, it has been suggested that separate sulfotransferases are involved in the sulfation of *N*-acetyl-*N*-hydroxy-2-aminofluorene and *N*-acetyl-*N*-methyl-4-aminoazobenzene,[38] but the evidence is not convincing.

The sulfotransferase using *N*-hydroxy-*N*-acetyl-2-aminofluorene has been considerably purified from male rat liver:[39] the final preparation had a specific activity of 2.0 μmol.mg^{-1}.min^{-1} with the above acceptor and 0.34 μmol.mg^{-1}.min^{-1} with 4-nitrophenol. The latter specific activity is slightly greater than those of the two specific phenol sulfotransferases of rat liver[49] (see Section IIIB) which are devoid of *N*-hydroxyarylamine sulfotransferase activity. During the preparation three incompletely resolved peaks of activity were obtained during chromatography on DEAE-cellulose: all three were taken together for the remainder of the preparation, and rechromatography, under identical conditions, at the final stage gave only a single peak of sulfotransferase activity. This suggests that the multiple peaks were not caused by aggregation but perhaps by the association of a single *N*-hydroxyarylamine sulfotransferase with other proteins or even with other sulfotransferases because the phenol sulfotransferase activity showed similar multiple peaks in the early stages of the preparation. Its behavior in the later stages was not commented upon. Gel electrophoresis of the most highly purified preparation showed that the *N*-hydroxyarylamine sulfotransferase activity was associated with the major protein band, although several other proteins were undoubtedly present.

The *N*-hydroxyarylamine and phenol sulfotransferase activities were closely associated throughout the preparations, but at the final stage neither estrone, dehydroepiandrosterone, testosterone, nor corticosterone were acceptors while serotonin and L-tyrosine methyl ester were very poorly sulfated. Despite the close association of the *N*-hydroxyarylamine and phenol sulfotransferase activities during the purification of the former, it was concluded[39] that these were due to two different enzymes which would agree with the findings of Sekura and Jakoby[49] with the phenol sulfotransferases, sulfotransferases I and II, of rat liver (see Table 3). On the other hand, Jakoby[81a] has since isolated from rat liver a second pair of phenol sulfotransferases which will sulfate hydroxylamine derivatives. However, these enzymes, unlike that of Wu and Straub,[39] will also use tyrosine methyl ester as acceptor. Once again, further investigations are required.

In its general properties the *N*-hydroxyarylamine sulfotransferase of rat liver resembled the other sulfotransferases from mammalian livers: its molecular weight was 68,000, made up of two similar subunits; its $s^{\circ}_{20,w}$ was 4.4 S and its isoelectric point was 5.7. Its pH optimum was 6.3, it was marginally activated by Mg^{2+} but inhibited by other divalent cations, and it was stabilized by thiols and inhibited by thiol reagents, particularly by *N*-ethylmaleimide or 4-chloromercuribenzoate. There have been suggestions[27] that *N*-hydroxyarylamine sulfotransferase undergoes changes on storage, analogous to those undergone by phenol sulfotransferase,[48] through oxidation of the enzyme.

Apart from the determination of the pH optima, all of which lie in the region of 6.3 to 7.0, scarcely any kinetic studies have been made. A figure of 0.25 m*M* has been quoted for the K_m of *N*-hydroxyphenacetin,[45] but this figure is difficult to interpret because of the method of assay which involved the transfer of sulfate from 4-nitrophenyl sulfate to the acceptor.

One of the most interesting features of *N*-hydroxyarylamine sulfotransferase is its distribution: some values for the livers of different species are given in Table 7. With *N*-acetyl-*N*-hydroxy-2-aminofluorene as acceptor by far the highest activity is found in the liver of the male rat,[38,39] and this correlates with the very high carcinogenicity of the acceptor in this animal, as well as providing further evidence for the separate identity of *N*-hydroxyarylamine and phenol sulfotransferases because the latter activity is not much lower in female than in male rat liver (see Section IIIE). Other tissues in the male rat showed only very low activities.[38] Although the results with *N*-hydroxy-*N*-methyl-4-aminoazobenzene are not as striking, they again correlate with the hepatocarcinogenicity of this compound in the male rat.[38] Only with 3-hydroxyxanthine have studies been made of the development of *N*-hydroxyarylamine sulfotransferase activity.[77] In the rat, the sulfotransferase activity could be detected, at about 25% of the adult level, in fetal livers at 21 days gestation, and after birth the activity slowly increased to adult levels which were reached at an age of about 6 weeks. In the mouse also the fetal *N*-hydroxyarylamine sulfotransferase activity was low.[77]

Table 7

THE SULFATION OF SOME N-HYDROXYARYLAMINES BY EXTRACTS OF THE LIVERS OF VARIOUS SPECIES

Species	AAF nmol. min^{-1}		MAB nmol.min.$^{-1}$.mg^{-1}		HOX nmol.min^{-1}.mg^{-1}	
	Male	Female	Male	Female	Male	Female
Rat	2.9	0.50	3.6	1.1	1.1	0.81 (0.99[a])
Rabbit	0.25	—	1.9	—	—	—
Mouse	0.06	—	1.1	—	—	1.1[a]
Hamster	0.06	—	0.2	—	—	—
Guinea pig	0.04	—	1.9	—	—	—

Note: The data for N-hydroxy-N-acetyl-2-aminofluorene (AAF), N-hydroxy-N-methyl-4-aminoazobenzene (MAB), and 3-hydroxyxanthine (HOX) are from References 38, 40, and 78, respectively. For the latter two compounds the rates are referred to the amount of protein in the assay, but for the first it is referred to an arbitrary volume of liver extract so that it is not directly comparable to the others.

[a]Pregnant animals.

X. ARYLAMINE SULFOTRANSFERASE

The existence of an arylamine sulfotransferase was first shown by Roy[160] who demonstrated that such an enzyme in the cytosol of rat liver could use aniline or 1- and 2-naphthylamine, but not benzylamine, as acceptors for the sulfate of PAPS. With 2-naphthylamine the product was 2-naphthyl sulfamate[161] which had recently been shown to be a metabolite of 2-naphthylamine in the rat.[162] One of the most striking features of the arylamine sulfotransferase activity was the modification of its behavior by 17-oxosteroids: 50 μM dehydroepiandrosterone, for example, activated the arylamine sulfotransferase of rat liver some twofold, whereas it inhibited the enzyme from guinea-pig liver by some 90%. Quite detailed kinetic studies of these effects were made,[163,164] and a common explanation of both the activation and the inhibition was given in terms of partially competitive relationships between the steroid and 2-naphthylamine: these would allow either activation or inhibition depending upon the magnitudes of the dissociation constants of the various enzyme complexes. An explanation in terms of allosteric effects is also possible[165] and particularly pertinent with the guinea-pig enzyme which gives sigmoidal substrate curves.[163] Whatever the detailed interpretation of these effects, it is clear that the arylamine sulfotransferases had high affinities for 17-oxosteroids, the apparent values of the K_i for 3β-methoxyandrost-5-en-17-one being 1.5 and 0.2 μM for the rat and guinea-pig enzymes, respectively.

Unfortunately, later studies[28] of the guinea-pig liver sulfotransferases have complicated the situation because two peaks of arylamine sulfotransferase activity were found during chromatography on DEAE-Sephadex. One of these was associated with estrone sulfotransferase and the other with androstenolone sulfotransferase. Moreover, it appeared that the arylamine sulfotransferase activities were intrinsic to these steroid sulfotransferases. The two arylamine sulfotransferases had very similar properties: the pH optima were 6.5 and 7.8 in the estrone and androstenolone sulfotransferase fractions, respectively, both required 2 mM Mg^{2+} to show their full activity, and both were inhibited by about 50% by 2 μM 3β-methoxyandrost-5-en-17-one which had no effect on the associated steroid sulfotransferase activities.[28] More recently, preparations of these steroid sulfotransferases from other sources have been obtained[15,22,87] which do not show arylamine sulfotransferase activity so that their association in the guinea pig may be due only to rather powerful interaction between the different sulfotransferases.

It is obvious that the arylamine sulfotransferases have some interesting properties, particularly their sensitivity to 17-oxosteroids, but once again any further development must wait their preparation in a more highly purified form because only then can their relationships with other sulfotransferases be established.

The distribution of arylamine sulfotransferase has not been studied. Apart from its occurrence in mammalian liver, it has been detected in sheep intestinal mucosa[166] and in chick embryo,[110] but studies of the metabolism of xenobiotics suggest that it has a much wider distribution than that indicated by those few results.[8] Despite this, sulfamate formation does not seem to be a particularly important metabolic pathway in mammals, and few examples are known. One is the formation of the N^4-sulfamate of 4-amino-5-chloro-N-(2-(diethylamino)ethyl)-2-methoxy-benzamide (metoclopramide: an antiemetic) in the rabbit,[167] and another is the formation of the sulfamates of certain sulfonamides, such as the N^4-sulfamate of sulfathiazole, in man.[168]

In the rat the arylamine sulfotransferase activity of female liver is about double that of the male.[160] No such sex difference exists in the guinea pig.[160] An interesting point is that while guinea-pig liver has a much greater arylamine sulfotransferase activity than has rat liver,[160] the formation of 2-naphthyl sulfamate as a metabolite of 2-naphthylamine is much more important in the latter species.[162] This could reflect either the different steroid effects in the two species—activation in the rat, inhibition in the guinea pig—or the possibility that the liver is not necessarily the most important organ for the conjugation of xenobiotics.[169]

XI. VITAMIN A AND THE SULFOTRANSFERASES

There have been numerous reports of vitamin A having an influence on sulfate metabolism.[60] Most of the studies have been made in vivo and have been concerned more with the activation of sulfate (Chapter 4, Section VIA) than with the sulfotransferases, but there has been some investigation of the latter. Subba Rao and Ganguly[170] showed that the activity of phenol sulfotransferase was low, about 60% of normal, in extracts of the livers of rats deficient in vitamin A, and the addition of retinoic acid (5 μg/ml; about 1.6 μM) in vitro restored the activity to normal. Retinol in the same concentration had a lesser effect. Similar claims were made by Carroll and Spencer[76] who reported that several types of sulfotransferase activity in the cytosol of fetal rat liver were stimulated by the addition, in vitro, of retinoic acid (0.25 μg/ml or retinol (0.8 μg/ml). This led them to suggest that the low sulfotransferase activity in fetal rat liver was not caused by a lack of the enzyme itself but rather of an essential "vitamin A" cofactor.[76] Subsequently, Carroll[56] reported that attempts to repeat this work were unsuccessful, provided that the conditions were such that the vitamin A was stable, and suggested that the earlier results were caused by peroxides of vitamin A oxidatively destroying an inhibitor present in the crude preparations of the sulfotransferases which were used.

There is therefore, little evidence for the view that vitamin A can activate sulfotransferases in vitro, and indeed Adams and Ellyard[92] clearly showed that 0.1 mM retinoic acid, like certain fatty acids (see Section IVB4), was an inhibitor of estrone sulfotransferase. This is not to say that a deficiency of vitamin A does not affect the levels of the sulfotransferases in an animal: it may do so.[170,171] However, this need not necessarily be due directly to a deficiency of vitamin A but to other effects thereof, such as an induced protein deficiency, as is the case with the effect of a deficiency of vitamin A on the level of ATP sulfurylase in animals.[172,173]

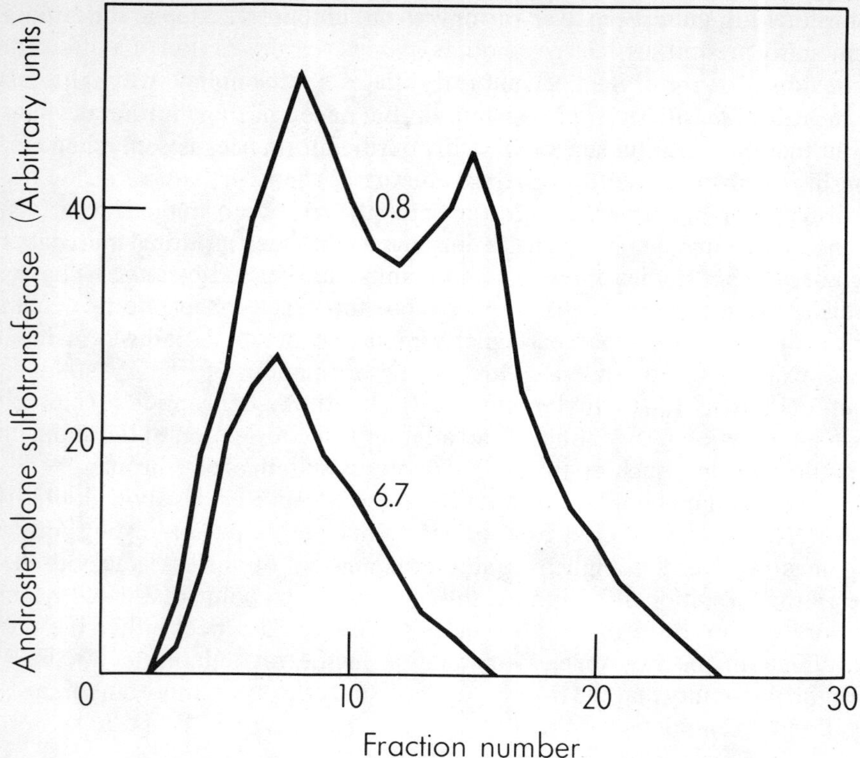

FIGURE 3.   The effect of estrone sulfotransferase on the elution of androstenolone sulfotransferase from a column of DEAE-Sephadex under the conditions specified in Reference 28. The ratios of androstenolone sulfotransferase to estrone sulfotransferase were 0.8 in the upper curve and 6.7 in the lower curve, as indicated on the figure.

XII. SOME GENERAL COMMENTS

Although there is now available a large amount of information on the sulfotransferases, much of it obtained only within the last few years, it should be obvious from the previous sections that there is still much which is not understood about them.

One of the most fundamental problems is that of knowing how many sulfotransferases exist in animal tissues, and this in turn depends finally upon the separation of the different sulfotransferase activities. There have been many indications of quite strong associations between different types of sulfotransferase activity: for example, phenol and arylamine sulfotransferases with estrone and androstenolone sulfotransferases;[28] phenol sulfotransferase with androstenolone sulfotransferase;[48] and phenol sulfotransferase with N-hydroxyarylamine sulfotransferase.[39] Although it is not impossible that these associations are only apparent and simply reflect multiple specificities of the sulfotransferases, a more likely explanation is that they show the existence of protein-protein interactions between specific enzymes. Evidence for such an interaction between estrone and androstenolone sulfotransferase activities has been obtained.[174] Figure 3 shows how the elution pattern of the androstenolone sulfotransferase of guinea-pig liver varies with the amount of estrone sulfotransferase simultaneously present: with large amounts of the latter the elution of androstenolone sulfotransferase is retarded. Reciprocal effects were noted with the estrone sulfotransferase activity. Further examples can be seen in the appropriate figures of References 28 and 113. This suggested that the two sulfotransferases interacted in some way, and as they were inseparable by chromatography on Sephadex G-200, any such interaction must have occurred without change in molecular weight. The only simple way in which this could arise would be through a disulfide exchange as in Equation 6 where And.S– and Oes.S– represent protein units showing androstenolone and estrone sulfotransferase activities, respectively. Obviously such a scheme could account

$$\text{And.S–S.And} + \text{Oes.S–S.Oes} \rightleftharpoons 2 \text{ And.S–S.Oes} \tag{6}$$

for the association of the different sulfotransferase activities to an extent varying with their individual concentrations, and also for changes in the association by the addition of thiols. Further evidence for the existence of such interactions was obtained by prolonged treatment of a mixture of estrone and androstenolone sulfotransferases with $0.05\ M\ SO_3^{2-}$ under aerobic conditions. Such treatment causes fission of disulfide bonds to thiols and thiosulfate esters (see Chapter 2, Section III): the former, under aerobic conditions, are oxidized to the disulfide which can again undergo sulfitolysis so that the fission of the disulfide eventually goes to completion (Scheme 7). Chromatography of

$$\text{R.S–S.R} + \text{HSO}_3^- \rightleftharpoons \text{R.SH} + \text{R.SSO}_3^- \tag{7}$$

such sulfite-treated mixtures of estrone and androstenolone sulfotransferases showed that the elution patterns did not vary with the relative proportions of the two enzymes, as would be expected from Scheme 7. These results, therefore, provide some evidence for an interaction between estrone and androstenolone sulfotransferases, but much further work is needed to clarify the situation.

Obviously related to the above problem is that of the specificities of the different sulfotransferases. This cannot be solved until better separation techniques are available and, if disulfide exchange can indeed cause complications, then attempts to isolate the enzymes in the form of their S-sulfonates might be useful. These should be relatively stable and less likely to interact: certainly they retain their enzymic activities. Their use might also provide further information about the relationships between thiol groups and specificities which have already been noted.

Another point of interest which has hardly been investigated is the role of Mg^{2+} in the sulfotransferase reactions. Many, but not all, of these are activated by Mg^{2+}, or by other similar ions, but in no case can it be said that such ions are essential for enzymic activity, and certainly there is no indication of any role they may play. Unfortunately there appears to be no information about the binding of Mg^{2+} to PAPS. Some years ago a value of 24 $l.\text{mol}^{-1}$ was given [175] for the apparent association constant of adenosine 5′-sulfatophosphate and Mg^{2+}: this is a very low value compared with that, say, for the reaction between ATP and Mg^{2+}. It would appear that before the role of Mg^{2+} in the sulfotransferase reaction can be usefully studied, its reaction with PAPS must be clarified.

REFERENCES

1. **Gregory, J. D. and Lipmann, F.**, The transfer of sulfate among phenolic compounds with 3', 5'-diphosphoadenosine as coenzyme, *J. Biol. Chem.*, 229, 1081, 1957.
2. **Schiff, J. A.**, Pathways of assimilatory sulfate reduction in plants and microorganisms, *Ciba Symp.*, 72, 49, 1980.
3. **Robinson, H. C.**, The reduction of inorganic sulphate to inorganic sulphite in the small intestine of the rat, *Biochem. J.*, 94, 687, 1965.
4. **Noir, B. A. and Nanet, H.**, A study of the ethyl anthranilate azo derivatives of bilirubin sulphate. Confirmation of the existence of bilirubin sulphate conjugates in bile, *Biochim. Biophys. Acta*, 372, 230, 1974.
5. **Butenandt, A., Biekert, E., Koga, N., and Traub, P.**, Uber ommochrome. XXI. Konstitution und Synthese des Ommatins D, *Z. Physiol. Chem.*, 321, 258, 1960.
6. **Boyer, G. L., Schantz, E. J., and Schnoes, K.**, Characterization of 11-hydroxysaxitoxin sulphate, a major toxin in scallops exposed to blooms of the poisonous dinoflagellate *Gonyaulax tamerensis*, *Chem. Commun.*, 889, 1978.
7. **Jutzi, H., Siegrist, H. P., Burkart, T., Wiesmann, U., and Herschkowitz, N.N.**, Diminished cerebroside-sulphotransferase activity in the Jimpy mouse mutant due to altered lipid composition in microsomal membranes, *Biochim. Biophys. Acta*, 552, 413, 1979.
8. **Smith, J. N.**, The comparative metabolism of xenobiotics, in *Comparative Biochemistry and Physiology III*, Lowenstein, O., Ed., Academic Press, New York, 1968, 172.
9. **Singer, S. S.**, Enzymatic sulfation of steroids. VI. A simple, rapid method for the routine enzymatic preparation of 3'-phosphoadenosine 5'-phosphosulfate, *Anal. Biochem.*, 96, 34, 1979.
10. **Dodgson, K. S. and Rose, F. A.**, Sulfohydrolases, in *Metabolic Pathways*, Vol. 7, 3rd ed., Greenberg, D. M. Ed., Academic Press, New York, 1975, 409.
11. **Spencer, B.**, Endogenous sulphate acceptors in rat liver, *Biochem. J.*, 77, 294, 1960.
12. **Adams, J. B.**, Enzymic synthesis of steroid sulphates. V. On the binding of estrogens to estrogen sulfotransferase, *Biochim. Biophys. Acta*, 146, 522, 1967.
13. **Spolter, L. and Rice, L. I.**, Enzymatic sulfation of Triton® X-100, *Biochim. Biophys. Acta*, 612, 268, 1980.
14. **Wengle, B.**, Studies on ester sulphates 16. Use of ^{35}S-labelled inorganic sulphate for quantitative studies of sulphate conjugation in liver extracts, *Acta Chem. Scand.*, 18, 65, 1964.
15. **Adams, J. B. and Poulos, A.**, Enzymic synthesis of steroid sulphates. III. Isolation and properties of estrogen sulphotransferase of bovine adrenal glands, *Biochim. Biophys. Acta*, 146, 493, 1967.
16. **Mattock, P. and Jones, J. G.**, Partial purification and properties of an enzyme from rat liver that catalyses the sulphation of L-tyrosyl derivatives, *Biochem. J.*, 116, 797, 1970.
17. **Borchardt, R. T. and Schasteen, C. S.**, Phenolsulfotransferase inactivation by 2, 3-butanedione and phenylglyoxal: evidence for an active site arginyl residue, *Biochem. Biophys. Res. Commun.*, 78, 1067, 1977.
18. **Davis, D. C.**, Radioisotopic assay for rat liver sulfotransferase activity, *Biochem. Pharmacol.*, 24, 975, 1975.
19. **Foldes, A. and Meek, J. L.**, Rat brain phenolsulfotransferase-partial purification and some properties, *Biochim. Biophys. Acta*, 327, 365, 1973.
20. **Chen, L.-J., Imperato, T. J., and Bolt, R. J.**, Enzymatic sulfation of bile salts. II. Studies on bile salt sulfotransferase activity from rat kidney, *Biochim. Biophys. Acta*, 522, 443, 1978.
21. **Sekura, R. D., Marcus, C. J., Lyon, E. S., and Jakoby, W. B.**, Assay of sulfotransferases, *Anal. Biochem.*, 95, 82, 1979.
22. **Ryan, R. A. and Carroll, J.**, Studies on a 3β-hydroxysteroid sulphotransferase from rat liver, *Biochim. Biophys. Acta*, 429, 391, 1976.
23. **Chen, L.-J., Bolt, R. J., and Admirand, W. H.**, Enzymatic sulfation of bile salts. Partial purification and characterisation of an enzyme from rat liver that catalyses the sulfation of bile salts, *Biochim. Biophys. Acta*, 480, 219, 1977.
24. **Hidaka, H. and Austin, J.**, Occurrence and distribution of serotonin *O*-sulfotransferase in human brain; a new radioisotopic assay, *Biochim. Biophys. Acta*, 268, 132, 1972.
25. **Rozhin, J., Soderstrom, R. L., and Brooks, S. C.**, Specificity studies on bovine adrenal estrogen sulfotransferase, *J. Biol. Chem.*, 249, 2079, 1974.
26. **Lööf, L. and Wengle, B.**, Enzymatic sulphation of bile salts in human liver, *Biochim. Biophys. Acta*, 530, 451, 1978.
27. **McDonald, J. J., Stöhrer, G., and Brown, G. B.**, Oncogenic purine *N*-oxide derivatives as substrates for sulfotransferase, *Cancer Res.*, 33, 3319, 1973.
28. **Banerjee, R. K. and Roy, A. B.**, The sulfotransferases of guinea pig liver, *Mol. Pharmacol.*, 2, 56, 1966.

29. **Banerjee, R. K. and Roy, A. B.**, Kinetic studies of the phenol sulphotransferase reaction, *Biochim. Biophys. Acta,* 151, 573, 1968.

30. **Yang, R. S. H. and Wilkinson, C. F.**, Sulphotransferases and phosphotransferases in insects, *Comp. Biochem. Physiol.,* 46B, 717, 1973.

31. **Roy, A. B.**, Die wirkung der Arylsulfatasen A und B auf Cholesterinsulfat, *Z. Physiol. Chem.,* 333, 166, 1963.

32. **Bernstein, S. and McGilvery, R. W.**, The enzymatic conjugation of *m*-aminophenol, *J. Biol. Chem.,* 198, 195, 1952.

33. **De Meio, R. H.**, Sintesis del *p*-nitrofenilsulfato por el higado de rata, *Acta Physiol. Lat. Am.,* 2, 251, 1952.

34. **Robbins, P. W. and Lipmann, F.**, Isolation and identification of active sulfate, *J. Biol. Chem.,* 229, 837, 1957.

35. **Hidaka, H., Nagatsu, T., and Yagi, K.**, A rapid and simple assay of serotonin sulfokinase activity, *Anal. Biochem.,* 19, 388, 1967.

36. **Van Kempen, G. M. J. and Jansen, G. S. I. M.**, Quantitative determination of phenosulfotransferase using 4-methylumbelliferone, *Anal. Biochem.,* 46, 438, 1972.

37. **Wong, K. P.**, A new method for measuring sulfotransferase, *Anal. Biochem.,* 62, 149, 1974.

38. **DeBaun, J. R., Miller, E. C., and Miller, J. A.**, *N*-Hydroxy-2-acetylaminofluorene sulfotransferase: its probable role in carcinogenesis and in protein-(methion-*S*-yl) binding in rat liver, *Cancer Res.,* 30, 577, 1970.

39. **Wu, S.-C. G. and Straub, K. D.**, Purification and characterization of *N*-hydroxy-2-acetylaminofluorene sulfotransferase from rat liver, *J. Biol. Chem.,* 251, 6529, 1976.

40. **Kadlubar, F. F., Miller, J. A., and Miller, E. C.**, Hepatic metabolism of *N*-hydroxy-*N*-methyl-4-aminoazobenzene and other *N*-hydroxy arylamines to reactivate sulfuric acid esters, *Cancer. Res.,* 36, 2350, 1976.

41. **Gugler, R., Rao, G. S., and Breuer, H.**, Reinigung und Charakterisierung einer 3′-Phosphoadenylylsulfat: Steroid-Sulfotransferase aus der Leber des Menschen, *Biochim. Biophys. Acta,* 220, 69, 1970.

42. **Rozhin, J., Huo, A., Zemlička, J., and Brooks, S. C.**, Studies on bovine adrenal estrogen sulfotransferase. Inhibition and possible involvement of adenine-estrogen stacking, *J. Biol. Chem.,* 252, 7214, 1977.

43. **Segal, H. L. and Mologne, L. A.**, Enzymatic sulfurylation of tyrosine derivatives, *J. Biol. Chem.,* 234, 909, 1959.

44. **Meek, J. L. and Neff, N. H.**, Biogenic amines and their metabolites as substrates for phenol sulphotransferase (EC 2.8.2.1) of brain and liver, *J. Neurochem.,* 21, 1, 1973.

45. **Mulder, G. J., Hinson, J. A., and Gillette, J. R.**, Generation of reactive metabolites of *N*-hydroxy-phenacetin by glucuronidation and sulfation, *Biochem. Pharmacol.,* 26, 189, 1977.

46. **Wortman, B.**, Enzymic sulfation of corneal mucopolysaccharides by beef cornea epithelial extract, *J. Biol. Chem.,* 236, 974, 1961.

47. **Bernstein, S. and McGilvery, R. W.**, Substrate activation in the synthesis of phenyl sulfate, *J. Biol. Chem.,* 199, 745, 1952.

48. **Barfold, D. J. and Jones, J. G.**, Thiol-dependent changes in the properties of rat liver sulphotransferases, *Biochem. J.,* 123, 427, 1971.

49. **Sekura, R. D. and Jakoby, W. B.**, Phenol sulfotransferases, *J. Biol. Chem.,* 254, 5658, 1979.

50. **Williams, R. T.**, Detox*ication Mechanisms,* Chapman and Hall, London, 1959.

51. **Van Kempen, G. M. J., Wolters, W. L., and Van Elk, R.**, Distribution of 3-methoxy-4-hydroxyphenylethyleneglycol sulphotransferase in brain fractions, *J. Neurochem.,* 24, 825, 1975.

52. **Pennings, E. J. M., Vrielink, R., Wolters, R. L., and Van Kempen, G. M. J.**, Inhibition of rat brain phenol sulphotransferase *in vitro* by noradrenaline and dopamine metabolites, *J. Neurochem.,* 27, 915, 1976.

53. **Jenner, W. N. and Rose, F. A.**, Studies on the sulphation of 3,4-dihydroxyphenylethylamine (dopamine) and related compounds by rat tissues, *Biochem. J.,* 135, 109, 1973.

54. **McEvoy, F. A. and Carroll, J.**, Purification from rat liver of an enzyme that catalyses the sulphurylation of phenols, *Biochem. J.,* 123, 901, 1971.

55. **Armstrong, L. M. and Carroll, J.**, Properties of a sulphotransferase from bovine kidney, *Biochem. Soc. Trans.,* 2, 743, 1974.

56. **Carroll, J.**, Phenolsulfotransferase in the developing rat, *Am. J. Clin. Nutr.,* 22, 978, 1969.

57. **Mattock, P., Barford, D. J., Basford, J. M., and Jones, J. G.**, The effect of substrate concentration and pH on the enzymic sulfation of L-tyrosyl derivatives, *Biochem. J.,* 116, 805, 1970.

58. **Dodgson, K. S.**, Conjugation with sulphate, in *Drug Metabolism—from Microbe to Man,* Parke, D. V. and Smith, R. L. Eds., Taylor and Francis, London, 1977, 91.

59. **Nemoto, N., Takayama, S., and Gelboin, H. V.**, Sulphate conjugation of benzo[*a*]pyrene metabolites and derivatives, *Chem. Biol. Interact.,* 23, 19, 1978.

60. **Roy, A. B. and Trudinger, P. A.,** *The Biochemistry of Inorganic Compounds of Sulphur,* Cambridge University Press, Cambridge, 1970.
61. **Barford, D. J. and Jones, J. G.,** The physiological role of L-tyrosine methyl ester sulphotransferase, *Biochem. J.,* 125, 76P, 1971.
62. **Vestermark, A. and Boström, H.,** On the sulphurylation of mono-, di-, and trihydric phenols, *Experientia,* 16, 408, 1960.
63. **Pennings, E. J. M., Vrielink, R., and Van Kempen, G. M. J.,** Kinetics and mechanism of the rat brain phenol sulphotransferase reaction, *Biochem. J.,* 173, 299, 1978.
64. **Borchardt, R. T., Wu, S. E., and Schasteen, C. S.,** Adenosine 5'-diphosphate dialdehyde: an affinity labelling reagent for phenol-sulfotransferase, *Biochem. Biophys. Res. Commun.,* 81, 841, 1978.
65. **Mulder, G. J. and Scholtens, E.,** Phenol sulphotransferase and uridine diphosphate glucuronyltransferase from rat liver *in vivo* and *in vitro.* 2,6-Dichloro-4-nitrophenol as selective inhibitor of sulphation, *Biochem. J.,* 165, 533, 1977.
66. **Pennings, E. J. M., Vrielink, R., and Van Kempen, G. M. J.,** Anomalous effect of probenecid on rat brain phenolsulphotransferase, *Biochem. Pharmacol.,* 25, 1687, 1976.
67. **Hart, R. F., Renskers, K. J., Nelson, E. B., and Roth, J. A.,** Localization and characterization of phenol sulfotransferase in human platelets, *Life Sci.,* 24, 125, 1979.
68. **Yang, R. S. H. and Wilkinson, C. F.,** Enzymic sulphation of *p*-nitrophenol and steroids by larval gut tissues of the Southern Armyworm (*Prodenia eridania* Cramer), *Biochem. J.,* 130, 487, 1972.
69. **Elmamlouk, T. H. and Gessner, T.,** Carbohydrate and sulfate conjugations of *p*-nitrophenol by hepatopancreas of *Homarus americanus, Comp. Biochem. Physiol,* 61C, 363, 1978.
70. **Kennedy, M. B.,** Products of biogenic amine metabolism in the lobster: sulfate conjugates, *J. Neurochem.,* 30, 315, 1978.
71. **Baker, J. T.,** Tyrian purple: an ancient dye, a modern problem, *Endeavour,* 33, 11, 1974.
72. **Foldes, A. and Meek, J. L.,** Occurrence and localisation of brain phenolsulphotransferase, *J. Neurochem.,* 23, 303, 1974.
73. **Boström, H. and Wengle, B.,** Studies on ester sulphates. 23. Distribution of phenol and steroid sulphokinase in adult human tissues, *Acta Endocrinol.,* 56, 691, 1967.
74. **Wengle, B.,** Distribution of some steroid sulphokinases in foetal human tissues, *Acta Endocrinol.,* 52, 607, 1966.
75. **Jansen, G. S. I. M., Vrensen, G. F. J. M., and Van Kempen, G. M. J.,** Intracellular localisation of phenol sulphotransferase in rat brain, *J. Neurochem.,* 23, 329, 1974.
76. **Carroll, J. and Spencer, B.,** Vitamin A and sulphotransferases in foetal rat liver, *Biochem. J.,* 96, 79P, 1965.
77. **Wengle, B.,** Studies on ester sulphates. 17. Sulphate conjugation in extracts of foetal and juvenile rat liver. *Acta Soc. Med. Ups.,* 68, 154, 1963.
78. **Anderson, L. M., McDonald, J. J., Budinger, J. M., Mountain, I. M., and Brown, G. B.,** 3-Hydroxyxanthine: transplacental effects and ontogeny of related sulfate metabolism in rats and mice, *J. Nat. Cancer Inst.,* 61, 1405, 1978.
79. **Jansen, G. S. I. M., Van Elk, R., and Van Kempen, G. M. J.,** Developmental patterns of sulfate activation and phenolsulphotransferase in rat brain, *J. Neurochem.,* 20, 9, 1973.
80. **Percy, A. K. and Yaffe, S. J.,** Sulfate metabolism during mammalian development, *Pediatrics,* 33, 965, 1964.
81. **Carroll, J. and Armstrong, L. M.,** Regulation of hepatic sulphotransferases, *Biochem. Soc. Trans.,* 4, 871, 1976.
81a. **Jakoby, W. B., Sekura, R. D., Lyon, E. S., Marcus, C. J., and Wang, J.-L.,** Sulfotransferases, in *Enzymatic basis of Detoxication* II, W. B. Jakoby, Ed., Academic Press, New York, 1980, 199.
82. **Wengle, B. and Boström, H.,** Studies on ester sulphates. 14. The *in vitro* formation of steroid disulphates in rat liver extracts, *Acta Chem. Scand.,* 17, 1203, 1963.
83. **Hirschmann, H. and Williams, J. S.,** The isolation of 5α-pregnane-3β,20β-diol 20-sulfate and its hydrolysis to uranediol (17α-methyl-D-homo-5α-androstane-3β,17aβ-diol), *J. Biol. Chem.,* 238, 2305, 1963.
84. **Levitz, M., Katz, J., and Twombly, G. H.,** The biosynthesis of labeled oestriol 3-sulfate 16-glucosiduronate, *Steroids,* 6, 553, 1965.
85. **Nose, Y. and Lipmann, F.,** Separation of steroid sulfokinases, *J. Biol. Chem.,* 233, 1348, 1958.
86. **Adams, J. B., Ellyard, R. K., and Low, J.,** Enzymic synthesis of steroid sulphates. IX. Physical and chemical properties of purified oestrogen sulphotransferase from bovine adrenal glands, the nature of its isoenzymic forms and a proposed model to explain its wave-like kinetics, *Biochem. Biophys. Acta,* 370, 160, 1974.
87. **Adams, J. B. and Low, J.,** Enzymic synthesis of steroid sulphates. X. Isolation of oestrogen sulphotransferase from bovine placenta and comparison of its properties with adrenal oestrogen sulphotransferase, *Biochim. Biophys. Acta,* 370, 189, 1974.

88. **Adams, J. B. and Chulavatnatol, M.,** Enzymic synthesis of steroid sulphates. IV. The nature of the two forms of oestrogen sulphotransferase of bovine adrenals, *Biochim. Biophys. Acta,* 146, 509, 1967.

89. **Adams, J. B., Dodsworth, I., and Jackson, D. E.,** Enzymic synthesis of steroid sulphates. XI. Study of the oestrogen binding site of oestrogen sulphotransferase by affinity labelling with 4-mercuri-17β-oestradiol, *Biochim. Biophys. Acta,* 384, 423, 1975.

90. **Horwitz, J. P., Neenan, J. P., Misra, R. H., Rozhin, J., Huo, A., and Philips, K. D.,** Studies on bovine adrenal oestrogen sulfotransferase. III. Facile synthesis of 3′-phospho- and 2′-phosphoadenosine 5′-phosphosulfate, *Biochim. Biophys. Acta,* 480, 376, 1977.

91. **Horwitz, J. P., Misra, R. S., Rozhin, J., Neenan, J. P., Huo, A., Godefroi, V. C., Philips, K. D., Chung, H. L., Butke, G., and Brooks, S. C.,** Studies on bovine adrenal oestrogen sulfotransferase. IV. Synthesis and assay of analogues of adenosine 3′, 5′-diphosphate as inhibitors of bovine adrenal estrogen sulfotransferase, *Biochim. Biophys. Acta,* 525, 364, 1978.

92. **Adams, J. B. and Ellyard, R. K.,** Enzymic synthesis of steroid sulphates. VIII. Inhibition of estrogen sulphotransferase by retinoic acid and free fatty acids. *Biochim. Biophys. Acta,* 260, 724, 1972.

93. **Holcenberg, J. S. and Rosen, S. W.,** Enzymatic sulfation of steroids by bovine tissues, *Arch. Biochem. Biophys.,* 110, 551, 1965.

94. **Adams, J. B.,** Presence of oestrogen sulphokinase in chick embryonic cartilage, *Nature (London),* 197, 1007, 1963.

95. **Raud, H. R. and Hobkirk, R.,** In vitro biosynthesis of steroid sulfates by cell-free preparations from tissues of the laying hen, *Can. J. Biochem.,* 46, 749, 1968.

96. **Creange, J. E. and Szego, C. M.,** Sulphation as a metabolic pathway for oestradiol in the sea urchin *Strongylocentrotus franciscanus, Biochem. J.,* 102, 896, 1967.

97. **Wengle, B.,** Studies on ester sulfates 21. On sulphate conjugation in foetal human tissue extracts, *Acta Soc. Med. Ups.,* 69, 103, 1964.

98. **Boström, H., Franksson, C., and Wengle, B.,** Studies on ester sulphates 22. Sulphate conjugation in adult human adrenal extracts, *Acta Endocrinol.,* 47, 633, 1964.

99. **Pack, B. A. and Brooks, S. C.,** Cyclic activity of estrogen sulfotransferase in the gilt uterus, *Endocrinology,* 95, 1680, 1974.

100. **Adams, J. B.,** Enzymic synthesis of steroid sulfates. II. Presence of steroid sulfokinase in human mammary carcinoma extracts, *J. Clin. Endocrinol. Metab.,* 24, 988, 1964.

101. **Godefroi, V. C., Locke, E. R., Singh, D. V., and Brooks, S. C.** The steroid alcohol and estrogen sulfotransferases in rodent and human mammary tumours, *Cancer Res.,* 35, 1791, 1975.

102. **Dao, T. L. and Libby, P. R.,** Conjugation of steroid hormones by breast cancer patients and selection of patients for adrenalectomy, *Surgery,* 66, 162, 1969.

103. **Roy, A. B.,** Sulfate conjugation enzymes, in *Handbuch der experimentellen pharmakologie,* Vol. 28/2. Brodie, B. B. and Gillette, J., Eds., Springer-Verlag, Berlin, 1971, 536.

104. **Adams, J. B. and Edwards, A. M.,** Enzymic synthesis of steroid sulphates. VII. Association-dissociation equilibria in the steroid alcohol sulphotransferase of human adrenal gland extracts, *Biochim. Biophys. Acta,* 167, 122, 1968.

105. **Adams, J. B. and McDonald, D.,** Enzymic synthesis of steroid sulphates. XII. Isolation of dehydroepiandrosterone sulphotransferase from human adrenals by affinity chromatography, *Biochim. Biophys. Acta,* 567, 144, 1979.

106. **Banerjee, R. K. and Roy, A. B.,** The formation of cholesteryl sulphate by androstenolone sulphotransferase, *Biochim. Biophys. Acta,* 137, 211, 1967.

107. **Roberts, K. D., Bandi, L., Calvin, H. I., Drucker, W. D., and Lieberman, S.,** Evidence that steroid sulfates serve as biosynthetic intermediates. IV. Conversion of cholesterol sulfate *in vivo* to urinary C_{19} and C_{21} steroidal sulfates, *Biochemistry,* 3, 1983, 1964.

108. **Baulieu, E.-E., Corpechot, C., Dray, F., Emiliozzi, R., Lebeau, M.-C., Mauvais-Jarvis, P., and Robel, P.,** An adrenal-secreted "androgen": dehydroisoandrosterone sulfate. Its metabolism and a tentative generalization on the metabolism of other steroid conjugates in man, *Recent Prog. Horm. Res.,* 21, 411, 1965.

109. **Hochberg, R. B., Ladany, S., and Lieberman, S.,** Cholesterol sulfate: some aspects of its biosynthesis and uptake by tissues from blood, *Endocrinology,* 94, 207, 1974.

110. **Spencer, B. and Raftery, J.,** Sulphate activation and sulphotransferase in foetal guinea-pigs and in developing hen's eggs, *Biochem. J.,* 99, 35p, 1966.

111. **Roy, A. B.,** The enzymic synthesis of steroid sulphates, *Biochem. J.,* 63, 294, 1956.

112. **Lewis, D. A.,** Androgen sulphate formation in male and female mice, *Biochem. J.,* 115, 489, 1969.

113. **Roy, A. B. and Banerjee, R. K.,** The steroid sulphotransferases, in *Proc. Second. Int. Congr. Hormonal Steroids,* Excerpta Medica, Amsterdam, 1966, 397.

114. **Singer, S. S., Giera, D., Johnson, J., and Sylvester, S.,** Enzymatic sulfation of steroids. I. The enzymatic basis for the sex difference in cortisol sulfation by rat liver preparations, *Endocrinology,* 98, 963, 1976.

115. **Singer, S. S.,** Enzymatic sulfation of steroids. III. The sulfation of corticosterone by the glucocorticoid sulfotransferases of rat liver cytosol, *Biochim. Biophys. Acta,* 539, 19, 1978.
116. **Singer, S. S.,** Partial purification and some properties of rat liver sulfotransferase I, a glucocorticoid sulfotransferase usually restricted to female rats, *Arch. Biochem. Biophys.,* 196, 340, 1979.
117. **Singer, S. S., Gebhart, J., and Hess, E.,** Enzymatic sulfation of steroids. V. Partial purification and some properties of sulfotransferase III, the major glucocorticoid sulfotransferase of liver cytosols from male rats, *Can. J. Biochem.,* 56, 1028, 1978.
118. **Singer, S. S. and Bruns, L.,** Enzymatic sulfation of steroids. VII. Hepatic cortisol sulfation and glucocorticoid sulfotransferases in old and young male rats, *Exp. Gerontol.,* 13, 425, 1978.
119. **Carlstedt-Duke, J. and Gustafsson, J.-A.,** Sexual differences in hepatic sulphurylation of deoxycorticosterone in rats, *Eur. J. Biochem.,* 36, 172, 1973.
120. **Gustafsson, J.-A., Carlstedt-Duke, J., and Goldman, A. S.,** On the hepatic sulfurylating activity in male pseudohermaphroditic rats, *Proc. Soc. Exp. Biol. Med.,* 145, 908, 1974.
121. **Singer, S. S. and Sylvester, S.,** Enzymatic sulfation of steroids. II. The control of the hepatic cortisol sulfotransferase activity and of the individual hepatic steroid sulfotransferases of rats by gonads and gonadal hormones, *Endocrinology,* 99, 1346, 1976.
122. **Singer, S. S.,** Enzymatic sulfation of steroids. IV. Control of the hepatic glucocorticoid sulfotransferase activity and the individual glucocorticoid sulfotransferases from male and female rats by adrenal glands and corticosteroids, *Endocrinology,* 103, 66, 1978.
123. **Singer, S. S., Kutzer, T., and Lee, A.,** Enzymatic sulfation of steroids. VIII. Control of hepatic cortisol sulfation and glucocorticoid sulfotransferases of rats by the pituitary gland, *Endocrinology,* 104, 571, 1979.
124. **Singer, S. S., Hess, E., and Sylvester, S.,** Hepatic cortisol sulfotransferase activity in several types of hypertension in male rats, *Biochem. Pharmacol.,* 26, 1033, 1977.
125. **Ghosh, P. C., Lockwood, E., and Pennington, G. W.,** Abnormal excretion of corticosteroid sulphates in patients with breast cancer, *Br. Med. J.,* 1, 328, 1973.
126. **Palmer, R. H.,** The formation of bile acid sulfates: a new pathway of bile acid metabolism in humans, *Proc. Natl. Acad. Sci. U.S.A.,* 58, 1047, 1967.
127. **Sommerfield, J. A., Gollan, J. L., and Billing, B. H.,** Synthesis of bile acid monosulphates by the isolated perfused rat kidney, *Biochem. J.,* 156, 339, 1976.
128. **Starka, L., Döllefeld, E., and Breuer, H.,** Biogenese von Freiem und Sulfatiertem 7α-hydroxyan-drostenolon in Zellfractionen der Rattenleber, *Z. Physiol. Chem.,* 348, 293, 1967.
129. **Chen, L.-J, Thaler, M. M., and Golbus, M. S.,** Enzymatic sulfation of bile salts. III. Enzymatic sulfation of taurolithocholate in human and guinea pig fetuses and adults, *Life Sci.,* 22, 1817, 1978.
130. **Imperato, T. J., Chen, L.-J., Cantor, D. S., Bolt, R. J., and Michas, C. A.,** Bile salt sulfotransferase activity in human liver, *Gastroenterology,* 71, 912, 1976.
131. **Hammerman, K. J., Chen, L.-J., Fernandez-Corugedo, A., and Earnest, D. L.,** Sex differences in hepatic sulfation of taurolithocholate in the rat, *Gastroenterology,* 75, 1021, 1978.
132. **Gadacz, T. R., Allan, R. N., Mack, E., and Hoffman, A. F.,** Impaired lithocholate sulfation in the rhesus monkey: a possible mechanism for chenodeoxycholate toxicity, *Gastroenterology,* 70, 1125, 1976.
133. **Boström, H. and Wengle, B.,** Studies on ester sulphates. 19. On sulphate conjugation in adult human liver extracts, *Acta Soc. Med. Ups.,* 69, 41, 1964.
134. **Herrmann, I. and Repke, K.,** Konjugation von Cardenolidgeninen mit Schwefelsaure oder Glucuronsaure, *Arch. Exp. Pathol. Pharmakol.,* 248, 370, 1964.
135. **Shimada, K., Fujii, Y., and Nambara, T.,** Isolation of bufalin 3-sulphate from the skin of *Bufo vulgaris formosus, Tetrahedron Lett.,* 2767, 1974.
136. **Haslewood, G. A. D.,** *Bile Salts,* Methuen, London, 1967.
137. **Bridgewater, R. J. and Ryan, D. A.,** Sulphate conjugation with ranol and other steroid alcohols in liver homogenates from *Rana temporaria, Biochem. J.,* 65, 24P, 1957.
138. **Scully, M. F., Dodgson, K. S., and Rose, F. A.,** Sulphation of simple aliphatic alcohols and bile alcohols by the toad *Xenopus laevis, Biochem. J.,* 119, 29P, 1970.
139. **Vestermark, A. and Boström, H.,** Studies on ester sulfates. V. On the enzymatic formation of ester sulfates of primary aliphatic alcohols, *Exp. Cell Res.,* 18, 174, 1959.
140. **Boström, H. and Vestermark, A.,** Studies on ester sulphates. 7. On the excretion of sulphate conjugates of primary aliphatic alcohols in the urine of rats, *Acta Physiol. Scand.,* 48, 88, 1960.
141. **Buhler, D. R.,** The metabolism of chlorphenesin carbamate, *J. Pharmacol. Exp. Ther.,* 145, 232, 1964.
142. **Law, G. L., Mansfield, G. P., Muggleton, D. F., and Parnell, E. W.,** Dimetridazole: absorption, excretion and metabolism in turkeys, *Nature (London),* 197, 1024, 1963.
143. **Yagi, T.,** Sulfate esters in developing eggs, *J. Biochem. (Tokyo),* 59, 495, 1966.
144. **Vestermark, A. and Boström, H.,** On the enzymatic formation of ester sulphates of aliphatic polyols, *Acta Chem. Scand.,* 13, 2133, 1959.

145. **Cooke, B. A. and Taylor, W.,** The metabolism of progesterone by animal tissues *in vitro*. 5. Inhibition of conjugate formation by ethanol and propylene glycol during the metabolism of [4-^{14}C] progesterone by rat liver *in vitro, Biochem. J.,* 87, 214, 1963.

146. **Mohamram, M., Rucker, R. B., and Hodges, R. E.,** Formation in vitro of ascorbic acid 2-sulfate, *Biochim. Biophys. Acta,* 437, 305, 1976.

147. **Roy, A. B.,** L-Ascorbic acid 2-sulphate. A substrate for mammalian arylsulphatases, *Biochim. Biophys. Acta,* 377, 356, 1975.

148. **Le Boulch, N., Gulat-Marnay, C., and Raoul, Y.,** Dérivés de la vitamine D$_3$ des laits de femme et de vache: ester sulfate de cholecalciférol et hydroxy-25 cholecalciférol, *Int. J. Vitamin. Nutr. Res.,* 44, 167, 1974.

149. **Le Boulch, N. and Marnay-Gulat, C.,** Elimination urinaire du cholecalciférol sous forme d'ester sulfurique chez le rat, *Biochimie,* 53, 1219, 1971.

150. **Higaki, M., Takahashi, M., Suzuki, T., and Sahashi, Y.,** Metabolic activities of vitamin D in animals. III. Biogenesis of vitamin D sulfate in animal tissues, *J. Vitaminol.,* 11, 261, 1965.

151. **Higaki, M., Takahashi, M., Suzuki, T., and Sahashi, Y.,** Metabolic activities of vitamin D in animals. IV. Distribution of vitamin D sulfokinase in animal tissues and its isolation, *J. Vitaminol.,* 11, 266, 1965.

152. **Cormier, M. J., Hori, K., Karkhanis, Y. D., Anderson, J. M., Wampler, J. E., Morin, J. G., and Hastings, J. W.,** Evidence for similar biochemical requirements for bioluminescence among the coelenterates, *J. Cell. Physiol.,* 81, 291, 1973.

153. **Cormier, M. J., Hori, K., and Karkhanis, Y. D.,** Studies on the bioluminescence of *Renilla reniformis* VII. Conversion of luciferin into luciferyl sulfate by luciferin sulfokinase, *Biochemistry,* 9, 1184, 1970.

154. **Hori, K. and Cormier, M. J.,** Structure and chemical synthesis of a biologically active form of *Renilla* (Sea Pansy) luciferin, *Proc. Natl. Acad. Sci. U.S.A.,* 70, 120, 1973.

155. **Anderson, J. M. and Cormier, M. J.,** Lumisomes, the cellular site of bioluminescence in coelenterates, *J. Biol. Chem.,* 248, 2937, 1973.

156. **Stanley, P. E., Kelley, B. C., Tuovinen, O. H., and Nicholas, D. J.,** A bioluminescence method for determining adenosine 3'-phosphate 5'-phosphate (PAP) and adenosine 3'-phosphate 5'-sulfatophosphate (PAPS) in biological materials, *Anal. Biochem.,* 67, 540, 1975.

157. **Boyland, E. and Nery, R.,** Arylhydroxylamines. Phenylhydroxylamine-*N*- and *O*-sulphonic acids. II, *J. Chem. Soc.,* 5217, 1962.

158. **DeBaun, J. R., Smith, J. Y. R., Miller, E. C., and Miller, J. A.,** Reactivity in vivo of the carcinogen *N*-hydroxy-2-acetylaminofluorene: increase by sulfate ion, *Science,* 167, 184, 1970.

159. **Weisburger, J. H., Yamamoto, R. S., Williams, G. M., Grantham, P. H., Matsushima, T., and Weisburger, E. K.,** On the sulfate ester of *N*-hydroxy-*N*-2-fluorenylacetamide as a key ultimate hepatocarcinogen in the rat, *Cancer Res.,* 32, 491, 1972.

160. **Roy, A. B.,** The enzymic synthesis of aryl sulphamates, *Biochem. J.,* 74, 49, 1960.

161. **Roy, A. B.,** The enzymic synthesis of aryl sulphamates, *Biochim. Biophys. Acta,* 30, 193, 1958.

162. **Boyland, E., Manson, D., and Orr, S. F. D.,** The biochemistry of aromatic amines. 2. The conversion of arylamines into arylsulphamic acids and arylamine-*N*-glucosiduronic acids, *Biochem. J.,* 65, 417, 1957.

163. **Roy, A. B.,** The enzymic synthesis of aryl sulphamates. 2. The effect of 3β-methoxyandrost-5-en-17-one on arylamine sulphokinase, *Biochem. J.,* 79, 253, 1961.

164. **Roy, A. B.,** The enzymic synthesis of arylsulphamates. 3. The specificity and mechanism of the activation of rat-liver arylamine sulphokinase by 17-oxosteroids, *Biochem. J.,* 82, 66, 1962.

165. **Roy, A. B.,** Possible allosteric effects with arylamine sulphokinase, *J. Mol. Biol.,* 10, 176, 1964.

166. **Kent, P. W. and Pasternak, C. A.,** Sulphate activation by intestinal mucosal enzymes, *Proc. IV Int. Cong. Biochem.,* 4, 74, 1958.

167. **Arita, T., Hori, R., Ito, K., and Ichekawa, K.,** Transformation and excretion of drugs in biological systems. III. Separatory determination of metaclopramide and its N^4-glucuronide and N^4-sulfonate in rabbit urine and bile, *Chem. Pharm. Bull.,* 18, 1670, 1970.

168. **Parke, D. V.,** *The Biochemistry of Foreign Compounds,* Pergamon Press, Oxford, 1968, 180.

169. **Powell, G. M., Miller, J. J., Olavesen, A. H., Curtis, C. G.,** Liver as a major organ of phenol detoxication?, *Nature (London),* 252, 234, 1974.

170. **Subba Rao, K. and Ganguly, J.,** Studies on metabolism of vitamin A. 6. The effect of vitamin A deficiency on the activation of sulphate and its transfer to *p*-nitrophenol in rat liver, *Biochem. J.,* 90, 104, 1964.

171. **Sudhakaran, P. R. and Kurup, P. A.,** Vitamin A and glycosaminoglycan metabolism in rats, *J. Nutr.,* 104, 871, 1974.

172. **Levi, A. S., Geller, S., Root, D. M., and Wolf, G.,** The effect of vitamin A and other dietary constituents on the activity of adenosine triphosphate sulphurylase, *Biochem. J.,* 109, 69, 1968.

173. **Geisen, R. L., Rogers, W. E., and Johnson, B. C.,** Comparative effects of vitamin-A deficiency and controlled food consumption on adenosine 5′-triphosphate: sulfate adenylyltransferase, *Biochim. Biophys. Acta,* 165, 448, 1968.

174. **Banerjee, R. K.,** Studies on Sulphotransferases, Ph.D. thesis, Australian National University, Canberra, 1967.

175. **Yount, R. G., Simchuk, S., Yu, I., and Kottke, M.,** Adenosine-5′-sulfatopyrosphosphate, an analogue of adenosine triphosphate. 1. Preparation, properties and mode of cleavage by snake venoms, *Arch. Biochem. Biophys.,* 113, 288, 1966.

176. **Lyon, E. S. and Jakoby, W. B.,** The identity of alcohol sulfotransferases with hydroxysteroid sulfotransferases, *Arch. Biochem. Biophys.,* 202, 474, 1980.

177. **Borchardt, R. T. and Schasteen, C. S.,** Personal communication.

178. **Horwitz, J. P., Misra, R. S., Rozhin, J., Helmer, S., Bhuta, A., and Brooks, S. C.,** Studies on bovine adrenal estrogen sulfotransferase. V. Synthesis and assay of analogs of 3′-phosphoadenosine 5′-phosphosulfate as cosubstrates for estrogen sulfurylation, *Biochim. Biophys. Acta,* 63, 85, 1980.

179. **Singer, S. S. and Burns, L.,** Enzymatic sulfation of steroids. XI. The extensive purification and some properties of hepatic sulfotransferase III from female rats, *Can. J. Biochem.,* 58, 660, 1980.

180. **Jakoby, W. B.,** Personal communication.

Chapter 6

SULFATION IN VIVO AND IN ISOLATED INTACT CELL PREPARATIONS

G. J. Mulder

TABLE OF CONTENTS

I. INTRODUCTION

In this chapter only the sulfate conjugation of low-molecular weight substances, both endogenous and exogenous, will be considered. The sulfation of endogenous macromolecules such as glycosaminoglycans falls outside the scope of this book, although much work has been done on the chemical characterization of these highly sulfated compounds, and on the incorporation of [^{35}S]-sulfate into tissue in vivo and in tissue slices of cell preparations.[1-13] Similarly, sulfated lipids (for instance cerebroside sulfate) will not be covered; recent reviews on sulfolipids are available.[14,15]

II. INVENTORY OF SUBSTRATES

A. Identification and Separation of Sulfate Conjugates in Biological Material

The first sulfate conjugates were detected in urine samples after feeding substrates of sulfation to animals. Until the early 1950s, these sulfate conjugates were determined indirectly, by the increase of the amount of "ethereal," esterified sulfate as compared with the control situation, in which no compounds were administered. This ethereal sulfate was determined by the difference in inorganic sulfate content between acid-hydrolyzed and nonhydrolyzed urine;[16-18] inorganic sulfate was determined either gravimetrically or turbidimetrically. Clearly, the specificity of these methods is very limited; yet, many of the original findings have been confirmed later with more specific methods.

Around 1952 arylsulfatase was introduced for the more specific enzymatic hydrolysis of arylsulfate ester conjugates.[19] The problem, however, was (and often still is) that the sulfatase preparations are contaminated by β-glucuronidase activity. Therefore, the activity of the latter must be selectively inhibited when for analytical purposes specific hydrolysis of only sulfate conjugates is required. With many β-glucuronidase preparations with an acid pH optimum, such as β-glucuronidase from rat preputial gland or from *Helix pomatia,* glucaro-1,4-lactone can be used as a highly effective and specific inhibitor of β-glucuronidase. With other glucuronidases this inhibitor may be less effective, and complete inhibition should always be checked with the reference compound, to make an unequivocal conclusion about the presence and amount of an arylsulfate conjugate possible. Thus, in some publications it is not clear whether the animals used did not synthesize the sulfate conjugate of the administered compound, or whether the bacterial β-glucuronidase, used in the analysis, was contaminated with arylsulfatase (see Reference 20). If the sulfate conjugate contributes only a small percent of the total amount of conjugates in a sample, it is obviously important to ascertain that a low percentage of hydrolysis in the presence of glucaro-1,4-lactone is not due to a small residual β-glucuronidase activity. Recently, more specific sulfatase preparations have become available, for instance the *Aerobacter aerogenes* sulfatase, which contains only minimum amounts of glucuronidase activity.

Substrate specificity of arylsulfatase may cause some additional confusion: it has been shown that sulfate conjugates of some types of phenols with a substituent group *ortho* to the sulfate ester position are hydrolyzed only very slowly, probably due to steric hindrance by the *ortho*-substituent.[21] Therefore, sulfate conjugates of such phenols have a chance to escape detection when the sulfate fraction is analyzed with an arylsulfatase preparation. Often, the identity of a conjugate as a sulfate ester is established by subjecting a sample of urine or bile to hydrolysis by a mixed arylsulfatase/β-glucuronidase preparation. If hydrolysis is inhibited by glucaro-1, 4-lactone, it is assumed to be a glucuronide conjugate, and if not, it is supposed to be an arylsulfate ester. Although usually this conclusion is justified, it seems advisable to separate first the components present in a sample by for instance, thin-layer chromatography, and then to perform these specific hydrolysis reactions on the separate spots from the plate. In that case the conclusions will certainly be more quantitatively reliable and less subject to errors. Moreover, some drugs or their metabolites may inhibit one of the hydrolyzing enzymes: the pentachlorophenol metabolite tetracholorohydroquinone was shown to inhibit β-glucuronidase.[22] If the conjugates are separated beforehand, less confusion will result from such an (unexpected) effect, and most likely it will be noted earlier.

Similar problems as discussed above for arylsulfatases apply to steroid sulfatases; this has extensively been discussed by Roy.[23]

Separation of the various metabolites before identification was achieved first by paper chromatography, and later by thin-layer chromatography. Usually the glucuronide and sulfate conjugates can be readily separated because the glucuronide conjugates are more water-soluble and less lipid-soluble than their sulfated counterpart. In the same run, the unconjugated substrates can mostly also be separated. Recently, high-performance liquid chromatography has become a rapid and very effective tool in separation of the conjugates; they can usually be quantitated directly by their UV absorption or fluorescence.

A very generally applicable way of identifying a sulfate conjugate in experimental animals is by incorporation of [^{35}S]-labeled sulfate into the substrate. A high dose of [^{35}S]-sodium sulfate can be injected intravenously immediately before the substrate to be studied, and urine and bile can be screened for radioactive metabolites of the substrate. This will confirm beyond doubt the identity of a sulfate conjugate because under normal conditions inorganic sulfate in blood is not converted to other forms of sulfur-containing compounds, such as glutathione or taurine, if nonruminants are used (see Chapter 3, Section V), certainly not when the radio-label is injected immediately before the substrate to be studied.

Whereas arylsulfates are usually identified by enzymatic hydrolysis with an arylsulfatase preparation, steroid sulfate conjugates are in general characterized by their relatively specific hydrolysis through solvolysis.[24-28] Many variations in procedure have been reported, but the principle is the same: acid hydrolysis under relatively mild conditions (see Chapter 2, Section IIB3). The conjugate is, e.g., dissolved in ethanol, acidified with 2 N HCl, and diluted with acetone. After a couple of days at room temperature, the sulfate conjugate is completely hydrolyzed and, in part, converted into an ethyl-ether; the latter can be hydrolyzed, after evaporation to dryness, by refluxing for 2 hr in 5% methanolic KOH. The efficiency of various solvolysis procedures has been compared by Aso et al.[29] The identity of a particular steroid sulfate can only be proven by comparison with a chemically synthesized authentic sulfate conjugate. When the steroid is administered in a radiolabeled form, or when the animal is given a high dose of [^{35}S]-sodium sulfate, (endogenous) steroids are conjugated with [^{35}S]-labeled sulfate; these conjugates may be identified by recrystallization with an unlabeled reference compound until constant specific radioactivity. This is a very unambiguous, general way of establishing the identity of the conjugate. Recently, sulfate conjugates have been derivatized for electron impact mass spectrometry by converting them into sulfate diesters with n-propyl-iodide.[30] Alternative mass spectrometric procedures are being developed for sulfate conjugates[31] (see Chapter 2, Section IIB1 and IIB4).

Bile salts, a special class of steroids, also give rise to sulfate conjugates at (one of) the secondary alcoholic OH group(s). Usually these are similarly identified by solvolysis after an initial separation from other conjugates or unconjugated material.[32-35] Especially in the older literature on bile salts, the presence of sulfate conjugates of the bile salts may have caused artifacts when the sulfated glycine and taurine conjugates were split by hydrolysis in strong alkali:[32] a part of the sulfate ester present will also be hydrolyzed, but also the C–O bond of the ester linkage will be attacked, leading to inversion of the alcoholic OH group on the ring, or to its elimination with the formation of a double bond in the ring. These complications may be prevented by using instead, enzymatic methods to remove glycine and taurine, with, e.g., choloylhydrolase.[36] Alternatively, the bile salts can first be desulfated by solvolysis, and, after that, the glycine or taurine group can be removed by alkaline hydrolysis in order to leave the steroid nucleus intact. Van Berge-Henegouwen et al.[34] have compared various methods and present a simple hydrolysis/solvolysis procedure.

Sulfate conjugates of steroids and bile salts are much more water soluble than the nonsulfated counterparts and therefore, can easily be separated by column chromatography, thin-layer chromatography, or even diethylether extraction from the unconjugated substrates.[37-44] Parmentier and Eyssen[44] described the thin-layer chromatography of 33 bile-salt sulfates, representing most of the possible sulfate esters of the common bile salts. Often Sephadex LH-20 or its diethylaminohydroxypropyl derivative is used for column chromatography to separate mono- and disulfate conjugates of steroids and bile salts.[45] Bile and urine samples can be rapidly prepurified and an Amberlite® XAD-2 column;[40,42,46,47] even better results have been reported with XAD-7.[48-50] Radioimmunoassays for sulfated steroids have become available for those compounds that are of clinical or pathological significance.[51-53] Thin-layer chromatography is still a much-used method for separation of the conjugates,[32,54,55] but recently, high performance liquid chromatography has been applied.[56-58]

B. Xenobiotics as Substrates

After the original report by Baumann in 1876, sulfate conjugates of numerous compounds have been detected when these compounds were fed to animals. Compounds containing an alcoholic or phenolic-OH group, or –NH and N–OH groups are potential substrates for the sulfotransferases in vivo.

R.T. Williams and his group were the first who studied the fate of a great number of xenobiotics in mammals in a systematic way. At first, Williams worked only on glucuronic acid conjugates, but soon he started work on the often competing sulfate conjugation that consumed part of many substrates and thereby limited their glucuronidation. In 1938 he reported on the metabolism of a series of monosubstituted phenols after oral administration of equimolar amounts to rabbits;[59] most of the 12 *ortho-*, 9 *meta-*, and 11 *para*-substititued phenols were sulfated to a smaller or greater percentage. Although at that time Williams used the very indirect determination of the increase of "ethereal sulfate" in urine as a measure of excretion of the sulfate conjugate when the phenol had been fed to the rabbit, several of these results have since been confirmed with other methods. Williams has reviewed the metabolism of phenols in 1964.[60] Table 1 shows a summary of some of his data, which usually were determined at only one dose level; as will be discussed in section IVD, the dose is important in the ratio between sulfation and glucuronidation of a compound. Since in vivo often other conjugation and oxidation reactions occur simultaneously with the sulfation of these phenols, it is impossible to analyze the data in terms of influence of substituents in the ring on one metabolic reaction only: if there is some balance between three or four reactions, a change in one of them may affect the others as well, and one needs detailed evidence to pinpoint the primary cause. Therefore, the conclusions on the influence of substituents in the phenol drawn in the original publication by Williams[59] were not repeated in his later review,[60] when a much wider insight had been gained in the various routes of drug metabolism. Nevertheless, an important factor seems to be the acidity of

Table 1
SULFATION AND GLUCURONIDATION OF SOME SUBSTITUTED PHENOLS IN THE RABBIT AFTER ORAL ADMINISTRATION[a]

Substituent in the phenol ring	Percentage of the dose excreted as	
	Sulfate	Glucuronide
o-Chloro	19	82
m-Chloro	21	78
p-Chloro	13	88
o-Amino	15	70
m-Amino	15	60
p-Amino	12	62
o-Methyl	15	72
m-Methyl	10	60
p-Methyl	15	61
p-Methoxy	13	69
o-Acetylamino	20	39
p-Acetylamino	13	63
o-Formylamide (CONH$_2$)	13	76
m-Formylamide	19	60
p-Formylamide	23	15
o-Nitro	11	71
m-Nitro	19	78
p-Nitro	16	65
Dimethyl (2,3-; 2,4-; 2,5-; 2,6-; 3,5-)	13—16	46—65
3,4-Dimethyl	8	65
4-Chloro-3,5-dimethyl	23	58

[a] Dose level: 0.15—0.30 g/kg orally.

With permission from Williams, R. T., *Biochemistry of Phenolic Compounds,* Harborne, J. B., Ed., Academic Press, New York, 1964, chap. 6. Copyright by Academic Press Inc. (London) Ltd.

the phenol: strongly acidic phenols are sulfated only to a low extent, or not at all.[60] For instance, pentachlorophenol and certain other tetra- and trichlorophenols are not sulfated and usually glucuronidated to only a minor extent.[61,62] Certain sulfonic acid derivatives were similarly not sulfated.[63] However, some caution is indicated, because the arylsulfatase preparations used for the identification of sulfate conjugates may not have hydrolyzed some *ortho*-substituted sulfate esters; in those cases, ironically, the older method in which the "ethereal sulfate" fraction was determined, gives more information.

It is to be expected that steric hindrance at the phenolic –OH group to be conjugated may play a role as well. It might contribute to the lack of sulfation of for instance, pentachlorophenol, although limited glucuronidation of this compound does occur.[62] Moreover, 2,6-dimethylphenol is sulfated in the rabbit (Table 1); since the methyl-group is of about equal size as the chloride atom, this suggests that for groups of this size steric hindrance may be not as important as acidity of the phenol. Similarly, in the rat and cat 2,6-dimethoxyphenol is readily sulfated.[64] Dacre[65] showed that the presence of two *tert*-butyl groups in the *ortho* positions prevented the sulfation of the antioxidant 3, 5-*di*-(*tert*-butyl)-4-hydroxytoluene, whereas the presence of only one such group in 2-*tert*-butyl-4-methoxyphenol still permitted sulfation to take place.[66] Since no in-depth study on the effect of steric hindrance in available, no clear-cut conclusions on its importance can be reached.

That other factors play a role is suggested by the fact that salicylic acid is not conjugated with sulfate, whereas salicylamide is. Since in man the rate of elimination of salicylic acid is limited by its rate of metabolism,[67,68] this indicates that the lack of sulfation of this compound is not due to a very rapid competing reaction that takes the substrate away before measurable sulfation can occur; it may be due to substrate specificity of the sulfotransferase.

The metabolism of many phenols, both monohydric and polyhydric, has been discussed by Williams in his 1964 review.[60] In brief, unless steric hindrance of high acidity prevents it, all phenols are sulfated to some extent, dependent on dose and species used (see Section IV of this chapter).

Another chemical group that may accept the sulfate group is the alcoholic hydroxyl group. Thus 3,5-*di*(*tert*-butyl)-4-hydroxytoluene, that (probably for steric reasons) is not sulfated at the phenolic group, is oxidized, *inter alia,* to the primary alcohol in one of the *tert*-butyl groups. This compound then can be sulfated at the newly introduced alcoholic hydroxyl group.[65] Similarly, the drug chlorphenesin carbamate was reported to be sulfated at a secondary alcohol group.[69] Many steroids and steroid-like drugs are sulfated at secondary alcohol groups in the steroid nucleus; these are discussed in Sections IID and IIE. Even simple short-chain alcohols like ethanol are excreted in the rat as sulfate conjugate.[70]

Finally, hydroxylamines and hydroxamic acids may be converted to sulfate conjugates that are often very unstable; this will be discussed at length in Chapter 8. Both *N–O*-sulfates and sulfamates may be formed; the group of Boyland has extensively studied the fate of 2-naphthylamine in various species, especially the formation of sulfate conjugates and their chemical reactivity (see Reference 71).

Figure 1 shows a number of chemical structures of compounds that are sulfated, sometimes in various positions. Many more examples can easily be found in the literature; data on the metabolic fate of many xenobiotics is compiled by Hathway.[72]

In spite of the very hydrophilic sulfate group, still most sulfate esters are highly protein-bound in plasma.[73,74]

Usually the sulfation of phenolic compounds leads to sulfate conjugates that are much less toxic than the parent compounds. If the conjugate is chemically and metabolically stable, it may be rapidly excreted in urine or bile (see Chapter 7). However, in some cases the sulfate conjugate is chemically reactive, although this has not yet been shown to occur with phenolic sulfate conjugates. The finding, however, that a glucuronide conjugate of benzo*(a)*pyrene may generate a chemically reactive intermediate when it was split by β-glucuronidase activity[75] suggests that the same might apply also to sulfate conjugates. The generation of reactive sulfate conjugates takes place especially with *N*-hydroxylarylamines. This is discussed in Chapter 8.

C. Ascorbic Acid Sulfate

Around 1970 the sulfate ester at the 2-position of ascorbic acid was identified as a physiological metabolite in several animal species. It was found first in the brine shrimp *Artemia salina*[76] and later also in many tissues and body fluids of mammals like liver, spleen, adrenals, bile, and urine.[77-80] Athough the compound was identified in human urine,[77] it could not be detected in ultrafiltrate from human blood;[81] the urinary ascorbic acid-2-sulfate levels in man (μg/mg creatinine) correlated negatively with the age of the subjects.[82]

After this sulfate conjugate had been discovered, much attention was paid to its potential role in physiological processes, and to its potential physiological role as a sulfate donor. Somewhat controversial results have so far been reported.

Chemically, sulfate esters at the 2- and 6-positions of ascorbic acid can easily be prepared by sulfation with for instance, pyridine-SO_3 complex.[78,81,83-86] Separation of

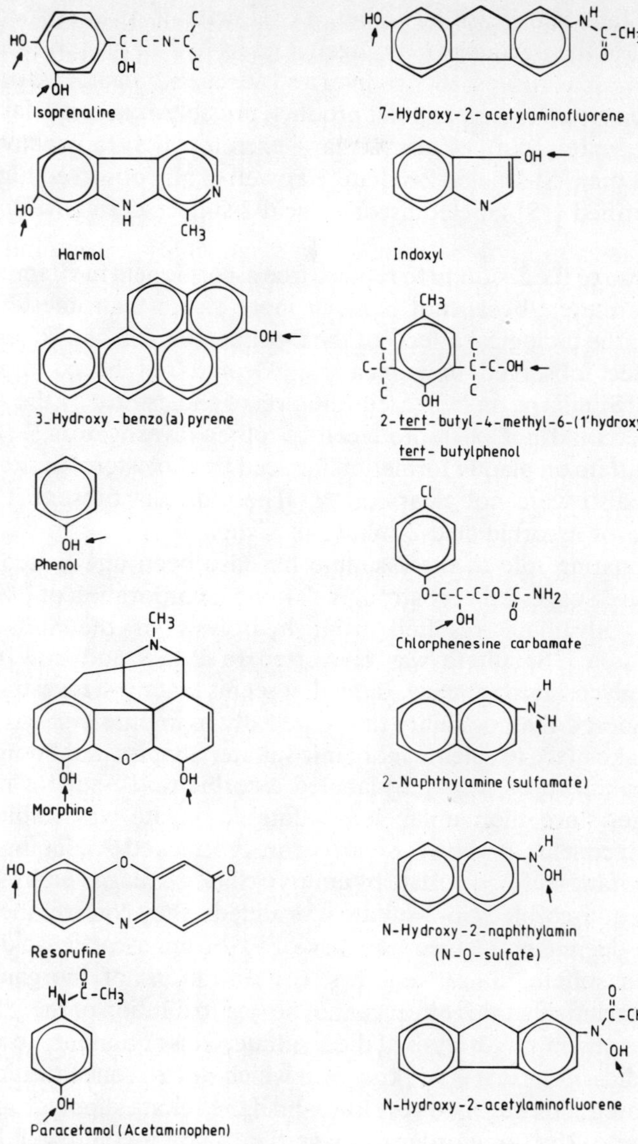

FIGURE 1. Chemical structure of some substrates for sulfation (xenobiotics). The acceptor group is indicated by an arrow.

ascorbic acid and its sulfate derivatives can be achieved by thin-layer chromatography or by high performance liquid chromatography.[83,87-89] Ascorbic acid-2-sulfate can be determined within 6 min by high performance liquid chromatography (hplc) of an urine sample; free and conjugated ascorbic acid can be estimated by various chemical methods.[90-92]

The mechanism of synthesis of the sulfate conjugate of ascorbic acid is not known so far (see Chapter 5, Section VI). Rat liver and colon homogenates required PAPS as intermediary sulfate donor for the synthesis of ascorbic acid sulfate.[93] Although no quantitative data are available on the percentage of a dose of ascorbic acid that is sulfated in vivo at various doses, it seems a minor part. The major metabolite in man is oxalate, and much of the dose is excreted unchanged in the urine.[94-97] The concentration of the 2-sulfate in liver was 0.4 mM in the rat after daily administration of 1 mg of ascorbic acid subcutaneously.[87]

The biological fate of the 2-sulfate when it is injected in various species, is mainly urinary excretion of the unchanged conjugate and its hydrolysis products.[81,92,94,95,97] It is also taken up by various tissues, such as liver and adrenals.[92] In at least one species, the guinea pig, it is converted to a more polar product, possibly a carboxyl derivative, which accounts for the major part of the urinary excreted [35S]-radioactivity after oral administration of the [35S]-labeled 2-sulfate.[98] Powell et al.[99] observed high secretion of an as yet unidentified [35S]-labeled ascorbic acid-2-sulfate derivative into the gastric lumen in the rat.

The potential use of the 2-sulfate to replace free ascorbic acid in vitamin preparations has drawn some interest because it is much more stable than unesterified ascorbic acid.[100] However, the biological effects of the 2-sulfate are still controversial. Thus, an antiscorbutic effect observed in guinea pigs[101] could not be confirmed by other investigators.[102,103] Similarly, an increased sulfation of cholesterol by the administration of the 2-sulfate[104] could not be reproduced by other investigators.[105] The beneficial effects of the 2-sulfate on plaque formation induced by cholesterol in the aorta, and on hyperlipidaemia also were not clear-cut.[106-109] Therefore, at present it is difficult to evaluate the role of ascorbic acid-2-sulfate in vivo.

The sulfate-donating role of the 2-sulfate has also been questioned. The data of Shapiro and Poon[110] suggested very strongly that the incorporation of [35S]-sulfate from ascorbic acid-2-[35S]-sulfate resulted from hydrolysis of the sulfate conjugate, whereupon the free [35S]-sulfate was converted to PAPS and only then used for incorporation in glycosaminoglycans. Indeed, it seems that most investigators have not sufficiently considered the possibility that especially in impure systems, hydrolysis of the sulfate may take place to release inorganic sulfate. Shapiro and Poon suggest that a spontaneous breakdown of their [35S]-labeled ascorbic acid-2-sulfate may be due to radiation damage, since their unlabeled sulfate conjugate was stable and did not decompose. Their conclusions however, are strongly attacked by Hatanaka et al.[111] who measured incorporation of [35S]-sulfate by embryo chick cartilage epiphyses when either inorganic sulfate or ascorbic acid-2-sulfate was added. They confirm the finding[110] that inorganic sulfate decreases the incorporation of [35S] from ascorbic acid-2-[35S]-sulfate into chrondroitin sulfate. Since very low concentrations of inorganic sulfate are effective, they conclude that this effect cannot be due to dilution of the [35S]-sulfate pool resulting from the possible hydrolysis of the 2-sulfate. This argument, however, may not be completely valid, because it is not known at which sulfate concentration chondroitin sulfation is saturated; this might be very low, and if the sulfate supply from hydrolysis of the 2-sulfate were of the same order of magnitude, then it could well be that even a relatively low concentration of inorganic sulfate could dilute the [35S]-sulfate pool considerably. However, a more important difference is that their 2-[35S]-sulfate was much more stable than that of Shapiro and Poon:[110] they did not find the breakdown reported by the other investigators. Therefore, a final conclusion as to the importance of the 2-sulfate as direct or indirect sulfate donor requires more clarification.

Ascorbic acid-2-sulfate inhibits dopamine β-hydroxylase from bovine adrenals competitively in respect to ascorbate. The authors[112] speculate about a role of this compound in the regulation of the biosynthesis of noradrenaline. The concentration required for inhibition, however, is rather high: a K_i of 3.44 mM was found.

Several arylsulfatases can hydrolyze the sulfate ester of ascorbic acid. A sulfatase preparation from liver of a marine gastropod, *Charonia lampas*, hydrolyzed the 2-sulfate more rapidly than the 6-sulfate.[84] Roy[113] determined properties of hydrolysis of the 2-sulfate by arylsulfatase A and B from ox liver and brain, respectively. Both enzymes had an acid pH optimum (around pH 4.8) and both were strongly inhibited by inorganic sulfate, with a K_i of 0.1 to 0.6 mM. The inhibition was competitive with ascorbic acid 2-sulfate, which had a K_m of 21(A) and 8(B) mM, respectively. An arylsulfatase A from rabbit kidney also hydrolyzed the 2-sulfate, but arylsulfatase B from the same source failed to do so.[114] Human arylsulfatase A similarly hydrolyzed ascorbic acid-2-sulfate, whereas arylsulfatase B from the same source did not[115] The various assay procedures in measurement of ascorbic acid-2-sulfate hydrolysis have been critically investigated.[116]

D. Bile Salts as Substrates

The fact that bile salts are conjugated with glycine and taurine at the C_{24} carboxyl group had already been known for a long time before the first report on a sulfate conjugate of lithocholic acid, at the only secondary alcohol group in the 3-position, appeared. Palmer[117] proved that certain until then-unidentified lithocholate metabolites were sulfate conjugates: by solvolysis sulfate was released, and recrystallization of one of the unknown conjugates with authentic, chemically synthesized lithocholate-3-sulfate proved its identity beyond doubt. That these sulfate conjugates also occurred in man was proven when [^{14}C]-labeled lithocholate was administered orally to some patients and the gall bladder bile, obtained at cholecystectomy, was collected. In these bile samples the sulfate esters of both glycolithocholate and taurolithocholate were identified. In more detail, chemical properties and occurrence of lithocholate-3-sulfate were reported by Palmer and Bolt.[32,118] Sulfation made the lithocholate conjugates much more polar and water soluble.[119,120] Lithocholate-3-sulfate was found as a natural component of bile both in man and rat; toxicologically this was an interesting finding, because lithocholate and its taurine and glycine conjugates are highly toxic. It appeared that sulfation might be a detoxifying reaction, especially since Palmer[118] found that the sulfated lithocholate conjugates could be excreted in urine relatively rapidly, whereas other bile salt conjugates are only excreted very slowly, even when the bile duct is obstructed.[121] Further, their absorption from the gut was slower that that of the nonsulfated conjugates. In everted sacs of guinea-pig intestine and in isolated perfused segments of the small intestine with an intact blood supply, active transport of sulfated tauro- and glycolithocholate in the ileum was observed.[122] This transport was strongly inhibited by nonsulfated taurocholate. It seems that sulfation of potentially toxic lithocholate conjugates can curtail their intestinal absorption, and enhance their fecal elimination. In addition, the sulfate conjugates appeared not to lose their sulfate group in the gut or during absorption, so that they remained nontoxic even when reabsorbed. The urinary excretion of the sulfated bile salts turned out to be of much clinical importance since in patients with biliary obstruction, the accumulation of bile salts constitutes a danger; in these patients the sulfated conjugates can be excreted at a relatively high rate in urine.[123-128] In the rhesus monkey, which has a low sulfating activity towards lithocholate, the protective action of sulfation clearly is demonstrated. This species is much more sensitive to the toxic action of chenodeoxycholate than many other species.[129] This is due to the fact that chenodeoxycholate is converted by bacterial activity into lithocholate; because this is not sulfated at a sufficiently high rate in the rhesus monkey, it is highly toxic, since it cannot be rapidly excreted in urine. And therefore, its precursor chenodeoxycholate is toxic too. Yet, bile-salt sulfates may still be toxic; thus, glycolithocholate sulfate still can induce cholestasis in the rat.[129a]

In healthy subjects, only very minor amounts of sulfated bile salts are present in urine.[126] Cowan et al.[130-132] extensively investigated the metabolism of administered lithocholate and its various conjugates in healthy human volunteers in whom they collected bile by intubation with a double lumen tube with an occlusive balloon, that was positioned immediately proximal to the ligament of Treitz. Most of the administered dose, approximately 60%, was excreted in bile as sulfate conjugate. In urine almost nothing was excreted.

Pharmacokinetics of chenodeoxycholate and cholate and their sulfate conjugates have been studied by i.v. injection of the [^{14}C]-labeled bile salts or their sulfates in patients with cirrhosis of the liver.[133] The halflives of the sulfate conjugates were only 30 to 15% of those of the nonsulfated compounds, reflecting the more rapid elimination of the conjugates. Chenodeoxycholate was more rapidly sulfated than cholate, and this presumably is the reason for the more rapid turnover and elimination of chenodeoxycholate as compared with cholate. In general, monohydroxy bile salts are sulfated to a higher degree than dihydroxy bile salts (such as chenodeoxycholate); trihydroxy bile salts (cholate) are least sulfated.[125,127,134] Bile salts with more than one hydroxyl group may give rise to mono- and disulfate conjugates. This is illustrated in Table 2 which shows the sulfate conjugates that are present in normal bile from rat, cat, and rabbit. Usually the position of the hydroxyl group that has been conjugated with sulfate is not determined; the presence of a sulfate group is only shown by solvolysis. In monohydroxy bile salts such as lithocholate the sulfate ester is of course in the only possible position, the 3-hydroxy group. Interestingly, in the isolated perfused rat kidney the 7-hydroxy group of chenodeoxycholate is first sulfated and not the 3-hydroxy group.[135] The same was found by Parmentier et al.,[136] who identified cholate-7-sulfate as a major component of the fecal bile salts of the mouse.

Species differences in the occurrence of the various sulfated bile salts in bile are illustrated in the data collected in Table 2.[45,137] These differences may be due to many factors, such as differences in the production of the substrates for sulfation. The data also suggest a sex difference (see also Chapter 5, Section IVE): in the male cat more sulfation was found than in the female, whereas in the rat the reverse was observed. In the rabbit there seemed to be no big differences. The sex difference in the rat was confirmed when taurolithocholate was infused.[138] Male rats sulfated 3.0% of the dose, whereas females converted 7.7% to this conjugate. Oophoroectomy in the females decreased this to 4.2%, and substitution therapy with estrogens restored this level to 9.0%. Table 2 shows that the composition of the sulfated bile salt fraction in the rat changes upon prolonged collection of bile, probably as a result of changes in the composition of the supply of bile salts upon cannulation and interruption of the enterohepatic circulation.

Even fetal human liver is able to sulfate bile salts: in meconium obtained from full-term newborn infants large amounts of these sulfated bile salts were found.[139,149] Indeed, in human fetal livers the bile-salt sulfotransferase is present, be it at a low activity.[141] In pregnancies complicated by maternal intrahepatic cholestasis, the bile-salt levels in both maternal and fetal blood were elevated, as was the concentration in the amniotic fluid. Since the fetus swallows considerable amounts of this fluid, increased amounts of the bile salts were found in meconium in cholestasis.[140] In pregnant sheep, further evidence was obtained that the fetus could sulfate exogeneously administered lithocholate, most likely in its liver.

Under normal conditions, the liver takes up and eliminates the bile salts extremely efficiently; therefore, disturbances in bile-salt metabolism can be expected during various liver diseases. Often, a greatly increased urinary excretion of especially sulfated bile salts is observed: acute hepatitis,[40,126] obstructive jaundice,[126] or the cholestatic syndrome[127,128,142] give rise to great increases, whereas during cirrhosis and chronic hepatitis, much smaller increases are observed.[40,125,126] In agreement with this, serum levels of the sulfated bile salts are also elevated in these diseased states,[40,126,127,143] though not in all patients.[33] As was to be expected, a decrease of kidney function will affect serum bile-salt sulfate concentration: in a patient with anuria dramatically high concentrations were found.[143] The increase in the degree of sulfation in liver disease may reflect a decreased rate of biliary elimination of the nonsulfated bile salts. As a

Table 2
SULFATED BILE SALTS IN BILE OBTAINED FROM VARIOUS SPECIES[a,b]

Bile salts (cholanoates)	Rabbit Male (µg/ml)	Rabbit Female (µg/ml)	Cat Male (µg/ml)	Cat Female (µg/ml)	Rat: 1—12 hr Male (nmol/12 hr)	Rat: 1—12 hr Female (nmol/12 hr)	Rat: 48—60 hr Male (nmol/12 hr)	Rat: 48—60 hr Female (nmol/12 hr)	Trivial name of bile salt
3α, 7α, 12α-trihydroxy-5α	—	—	17	7	—	25	1	23[c]	Allocholate
3α, 7α, 12α-trihydroxy-5β	tr	tr	3	7					Cholate
3β, 7α, 12α-trihydroxy-5α	nd	nd	nd	nd	—	40	17	84[c]	—
3α, 6β, 7α-trihydroxy-5β	nd	nd	nd	nd	—	17	6	7[c]	α-Muricholate
3α, 6β, 7β-trihydroxy-5β	nd	nd	nd	nd	—	tr	—	—	β-Muricholate
3α, 12α-dihydroxy-5α	27	31	120	83	2	20	—	—	—
3β, 12α-dihydroxy-5β	5	7	22	15	nd	nd	nd	nd	—
3α, 12α-dihydroxy-5β	92	88	70	57	9	36	1	—	Deoxycholate
3α, 12β-dihydroxy-5β	22	17	tr	tr	nd	nd	nd	nd	—
3β, 12α-dihydroxy-5α	2	2	95	20	23	75	—	—	—
3α, 7α-dihydroxy-5α	nd	nd	nd	nd	—	167	—	275[c]	—
3α, 7α-dihydroxy-5β	nd	nd	nd	nd					Chenodeoxy-cholate
3β, 7α-dihydroxy-5α	nd	nd	nd	nd	—	67	—	—	
3α-hydroxy-5α	2	5	11	4	nd	nd	nd	nd	—
3α-hydroxy-5β	10	21	105	41	nd	nd	nd	nd	Lithocholate

[a] Data from References 45 and 137. Gall-bladder bile was obtained from rabbits and cats; rat bile was collected by bile duct cannulation during 1 to 12 hr and 48 to 60 hr after insertion of the cannula.
[b] nd = not determined; tr = a trace.
[c] Indicates that both mono and disulfates have been found.

consequence, there is ample opportunity for their sulfation, which facilitates their urinary elimination.

On the other hand, the kidney may play an important role in sulfation of the bile salts under diseased conditions, when for instance, the liver does not take up the bile salts from the blood any more. Bile salts sulfotransferase is present in the kidney (Chapter 5, Section IVE), and the percentage of bile salts in the urine that is sulfated is much higher than that in serum.[40,125,126,128] About 2 to 20% of the total bile-salt concentration in serum is in the form of sulfate conjugates; this may be higher during liver disease, where for instance, 50% was found sulfated in serum from cholestatic patients. In urine up to 80% of the bile salts may be sulfated. This implies that either the kidney preferentially excretes the sulfate conjugates, or that it actively sulfates the bile salts before eliminating them into the urine. Indeed, the isolated perfused kidney does sulfate bile salts.[134,135,144] Barnes et al.[144] perfused isolated rat kidneys with a protein-free dextran medium under carefully controlled conditions.[135] Because no protein was present, the problem of protein binding of the bile salts was circumvented; in fact, the presence of bovine serum albumin virtually completely prevents the metabolism of bile salts to polar metabolites.[135] When [14C]-labeled chenodeoxycholate and lithocholate were added to the perfusion medium, they were identified as sulfate conjugates in urine and perfusion medium. Their identity was confirmed by the incorporation of [35S]-labeled inorganic sulfate added to the perfusion medium. When low concentrations of the sulfate conjugates were added to the perfusion medium, they were only slowly eliminated in urine, because they were 90% reabsorbed from the urine. If, however, high concentrations of nonsulfated bile salts were present, the reabsorption of the sulfate conjugates was much decreased, and then the [35S]-labeled sulfate conjugates were rapidly excreted in the urine. The authors[144] concluded that the rapid urinary excretion of the sulfated bile salts most likely is due to competition for reabsorption in the kidney between sulfated and nonsulfated bile salts, with the latter having the highest affinity. This conclusion was confirmed by Czygan et al.[134] who used a similar perfused rat kidney system. They found higher sulfation rates for monohydroxy bile salts than for dihydroxy bile salts in this system. These findings underline the importance of the kidneys in the elimination of bile salts during liver disease, although many details have still to be filled in.

Interaction with drugs may affect sulfation of the bile salts at various levels. So far one such interaction has been reported: ethinylestradiol impairs the conversion of deoxycholate to taurocholate. The latter requires 7α-hydroxylation and taurine conjugation. Under these conditions the sulfation of infused deoxycholate in the rat is increased.[145] Most likely more interactions will be found, for instance with compounds that compete with bile salts for sulfation.

As with the xenobiotic substrates and steroids, also with bile salts, glucuronidation may compete for the same substrate; bile-salt glucuronides have been identified in humans and animals.[146-148]

Chemically, bile-salt sulfates can easily be synthesized in various positions by using sulfur-trioxide complexes or chlorosulfonic acid.[149-153] Several reactive derivatives of sulfated bile salts have been synthesized recently, that will be tested as affinity labels in the isolation of bile salt carriers from ileum and other tissues.[154]

E. Steroid Hormones and Related Compounds as Substrates

Steroid hormones are derived from cholesterol and comprise a great number of chemical structures of which a few are shown in Figure 2. Since the steroid hormones are further metabolized to very many metabolites by oxidation and reduction reactions, hydroxyl groups are introduced in various positions of the steroid nucleus, and therefore, a host of steroid hormone-derived sulfate conjugates is usually observed in various tissues or body fluids. An excellent review on all aspects of sulfate conjugation of steroids is the book *Chemical and Biological Aspects of Steroid Conjugation*, published in 1970.[155]

From a chemical point of view the first subdivision that can be made is between sulfate conjugates at the hydroxyl group in a primary (e.g., C_{21}), secondary (e.g., C_3, or C_{11}), or tertiary (C_{17}) alcoholic position in steroids with a saturated A ring, and the phenolic hydroxyl group in the steroids with an aromatic A ring such as C_3 in estradiol. The latter sulfate conjugates can be hydrolyzed by arylsulfatase, whereas the alcoholic sulfate conjugates may be hydrolyzed by so-called steroid sulfatases.[23,27,156] The alcoholic sulfate conjugates are usually identified by solvolysis (see Section IIA); the exact position of the conjugated hydroxyl group can be determined by derivatization of the free hydroxyl groups by, e.g., acetylation with acetic anhydride before solvolysis,[157,158] so that the only (or two in the case of a disulfate conjugate) free hydroxyl group after solvolysis can be identified in the mass spectrogram.

Tables 3 and 4 illustrate the complication pattern of steroid sulfate conjugates that may be found in human bile and intestinal contents of early and midterm fetuses.[159,160] As many as 29 components were identified, both as mono-and disulfate conjugates. Following intravenous administration of 4-[^{14}C]-labeled cortisol to several human volunteers, Kornel and Miyabo[161] identified 20 different metabolites of this compound in urine, that were present in sulfated form.

Usually glucuronide conjugates are also formed of the various steroids, and in addition to that, mixed glucuronide-sulfate diconjugates are often found in considerable amounts.[50,155,162-164] Similarly mixed conjugates with other sugars are found such as with N-acetylglucosamine.[165,166] Since there is such an overwhelmingly extensive literature on the various mono-, di-, and mixed-sulfate conjugates, formed in the

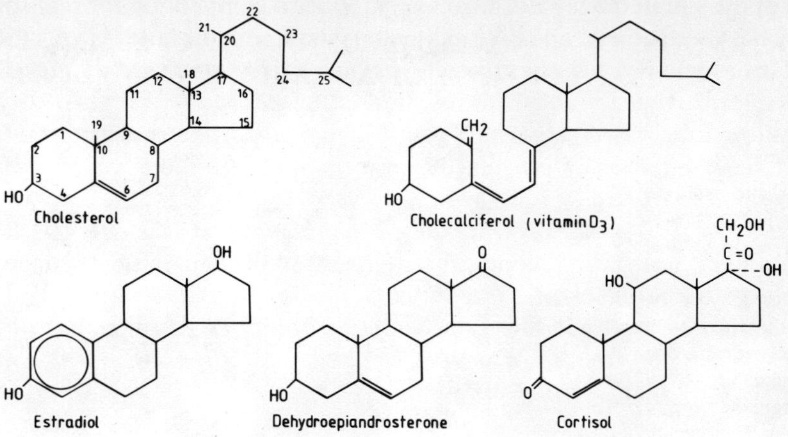

FIGURE 2.   Chemical structure of some substrates for sulfation (steroid hormones and analogues).

Table 3
SOME STEROID SULFATES IDENTIFIED IN HUMAN BILE

Steroid	Fistula bile[a] pool	N[b]	Gall-bladder[a] bile pool
Monosulfates			
3α-hydroxyandrost-5-en-17-one	2.1 ± 0.4[c]	11	4.6
Androsterone	9.3 ± 0.3	11	36.5
Etiocholanolone	2.6 ± 0.2	11	12.2
Dehydro*epi*androsterone	34.9 ± 1.1	11	97.0
Pregnenolone	7.5 ± 0.8	11	22.8
5α-pregnane-3α, 20α-diol	3.4 ± 0.4	9	37.0
5β-pregnane-3α, 20α-diol	2.5 ± 0.5	9	23.3
Pregn-5-ene-3β, 20α-diol	10.1 ± 0.4	11	17.1
Disulfates			
5α-androstane-3α, 17α-diol	10.1 ± 1.7	7	9.8
5α-androstane-3α, 17β-diol	23.2 ± 2.8	7	14.4
androst-5-ene-3β, 17α-diol	42.4 ± 5.1	7	105
androst-5-ene-3β, 17β-diol	33.1 ± 3.0	7	69.0
5α-pregnane-3α, 20α-diol	7.5 ± 1.3	6	54.0
5β-pregnane-3α, 20α-diol	4.0 ± 0.3	6	27.0
Pregn-5-ene-3β, 20α-diol	133 ± 7.1	7	254

[a] Quantitation of steroid sulfates in a fistula bile pool from men and in a gall-bladder bile pool from women. Values are expressed as µg of the free steroid/100 m*l* bile.

[b] N = number of determinations.

[c] Mean ± S.D.

From Laatikainen, T. and Vihko, R., *Steroids*, 14, 119, 1969. With permission.

various species investigated, it is outside the scope of this book to give a detailed account of all the various sulfate conjugates; the interested reader is referred to one of the many reviews on steroid metabolism.[155,167,168] In this section we will briefly review some of the topics of interest and illustrate them with only a few references.

First of all, sulfate conjugates of steroid metabolites may be formed by sulfation of the metabolite or by further metabolism of sulfate conjugates. Many sulfate conjugates are good substrates for both reduction and oxidation at the steroid nucleus. In this

Table 4
CONCENTRATIONS OF MONO- AND DICONJUGATES OF SOME STEROIDS IN INTESTINAL CONTENTS OF AN EARLY HUMAN FETUS[a]

Steroid	Monosulfate	Disulfate
Dehydroepiandrosterone	220[b]	—
5-Androstene-3β, 17α-diol	20	70
5-Androstene-3β, 17β-diol	20	40
16α-Hydroxydehydroepiandrosterone	440	210
16β-Hydroxydehydroepiandrosterone	80	310
3β, 17β-Dihydroxy-5-androsten-16-one	180	430
18-Hydroxyandrosterone	—	50
5-Androstene-3β, 16α, 17β-triol	50	20
5-Androstene-3β, 16β, 17α-triol	—	30
3α-Hydroxy-5β-pregnan-20-one	180	—
Pregnenolone	320	—
3β-Hydroxy-5, 16-pregnadien-20-one	790	—
3β, 15ξ-Dihydroxy-5, 16-pregnadien-20-one[c]	230	—
5α-Pregnane-3α, 20α-diol	—	130
5α-Pregnane-3β, 20α-diol	90	150
5β-Pregnane-3α, 20α-diol	500	590
5-Pregnene-3β, 20α-diol	390	160
3β, 16α-Dihydroxy-5β-pregnan-20-one	80	—
16α-Hydroxypregnenolone	240	190
17α-Hydroxypregnenolone	80	20
3α, 21-Dihydroxy-5β-pregnan-20-one	80	160
21-Hydroxypregnenolone	390	400
3β, 21-Dihydroxy-5, 16-pregnadien-20-one[c]	320	490
5α-Pregnane-3α, 20α, 21-triol	200	
5β-Pregnane-3α, 20α, 21-triol	—	420
5-Pregnene-3β, 20α, 21-triol	—	230
3ξ, 15ξ, 16ξ-Trihydroxy-5ξ-pregnan-20-one[c]	100	—
3ξ, 16ξ, 19-Trihydroxy-5ξ-pregnan-20-one[c]	130	—
3β, 11β, 21-Trihydroxy-5β-pregnan-20-one	310	10
Total	5440	4110

[a] The meconium was obtained from one fetus of 2.7 g (age 20 weeks, crown-rump length 20 cm).
[b] The values are expressed as μg of the steroid (unconjugated) in 100 g meconium (wet weight).
[c] Tentative identification of steroid.

From Huhtaniemi, I. and Vihko, R., *J. Endocrinol.*, 57, 143, 1973. With permission.

process the sulfate group is left in position, but may change the type of metabolism considerably.[155] Thus, female guinea-pig liver microsomes converted estrone and estradiol-17β under certain conditions to 16β-hydroxylated products, whereas the corresponding 3-sulfate conjugates of these compounds were predominantly converted to the 16α-hydroxylated products.[169] Ingelman-Sundberg et al.,[170] who did very extensive work on the metabolism in vitro of sulfated steroids, concluded that a hydrophilic sulfate group in the 18, 19, 21, or 27 position causes a slightly different part of the hydrophobic moiety of the steroid substrate to be exposed to the active site of cytochrome P_{450}. As a consequence, quite big differences in the metabolism by this monooxygenase may result: whereas human fetal liver microsomal preparations do not hydroxylate estradiol, estradiol-3-sulfate was both hydroxylated in the 15α and 16α positions. A 15β-hydroxylase (containing cytochrome P_{450}) that can hydroxylate 5α-androstane-3α,17β-diol-3,17-disulfate has been solubilized from rat liver microsomes.[171] A number of hydroxysteroid oxidoreductases were equally or more active with sulfated substrates than the corresponding unconjugated substrates[172] (see Chapter 7,

Section IA). However, in bovine adrenal cortex mitochondria a much higher affinity of cytochrome P_{450} was found for some unconjugated steroids than for their sulfated conjugates.[173] Although the role of the sulfate conjugates in the interconversion of the several steroids is not completely clear, an important role of these conjugates in steroid metabolism is certainly suggested by these and similar findings.[174] Thus, for instance, Ruokonen et al.[175,176] have pointed out that sulfated precursors may be important intermediates in the testicular biosynthesis of testosterone, and that steroid sulfatases may therefore be involved in the regulation of this process. Biosynthesis and metabolism of testosterone sulfate have been reviewed recently.[177]

Whereas sulfate conjugates may be further metabolized, glucuronide conjugates of the same steroid substrate usually are left intact in vivo. This can be shown by injection of both glucuronide and sulfate conjugates of the same compound. Thus, when Matsui and Hakozaki[178] injected the glucuronide or sulfate conjugate of androsterone into rats, they observed rapid excretion in bile of the unchanged glucuronide. However, the sulfate conjugate was futher metabolized to several more, oxidized sulfate conjugates and to disulfates. Similar in vivo findings were reported on testosterone and corticosterone.[179-181] Therefore, it may well be that only a limited number of free steroid hormones are substrates for sulfation, and that other steroid sulfate conjugates found in vivo are formed from these "primary" sulfates by further metabolism. An additional reason why the sulfate conjugates are much more further metabolized than the glucuronide conjugates may be that the sulfates are more slowly eliminated than the glucuronide conjugates.[161,178]

The fact that several organs release preferentially sulfated steroid hormones suggests that sulfatases play an important role in the effects of several steroid hormones. For instance, the human adrenal cortex excretes large amounts of dehydroepiandrosterone sulfate into the blood.[174] Similarly, the human testis secretes sulfated neutral steroids and this process is dependent on human choriogonadotropin (HCG).[182] Such sterol sulfates are avidly taken up by spermatozoa and have been suggested to affect membrane properties.[183] Therefore, sulfate conjugates of the steroids are not necessarily end products of catabolism, but rather are storage forms of these hormones that can be released when required by sulfatase action. To a certain extent the hormones are protected against some of the catabolic reactions as shown when the metabolism of estrone and estrone-3-sulfate are compared in the isolated perfused rat liver: the sulfate conjugate is cleared much more slowly than unconjugated estrone, and is metabolized also much slower.[184]

Usually the amounts of double conjugates formed are much smaller than those of the monoconjugates; possibly the monoconjugates are relatively poor substrates of the conjugating enzymes. As yet it is unclear how many sulfotransferases are involved in the various sulfation reactions of steroids and which factors govern substrate specificity and reaction rates at the various hydroxyl groups; this is more fully discussed in Chapter 5 (Section IV).

A factor which may contribute to the relatively slow elimination of sulfate conjugates of the steroids is that these conjugates are strongly protein-bound in blood, especially to albumin.[185-187] This strong protein binding may prevent their filtration in the kidney glomerulus and decrease their hepatic extraction rate. In the liver cytosol they may be bound very strongly to the hepatic cytosolic binding protein ligandin, as shown to be the case with estrone sulfate [188] and dehydroepiandrosterone sulfate.[189] Many of the sulfate conjugates are excreted in bile.[159,178,179,186,190-192] Although most of the biliary-excreted steroid sulfates are also found in urine, sometimes a sulfate is preferentially found in bile, and is lacking in urine, such as estrone-3-sulfate in the guinea pig.[190] In dog bile no sulfate conjugates of injected testosterone were found.[193] Many steroid sulfates are found in urine.[155,161,174,194] Even lower animals such as the starfish[195] and sea urchin[196] excrete steroid sulfates.

Although the hydrophilic sulfuric acid moiety makes them more water-soluble, steroid sulfates may still be rather lipophilic.[197,198] Thus estrone sulfate dissolves in egg phosphatidylcholine liposomes during equilibrium dialysis.[188]

Obviously, the amount of sulfated steroids of endogenous origin excreted in urine and bile is under complicated hormonal control.[199] Aso et al.[200] found a cyclic variation of pregnenolone sulfate in plasma of normal menstruating women, whereas the levels of dehydroepiandrosterone sulfate showed no such change. Many steps are involved, including various steroid (-sulfate) dehydrogenase activities and the supply of precursors of steroid hormones from, e.g., the adrenals or placenta/uterus. During pregnancy, healthy women excrete several steroid sulfate conjugates in urine that are not present in urine of non-pregnant women;[201] again this probably is due to an altered steroid pattern and not to any effect on sulfotransferases. Steroid sulfatases also play a role (see Chapter 7, Section III) as illustrated by the fact that pregnant women with a placental sulfatase deficiency excrete very high levels of steroid sulfates in urine.[202] Several other diseases have effects on the excretion of steroid hormones and their sulfate conjugates, such as congenital adrenal hyperplasia,[203] primary aldosteronism,[204] and mammary tumors,[205] to name just a few. Again many factors may determine the changes observed. Similarly, drugs may change the excretion of sulfated steroid hormones, as observed, e.g., with oral contraceptives[206] or ampicillin.[207] Many oral contraceptives are also sulfated to a high extent,[208] because they are steroid analogues; therefore, they may inhibit sulfation of endogenous steroid hormones competitively.

Some other steroid structures are also sulfated in vivo. A sulfate conjugate of 24-hydroxycholesterol has been found in human plasma[48] and in the feces of infants.[209] Similarly, sulfate conjugate(s) of vitamin D_3 have been isolated from normal milk (where it is the major form of vitamin D);[210] the metabolism of vitamin D_3-sulfate has been studied in the rat.[211]

F. Other Low-Molecular Weight Endogenous Substrates of Sulfation

Many substrates for sulfation are present in animals, derived both from food (xenobiotics) and from the metabolism of endogenous compounds. Thus, in 1960 Spencer[212] detected many radioactively labeled compounds in bile and urine when he administered [^{35}S]-labeled inorganic sulfate to rats, which presumably were sulfate conjugates of steroids and phenols (see Chapter 7, Section III A). Here some examples will be given of substrates that are formed by metabolism of endogenous compounds. No further discussion of substrates taken up from the natural environment[213,214] will be given, since these are to be considered as xenobiotics (albeit "physiological" ones when compared with recent additions to the natural environment such as dyes, food additives, insecticides, etc., etc.).

Several neurotransmitters in brain or their metabolites are excreted as sulfate conjugates. Although under normal conditions the main metabolism of 5-hydroxytryptamine (serotonin) is to 5-hydroxyindoleacetic acid or the corresponding alcohol, under conditions of increased serotonin supply especially the amount excreted as the sulfate conjugate increases;[215,216] this may occur when a serotonin-producing tumor is present or when monoaminooxidase, the main metabolizing enzyme is inhibited. Another important transmitter that is in part converted to the sulfate conjugate (at the phenolic-OH group) is noradrenaline (norepinephrine): 3-methoxy-4-hydroxyphenyl-glycol sulfate (MOPEG-sulfate) is a metabolite of noradrenaline that is excreted in the urine.[47,217,218,219] This metabolite is actively transported across the blood-brain barrier, unlike unconjugated MOPEG.[220] A corresponding sulfate conjugate is formed from a dopa and dopamine metabolite, 3-methoxy-4-hydroxyphenylethanol.[221] A 3-*O* and 4-*O*-sulfate ester of dopamine have been identified in urine of Parkinsonian patients receiving a dopa therapy.[222] These sulfate conjugates are not pharmacologically active, but in some cases may be further metabolized. Recently Buu and Kuchel[223,224] have shown that dopamine 3-*O*-sulfate is a substrate for purified bovine dopa β-hydroxylase; the K_m for the conjugate, however, is much higher than for the unconjugated substrate.

Besides these neurotransmitter metabolites, many more metabolic products containing a phenolic group may be eliminated from the body as sulfate conjugates. Some of these sulfate conjugates found, e.g. in the urine, may have been formed when they were part of a macromolecular structure. L-Tyrosine-*O*-sulfate is an example of such a compound, which may be formed when a protein is sulfated at one of its exposed tyrosine moieties (see Chapter 5, Section IIID1). When the protein is broken down, the tyrosine-*O*-sulfate is set free, and is excreted,[224,225] or may be hydrolyzed by more or less specific sulfatases.[226] Similarly, the sulfated glycosaminoglycans are catabolized in vivo which releases sulfated saccharides, that can subsequently be found in urine. Again in this case, the substrate for sulfation were not the sugars or uronic acids themselves, but the polymerized glycosaminoglycan.[227,228]

Another compound that has been claimed to be sulfated is bilirubin, the main metabolism of which is conjugation with glucuronic acid or related sugars.[229] Several reports have suggested that it is excreted as the (di)sulfate conjugate,[230-232] but such a structure has not been identified unequivocally so far.

Taurine is synthesized in mammals from cysteine.[233] However, synthesis from inorganic sulfate in the rat has been suggested recently by Robeson and Martin.[234] When they gave a cysteine-low diet to rats treated with zinc, they observed much enhanced incorporation of [^{35}S]-labeled inorganic sulfate into taurine. They explain these findings by the fact that the zinc in the diet induces metallothionein synthesis, which requires high amounts of cysteine. Only under these extreme conditions, they suggest, will the rat synthesize its taurine directly from inorganic sulfate.

Several sulfated lipids are synthesized by membrane-bound sulfotransferases; these will incorporate radiolabeled inorganic sulfate.[235-238]

III. SULFATE AVAILABILITY AND SULFATE DEPLETION IN VIVO

The sulfate required for sulfation is provided either by its absorption from the gut, or by sulfoxidation of cysteine. The sulfate supply from these sources may become rate-limiting in the conjugation process at high doses of substrates for sulfation. This was clearly demonstrated by the results of Bray et al,[239] who fed various phenolic compounds to rabbits in huge doses. The concomitant oral administration of a number of sulfate precursors increased the percentage of the dose that became sulfated, and, thereby, decreased the fraction that was glucuronidated. The most effective sulfate precursors in this study were cystine and sulfite: administration of these compounds caused a considerable increase in urinary inorganic sulfate. Much less effective were methionine and sodium thiosulfate, and sodium sulfate, surprisingly, had almost no effect at all. With 4-chlorophenol as substrate, the feeding of cystine increased the excretion of the sulfate conjugate to about three times the amount in controls, and there was a compensating decrease in the synthesis of the glucuronide conjugate. The amounts of some other phenyl sulfates were as much as doubled by cystine of sulfite feeding. Indeed, the doses of the phenols administered to the rabbits were so high, that they may very well have exhausted the available sulfate in the animals. Assuming a sulfate serum concentration of 2 mM[240] and a sulfate distribution space of 25% of body weight (Chapter 3, Section VI), about 500 µmol sulfate per kilogram body weight would be immediately available. The dose administered orally was about 2500 μmol/kg, and 10 to 20% of the dose was usually sulfated in the absence of an additional sulfate precursor. This certainly would require much or even all of the available sulfate. However, no data are available on the physiological rate of supply of inorganic sulfate in the rabbit, and therefore, it is not exactly known what the serum sulfate concentration may have been in these rabbits; it may have been much decreased, eventually to almost zero. Thus, feeding sulfate precursors in that situation may well increase sulfation, presumably by increasing sulfate availability. Direct proof of a depletion of inorganic sulfate, however, was not obtained because Bray et al. did not determine inorganic sulfate in serum in their rabbits. Surprisingly, later investigators also failed to do so in similar experiments on sulfate depletion by substrates of sulfation. Therefore, the evidence for sulfate exhaustion necessarily remained indirect, although the observation of an increase of sulfation by administration of sulfate or a sulfate precursor was confirmed by many other investigators, using very different experimental conditions.[241-249] This has led to a certain inaccuracy in the interpretation of various findings, and therefore, the available data will be discussed at some length.

One important assumption in all this work is that the sulfate concentration in plasma determines the sulfate availability and, by implication, the sulfation rate in the tissues, because intravenous administration of inorganic sulfate increased sulfation rate, notwithstanding the generally presumed poor membrane-permeating properties of the sulfate ion. This implies that there must be a rapid uptake in, for instance, the liver, a major site of sulfation for many compounds. The first study on the rate of availability of plasma sulfate for conjugation of a xenobiotic, phenol, was by Herbai,[250] who measured incorporation of [^{35}S]-labeled sulfate into phenyl sulfate, using [^{3}H]-labeled phenol in mice. He injected simultaneously [^{35}S]-phenol and a tracer dose of [^{35}S]-sulfate intravenously, and measured [^{3}H]/[^{35}S] ratios of phenyl sulfate excreted in urine, various times after injection of the mixture. This ratio was the same in phenyl sulfate collected during the first 15 min and in the next 60 min which indicated that the injected [^{35}S]-sulfate had rapidly mixed with the endogenous sulfate pool used for sulfate conjugation of phenol. That this equilibration was very rapid was confirmed by Mulder and Scholtens[251] in a study on sulfate conjugation of the phenolic drug harmol in the rat. [^{35}S]-labeled sodium sulfate (a tracer dose) and harmol were injected simultaneously into the femoral vein, and the incorporation of [^{35}S]-sulfate into harmol sulfate excreted in bile was followed. There was no lag phase in this incorporation: after 1 min (dead space of the bile ducts), harmol-[^{35}S]-sulfate (determined by radioactivity) and fluorimetrically determined harmol sulfate appeared in bile with the same time course. Therefore, the [^{35}S]-sulfate tracer had mixed with the endogenous sulfate pool directly available for sulfation (mainly in the liver) almost instantaneously. Further, when the specific radioactivity of sulfate in blood decreased, so did the amount of radioactivity of [^{35}S]-sulfate incorporated into harmol sulfate. These results suggest that the liver pharmacokinetically is part of the central compartment for sulfate distribution. In agreement with this, the sulfate concentration in rat-liver cytosol available for sulfation, was calculated to be of the same order of magnitude as the serum concentration, as determined in the isolated perfused rat liver at various sulfate levels in the perfusion medium.[252] As yet, the sulfate concentration and rate of sulfate uptake from blood in other tissues has not been studied in detail.

The above results show that at least for the liver there is a very rapid equilibration of the cellular sulfate pool with serum sulfate. Therefore, any change in blood sulfate levels would result in a corresponding change in availability of sulfate for sulfation in the liver. This would easily explain why administration of sulfate or a sulfate precursor enhanced the sulfation of substrates for sulfotransferases when these were given in very high doses.[239] Two different mechanisms may be involved in depletion of sulfate in blood. In the first place the K_m for sulfate in the overall sulfation process may be high relative to its physiological serum concentration (for instance a K_m equal to this concentration or higher). In that case any decrease in serum sulfate would result in a more or less equivalent decrease in sulfation rate. In the second place the K_m may be much smaller than the physiological sulfate concentration, for instance 10 μM. In that case even a major decrease of serum sulfate would not cause a decrease of sulfation rate unless sulfate were almost completely exhausted. It can easily be seen that if a high K_m is operative, administration of inorganic sulfate may do more than compensate for a loss of sulfate: it may cause an increased sulfation rate by an increased sulfate substrate concentration alone. Therefore, if administration of sulfate causes an increased sulfation of a substrate, this does not necessarily imply that sulfate had been exhausted by the substrate.

When the available data are reviewed with these two possibilities in mind, some results may have to be reinterpretated. This seems the case with the effect of sodium sulfite on harmol conjugation as observed by Slotkin et al.[253] They investigated the metabolism of harmol that was generated from intravenously injected harmine, ("methoxy-harmol") by oxidative demethylation in the rat and other animals. Harmol is subsequently mainly sulfated and glucuronidated, and the conjugates are excreted in urine and bile.[253,254] A decrease was observed in the ratio between harmol glucuronide and harmol sulfate (G/S ratio) excreted in urine when they administered sodium sulfite intraperitoneally at the same time as harmine (i.v.). They concluded that sulfite increased sulfation, but their results clearly show that rather than an increase in sulfation, sulfite caused a decrease in glucuronidation. In vitro it has been shown that high concentrations of sulfate indeed inhibit glucuronidation of harmol by UDP-glucuronosyltransferase.[255] Moreover, the dose of harmine was about 20 μmol/kg, and even if all of it were converted into harmol sulfate (which is certainly not the case), still only about 10% of the directly available sulfate pool would have been required (assuming a plasma concentration of 0.8 mM sulfate, and a sulfate space of 25% of body weight). Therefore, the effect of sodium sulfite cannot be a relief of sulfate depletion by harmol sulfation. More likely it is either an inhibition of glucuronidation of harmol, or (if the observed decrease of the glucuronide reflected an increase of harmol sulfate synthesis) an increase of sulfation due to a considerable increase of serum sulfate after the injection of sodium sulfite. If the intraperitoneal dose (0.47 mmol sulfite per kilogram) is rapidly absorbed, it would increase plasma sulfate (assuming rapid oxidation of sulfite to sulfate) by at most 1.9 mM; almost certainly, therefore, the plasma level of sulfate in the experiment will have been considerably above normal. The interpretation of the results is further complicated because in this study the precursor harmine was used (does sulfite administration affect oxidative demethylation of harmine to harmol?), and because the authors did not collect bile, in which a considerable part of the dose is excreted.[254]

Büch et al.[242] have determined the effect of intravenous administration of sodium sulfate on sulfation of a high dose of paracetamol (acetaminophen). After intraperitoneal injection of 1330 μmol/kg paracetamol in rats, the urinary excretion of free inorganic sulfate was very strongly decreased, with a concomitant, slightly higher, increase in the excretion of esterified sulfate, mainly paracetamol sulfate. Subsequently, sodium sulfate was administered intravenously to rats, leading to a transient plasma concentration of about 12 to 16 mM sulfate (the physiological level being about 0.8 mM!). A 70% increase of sulfation of paracetamol resulted, as compared to control rats that received no such sulfate injection. The authors conclude that sulfate was depleted in the control rats by the paracetamol injection and that the sulfate injection compensated this. About 100 to 160 μmol paracetamol sulfate was synthesized by the rats in this experiment. The 60 μmol free sulfate normally excreted in urine during the period of the trial was used for sulfation, and in addition to that a further 60 μmol of sulfate was available in the sulfate distribution space. Therefore, a depletion of sulfate is to be expected and indeed has been demonstrated.[256] The intravenous injection of sulfate may have prevented this depletion, and (in addition) it may have enhanced sulfation rate by the high resulting plasma sulfate concentration.[249] Büch et al.[242] further found that sodium thionite (i.v.) was even more effective than sulfate (Table 5). Intraperitoneal injection of DMSO enhanced sulfation too, as well as oral administration of cysteine. Rather surprising is the fact that in none of these experiments the glucuronidation of paracetamol decreased as its sulfation increased. The latter increase, therefore, resulted in a more complete recovery of the drug in the urine.

In a second series of experiments,[242] increasing doses of paracetamol were injected intraperitoneally in rats, and the effect of the high intravenous dose of sodium sulfate was determined (Table 6). At every dose level the sulfate injection increased the excretion of the sulfate conjugate. However, the effect of the administered sulfate diminished as the dose of paracetamol was increased, which implies that in addition to sulfate availability, other factors must play a role, such as saturation of the sulfotransferase with the substrate paracetamol at high dose. On the other hand, the rate of absorption from the peritoneal cavity may have become rate limiting at high dose. Another surprising finding was that phenobarbital pretreatment increased sulfation of paracetamol only after the intravenous injection of sulfate, to 170% of control. Since many interactions have to be considered in the analysis of effects of phenobarbital pretreatment, these interesting findings require more work before the mechanisms involved can be fully understood.

Several papers on sulfate availability as a rate-limiting factor in sulfation have been published by the group of Levy.[241,243,247,249,257-259] They advocate sulfate depletion by substrates of sulfation mainly because administration of cysteine or sulfate enhances sulfation of several drugs in human volunteers. Thus by treating their volunteers with 2 g of cysteine every hour, starting 3 hr before the administration of the drug salicylamide (7.3 mmol or 1000 mg orally), the percentage that became sulfated was almost doubled.[241,243] Assuming a plasma concentration of 0.3 mM and a sulfate distribution volume of 25% of body weight, the directly available sulfate pool in a 70-kg human being is about 5.5 mmol. In control subjects about 30% of the dose, i.e., 2.2 mmol, was sulfated. The urinary excretion of about 24 mmol inorganic sulfate per 24 hr implies that there is supplementation of about 1 mmol sulfate per hour, and therefore, the decrease in plasma sulfate by oral salicylamide must have been small. Indeed, Greiling and Schulder[260] showed that a much higher dose of salicylamide, about 2500 mg, caused only a 40% decrease in serum sulfate after 2½ hours in patients. In the above experiments cysteine may have increased serum sulfate considerably, and thereby have caused an increased rate of sulfation of salicylamide.

Paracetamol (which, as salicylamide, is both sulfated and glucuronidated in vivo) decreased the sulfation of salicylamide and increased its glucuronidation. Apparently, paracetamol has a higher affinity for sulfation than salicylamide, whereas its affinity for glucuronidation must be lower. The administration of cysteine seemed to abolish the effect of paracetamol on salicylamide sulfation, as measured once in one volunteer.[243] It is hard to evaluate the reliability and reproducibility of this finding without data on reproducibility of the conjugation pattern in that volunteer. Moreover, later the effect of cysteine could not be reproduced by this group[247] possibly because a different dose schedule for cysteine was used.

Table 5

EFFECT OF VARIOUS SULFATE PRECURSORS ON SULFATION AND GLUCURONIDATION OF PARACETAMOL IN THE RAT[a]

Sulfate precursor[b] (dose, route)	Paracetamol conjugate in urine[c]		Total recovery of paracetamol metabolites[c]
	Sulfate (μmol)	Glucuronide (μmol)	(μmol)
Controls	80 ± 7[d]	97 ± 20	209
Sodium sulfate (1 mmol, i.v.)	143 ± 32	74 ± 13	243
Sodium thiosulfate (1 mmol, i.v.)	166 ± 21	113 ± 15	305
DMSO (4 mmol, i.p.)	103 ± 17	77 ± 12	208
Cysteine (2 mmol, oral)	99 ± 13	90 ± 3	196

[a] The rats used were female rats of body weight 250 to 300 g; the dose of paracetamol was 1330 μmol/kg intraperitoneally (about 350 μmol per rat).

[b] Sodium sulfate and sodium thiosulfate were administered intravenously shortly after paracetamol; dimethylsulfoxide (DMSO) 10 min before paracetamol; and cysteine immediately before paracetamol.

[c] The amount excreted in urine collected during 4 hr after injection of paracetamol is given.

[d] The mean ± S.D. or S.E.M. of 18, 8, 4, 10, and 4 rats per group, respectively.

From Büch, H., Rummel, W., Pfleger, K., Eschrich, C., and Texter, N., *Naunyn-Schmiedeberg's Arch. Pharmacol.*, 259, 276, 1968. With permission of Springer-Verlag, Heidelberg.

Table 6

EFFECT OF AN INTRAVENOUS INJECTION OF SODIUM SULFATE ON SULFATION OF PARACETAMOL IN THE RAT

Dose[a]		Paracetamol sulfate in urine in 4 hr	
(μmol/kg i.p.)	(μmol/rat)[b]	Controls (μmol)	After 1 mmol sodium sulfate[a] (μmol)
500	125	48 ± 12[c]	92 ± 19
1330	330	80 ± 7	143 ± 32
2000	500	99 ± 20	129 ± 24
4000	1000	85 ± 36	110 ± 39

[a] The body weight of the rats was 250 to 300 g (females); sodium sulfate was given as an i.v. injection, increasing plasma sulfate to 14 to 16 m*M*, from the normal level of 0.8 mM.

[b] Calculated from the dose by assuming a body weight of the rats of 250 g.

[c] Mean ± S.D. or S.E.M. (not stated) for 10 to 18 rats per group.

From Büch, H., Rummel, W., Pfleger, K., Eschrich, C., and Texter, N., *Naunyn-Schmiedeberg's Arch. Pharmacol.*, 259, 276, 1968. With permission of Springer-Verlag, Heidelberg.

The oral administration of 3 g of ascorbic acid, presumably a substrate for sulfation, to human volunteers decreased considerably the urinary excretion of paracetamol sulfate: from 33% in controls to 23% of the dose, with a corresponding increase in paracetamol glucuronide.[247] The same was found for salicylamide.[257] The mechanism of this effect was supposed to be competition of ascorbic acid with paracetamol (or salicylamide) for the available sulfate: administration of sodium sulfate (but not of cysteine) abolished the effect of ascorbic acid.[247] The interpretation of these effects, however, is complicated by the fact that the percentage of ascorbic acid that is converted to the sulfate conjugate is unknown. In fact, the available data suggest that only a (very) minor percentage may be converted to the 2-sulfate conjugate (see Section IIC) in vivo.

Serum sulfate determination would have given the answer, but was not done. Even more important, however, is that the authors have not determined the effect of sodium sulfate alone on the metabolism of paracetamol. Since the sulfation of salicylamide in man can be enhanced by administration of cysteine[243] and that of paracetamol in the rat by giving sulfate,[242,249] it seems an obvious control experiment to test the effect of sodium sulfate on sulfation of paracetamol in the volunteers. Sulfate treatment may have increased the amount sulfated above the control, from, e.g., 30% of the dose to 40%, then ascorbic acid treatment might have decreased it again to the control level of 30%. Unfortunately, this control experiment is lacking and, therefore, these experiments permit no conclusion as to the mechanism. One might consider competition of paracetamol and ascorbic acid for sulfation. Further, effects of ascorbate and sodium sulfate on the rate of absorption of paracetamol from the gut like the retarding effect of acetylsalicylate[261,262] may affect the balance between sulfation and glucuronidation.

Recently, Galinsky et al.[263] reported in the rat an increased sulfation and decreased glucuronidation of paracetamol by concomitant administration of N-acetylcysteine in vivo. They suggest that N-acetylcysteine is a source of inorganic sulfate in the rat. Other groups have shown that N-acetylcysteine is used for the synthesis of glutathione in hepatocytes.[264]

Another drug that has been studied in man is tyramine. Urinary excretion of the sulfate conjugate of this drug was enhanced by the oral administration of sodium sulfate.[245] At most, 15% of the dose (0.7 mmol) was excreted as sulfate ester in urine. This requires about 0.10 mmol of the 5.5 mmol sulfate directly available for sulfation in a 70-kg man. It is obvious, therefore, that a 30% increase of sulfate conjugation of tyramine observed after oral administration of sodium sulfate (2.1 mmol) cannot have been due to depletion of sulfate by tyramine and replenishment by the oral sulfate dose. The most likely explanation seems that tyramine is sulfated during absorption in the mucosa. The administration of sodium sulfate may lead to a greatly increased sulfate concentration in the mucosa cells. This may increase a first-pass sulfation of tyramine in the mucosa (sse Section IVB).

Much more indirect evidence of enhancement of sulfation comes from experiments on the effect of sulfate feeding or sulfate withdrawal on the toxicity of compounds that are assumed to be detoxified or toxified by sulfation; the growth-inhibiting effect of indole in the rat was relieved by feeding the sulfate precursors cysteine or methionine.[244] Also, a decrease in the toxicity of paracetamol by huge doses of sodium sulfate was observed.[258] In both cases, sulfation leads to less toxic compounds, and sodium sulfate or cysteine feeding was supposed to increase the rate of sulfation, i.e., detoxification.

In spite of the fact that often a decreased serum sulfate has been postulated, only few investigators have actually measured serum sulfate after administration of high doses of a substrate of sulfation. Already in 1963, Greiling and Schulder[260] showed that therapeutic doses of salicylamide (50 mg/kg) caused a 40% reduction in serum sulfate after 2½ hr in patients. After 7 hr the sulfate levels were back at control levels. Acetylsalicylate and salicylate did not cause any reduction in serum sulfate: these drugs are not sulfated, whereas salicylamide is. Much later, Weitering et al.[265] showed that phenol at high doses (266 μmol/kg intravenously) decreased serum sulfate from 0.92 mM to 0.71 mM (the lowest point) 1 hr after phenol. Since sulfate conjugation required about 106 μmol/kg, the concentration of free sulfate should have decreased to about 0.50 mM; this clearly indicates that more sulfate is available than only the free sulfate in the sulfate distribution space. This extra sulfate may become available because urinary excretion of sulfate stops under these conditions.

Another unsolved question is the K_m for sulfate of the overall sulfation process (sulfate activation and sulfate transfer). In isolated perfused organs or with isolated cells and tissue cultures, the sulfate concentration can be varied, and the K_m can be determined. Recently, Mulder and Keulemans[252] reported sulfation and glucuronidation of harmol in the isolated perfused rat liver at three different concentrations of sulfate in the perfusion medium: 0.0, 0.65, and 1.30 mM. At low concentration, only the sulfate present in the liver was available in the system for sulfation. Since this is only a minor amount, they found low sulfation rates at zero sulfate in the perfusion medium. When increasing sulfate to 0.65 mM there was a big rise in sulfation and a corresponding decrease in glucurondiation. Upon further increase of the sulfate concentration in the perfusion medium from 0.65 to 1.30 mM, sulfation increases still further, indicating that the K_m for sulfate of the overall sulfation process was rather high, of the order of the plasma concentration. In these experiments the sulfate availability was not rate limiting at the two higher sulfate concentrations. These findings, therefore, would imply that any decrease of the plasma concentration of free sulfate would be followed by a decrease of sulfation rate in the rat (assuming that the overall K_m for sulfate is the same for every substrate of sulfation).

In isolated rat hepatocytes, a K_m for sulfate in overall sulfation of paracetamol of approximately 3mM was observed.[266] These data are still very incomplete, and more work is needed on the relationship between sulfate concentration and sulfation rate, in order to gain complete insight in the effects of sulfate depletion.

In summary, at high doses of substrates for sulfation, the plasma sulfate concentration may decrease and thereby cause a decreased sulfation rate. Inorganic sulfate or a sulfate precursor may compensate for that. High doses of a sulfate precursor or inorganic sulfate may lead to unphysiologically high sulfate plasma concentrations, which may increase sulfation presumably because of a relatively high K_m for sulfate. A first-pass sulfation in the mucosa may play a role when drugs are administered orally.

IV. SULFATION IN VIVO AND IN ISOLATED CELL PREPARATIONS

Sulfation of compounds with an appropriate acceptor group takes place in several organs, such as the liver, kidneys, and gut; the liver is (quantitatively) the main site of sulfation for most xenobiotics. In Section II of this chapter a survey has been given of the various compounds that may be sulfated in vivo. In this section the following aspects will be discussed:

A.   Species differences
B.   Extrahepatic sulfation
C.   Age and sex differences
D.   Dose dependence in vivo and in isolated hepatocytes
E.   Sulfotransferase and UDP-glucuronosyltransferase as determinants in the balance between sulfation and glucuronidation.

Most of the substrates for sulfation can also be converted by the competing glucuronide conjugation to β-D-glucuronides. It is obvious that the final outcome of the competition between the transferases for the same substrate is usually not determined by a single factor. Only in those cases when one transferase does not at all convert a potential substrate, and only the other accepts it, a single factor, namely, substrate specificity, determines the conjugation pattern. Unfortunately, so far only limited research has been done on this problem. Until recently in most cases data have been collected at only one dose level; since it has been known for a long time that metabolic patterns of drugs in vivo are highly dose dependent, it is hard to evaluate single-dose experiments in terms of competition between the two transferases.

Further competing reactions are *O*-methylation and conjugation with sugars (glucose, *N*-acetylglucosamine) and phosphate.

A. Species Differences

Conjugation with sulfate occurs in mammals, birds, reptiles, and amphibia. In liver slices from various fish species sulfation of phenol has been observed, but to a much lower rate than in rat liver slices.[267] With invertebrates (as far as investigated) ethereal sulfate formation occurs in arthropods, insects, and molluscs. Most work on species differences in a systematic way has been done by R. T. Williams and his group (Table 7). Thus, the metabolism of phenol has been investigated in 19 species, from man to chicken.[268] All species received comparable oral doses, except (understandably) the human volunteers; therefore, their conjugation pattern (at a much lower dose) cannot straightforwardly be compared with the animals (see Section IVD). Later, these observations were extended to even more, exotic species.[269-273] The results indicate that most species can convert phenol to both the sulfate and glucuronide conjugate, though there is a wide variation in the ratio between the conjugates. Usually only the urinary excretion of these is determined, and conjugates excreted in bile have not been collected in most of the studies. This may affect the outcome, because usually the glucuronides are excreted in bile to a higher extent than their sulfate counterparts (see Chapter 7, Section IV).

Of special interest are those species that lack, or are very deficient in one of the conjugations. All representatives of the Felidae have a highly deficient glucuronidation activity towards phenol, although the cat does conjugate some compounds with glucuronic acid (see review by Dutton),[274] possibly because these are extremely poor substrates of sulfation. On the other extreme, the pig has a very deficient sulfation capacity since, for instance, (almost) no phenyl sulfate is formed from phenol. The commonly used laboratory animals, rat and mouse, excrete about the same amounts of both conjugates whereas the guinea pig clearly prefers glucuronidation.

The preference of the cat for sulfation was further confirmed when harmol, quinol, 2, 6-dimethoxyphenol, 1-naphthol, 2-naphthol, morphine, phenacetin (a precursor of paracetamol), and phenolphthalein were used as substrates.[275-277] Only phenolphthalein and harmol were glucuronidated to a considerable extent, the other substrates being almost completely converted to the sulfate esters. In the pig, mainly glucuronidation was observed with 2-naphthol, phenacetin, and 4-hydroxyamphetamine, but 1-naphthol was converted to the sulfate ester to a high extent, confirming that the pig has the ability to conjugate with sulfate. Besides differences in amounts of the conjugating enzymes, different volumes of distribution of the lipid-soluble compounds between the species, and the rate of release of the accumulated compound from the fat tissues into the blood may play a role in these species differences.

Studies with harmol confirmed the preference for glucuronidation in the rabbit and guinea pig, whereas in the rat and mouse appreciable amounts of both conjugates were found.[275] Similarly, in rat, mouse, and hamster about equal amounts of the glucuronide and sulfate conjugates of paracetamol were formed at a dose of 330 μmol/kg (i.p.).[278] However, in isolated hepatocyte preparations, those from mouse liver had a lower sulfation rate than those from the rat.[279] In vivo, paracetamol can be generated from its precursor phenacetin by oxidative deethylation. When phenacetin is administered to various species, predominantly the glucuronide of paracetamol is found in urine in the rabbit, guinea pig, and the ferret, whereas in the rat this was the sulfate conjugate.[280] When paracetamol itself was administered orally or intraperitoneally to both Wistar and Sprague-Dawley rats at a low dose, the sulfate conjugate was indeed the most prominent metabolite of paracetamol.[281] In man, at a much lower dose level, about

Table 7
SPECIES DIFFERENCES IN THE CONJUGATION OF ORALLY ADMINISTERED PHENOL[a]

Species (n, sex)	Dose (μmol/ kg)	Radioactivity excreted in 24-hr urine (% of dose)	Phenyl sulfate[b] (%)	Phenyl glucuronide[b] (%)
Primates				
Man (3,m)	0.11	90	77	16
Rhesus monkey (2,f)	530	43	65	35
Squirrel monkey (3,f)	266	31	7	58
Capuchin (1,f)	266	73	14	65
Carnivores				
Ferret (3,f)	266	51	28	40
Cat (3,f)	266	59	87	—[c]
Lion (3,f)	108	77	99	—
Civet (1,f)	108	60	97	—
Genet (2,m)	108	48	99	—
Dog (1,f; 1,m)	266	58	50	18
Hyena (1,f; 1,m)	108	31	90	—
Miscellaneous				
Elephant (1,f)	108	49	73	25
Pig (3,f)	226	51	—	100
Hedgehog (2,m)	213	38	75	15
Fruitbat (2,f)	266	54	10	90
Rabbit (3,f)	266	48	45	46
Chicken (3,f)	266	57	78	22
Rodents				
Rat, Wistar (3,f)	266	95	54	42
Mouse, ICI (3×10,f)	266	66	46	35
Jerboa (3,f)	266	47	61	26
Gerbil (2,f)	266	55	42	35
Hamster (2,f)	266	75	26	43
Lemming (3,f)	266	40	35	39
Guinea pig (2,f)	266	64	18	88

[a] Data taken from References 268, 269, and 271.

[b] When the percentages in the last two columns add up to less than 100%, the remainder consisted of other metabolites, such as quinol conjugates; see original publications.

[c] Means not detectable.

equal amounts of both conjugates were excreted. Another precursor of paracetamol in vivo is aniline, which is converted into paracetamol by a two-step metabolism: first acetylation of the amino group and subsequently hydroxylation in the *para*-position. In addition to parahydroxylation, also *ortho*hydroxylation takes place, but to a much lesser degree. In the pig and sheep the major metabolite of aniline is the glucuronide conjugate of paracetamol, but in the rat it is the sulfate conjugate of this compound,[282] in agreement with the above findings.

A difference in metabolism of dopamine in dogs on one hand, and the rat and guinea pig on the other was pinpointed to a species difference in first-pass sulfation by the gut mucosa.[283]

It can be concluded from these findings that all species mentioned above have the capacity for sulfation and glucuronidation of xenobiotics. The cat, however, preferentially sulfates them, whereas the pig and the rabbit mainly conjugate with glucuronic acid. Caution is warranted, however, because all these findings were obtained in single-dose studies, disregarding dose-dependent shifts in conjugation ratio (see Section IVD). Reviews on species differences in drug metabolism have been published by Williams[284] and R. L. Smith.[285]

B. Extrahepatic Sulfation

In a quantitative sense the liver is the main site of sulfation, because of its high sulfotransferase activities and its size. Moreover, many xenobiotics are rapidly taken up by the liver. Yet, other organs are capable of sulfation of either specific endogenous compounds (such as steroid hormones in the adrenals or testis), or xenobiotics. In fact, most organs probably have the potential for sulfation of low-molecular weight compounds, since the sulfotransferases are widely distributed (Chapter 5, Section IIIE and IVB5 and C4); studies with tissue slices may confirm these findings.

However, as compared to the many data obtained in the isolated perfused liver or isolated hepatocytes (Section IVD), only few studies have been performed with other organs. Only the kidney, lung, and intestine will be discussed here, because such data on other organs are lacking.

Sulfation of phenolic compounds in the kidney has mainly been studied in the Sperber chicken preparation, where drugs are injected in a leg vein. The chick kidney has a portal system through which blood from the leg vein first enters the kidney. Drugs in this blood, therefore, may undergo first-pass metabolism in that kidney. Eventual metabolites can be collected in the urine from that kidney, and urine from the other kidney serves as control. In such a preparation, catechol,[286] morphine,[287] phenol, and 4-nitrophenol[288] are sulfated by the kidney; also glucuronidation occurs. In the isolated perfused rat kidney, lithocholate and chenodeoxycholate were sulfated.[135] These findings in the perfused organ were confirmed by experiments in isolated kidney cells.[289] The cell preparation converted paracetamol into the sulfate and glucuronide conjugates.

Cultures of hamster and rat lung formed various sulfated and glucuronidated metabolites from 3-hydroxybenzo(a)pyrene.[290,291] In short-term organ cultures of human periferal lung only sulfate conjugates were synthesized from both benzo(a)pyrene and 1-naphthol.[292] Therefore, the human lung seems to have a poorly developed glucuronidating capacity.

The gut contains most of the drug metabolizing enzymes.[293] In isolated epithelial intestinal (mucosa) cells from rat and guinea pig many phenolic compounds such as phenol, 1-naphthol, 7-hydroxycoumarin, and 4-hydroxybiphenyl are sulfated (and glucuronidated).[294,295] The highest activity was found at the oral end of the small intestine and the lowest activity at the aboral end. Interestingly, in isolated guinea-pig intestinal cells glucuronidation of 7-hydroxycoumarin was saturated at a lower substrate concentration than sulfation (see Section IVD).[295]

Isolated loops and gut sacks of the intestine from rat and guinea pig similarly conjugate several substrates with sulfuric acid, such as 7-hydroxycoumarin.[296] Possibly also sulfate conjugates are formed from paracetamol and morphine after instillation of these substances in the closed loop in rat intestine;[297] the main conjugates, however, were glucuronides of these compounds. 1-Naphthol formed only the glucuronide during first-pass conjugation in this system.

First-pass sulfation of several drugs during their absorption in the mucosa cells has clearly been demonstrated.[246,297-300] When Powell et al.[299] perfused the lumen of the small intestine of rats *in situ* and added [14C]-phenol to the perfusion medium, in portal blood samples only the sulfate and glucuronide conjugates of phenol could be demonstrated, indicating a complete first-pass metabolism of phenol. These results were confirmed with the drug isoprenaline that is excreted largely unchanged in urine both in man and dog when it is administered intravenously. However, if isoprenaline is given orally, it is excreted principally as sulfate conjugate.[298] These results were explained when it was shown that isoprenaline placed in an isolated dog-gut loop *in situ,* appeared to a small fraction as free isoprenaline in the venous effluent draining the loop, the major proportion being a sulfate conjugate.[300] Salicylamide increased the efflux of free isoprenaline in the venous effluent because its sulfation was inhibited competitively by salicylamide, or because the availability of sulfate in the gut became rate limiting. Indeed, feeding of cysteine in dogs treated with salicylamide decreased the effects of isoprenaline, presumably by increasing the availability of sulfate and, thereby, the inactivation of isoprenaline by its sulfation.[246] A local depletion in the gut mucosa of sulfate by first-pass sulfation can probably very efficiently be overcome by oral administration of sulfate, resulting in a high concentration of sulfate in the gut lumen and in the neighboring mucosa cells.

As yet it is not clear whether first-pass sulfation in the gut is of wider importance, for more drugs. A species difference in this respect has been reported: in the dog, dopamine is mainly sulfated at the 3-position after oral administration, whereas this conjugate was a minor metabolite in the guinea pig and the rat.[283] If the drug was administered intravenously in the dog, it was metabolized mainly by *O*-methylation and deamination, like in the other species. Supernatants from dog gut indeed actively synthesized the sulfate ester of dopamine in vitro, whereas similar supernatants from rat and guinea-pig gut could not catalyze this reaction.

The role of each of these organs in the sulfation of drugs in vivo is not yet clear, and will depend on the structure of the substrate. Only the role of first-pass sulfation in gut or liver can be shown by comparison of oral and intravenous administration of the drug. Differentiation between the role of the gut and the liver may be performed with the isolated loop preparation. For those drugs that are not actively taken up by the liver, extrahepatic sulfation may play an important role. A recent review on extrahepatic drug metabolism is available.[301]

C. Age and Sex Differences

Only a few data are available on the development of sulfation beyond the early postnatal period, as is the case with most drug-metabolizing activities.[302] Clearly, sulfation is present early in fetal development, in some cases at an even higher level than in adults. This has been found in mice,[303] rat, guinea pig,[304] rhesus monkey,[30] and man.[306] For man, this was confirmed in isolated human fetal hepatocytes.[307] Glucuronidation, on the other hand, is very low for most compounds in the early postnatal period in man and other species.[274,308] Miller et al.[306] found higher excretion of the sulfate conjugate or orally administered paracetamol in urine in newborns and 3 to 9-year-old children than in 12-year-old children and adults; glucuronidation of paracetamol was much lower in the newborns than in adults. In man therefore, sulfation can easily compensate for a relative deficiency in glucuronide formation, at least at moderate doses of the substrates. It is not clear whether developmental factors may also play a role in sulfatase activity. Some sulfate conjugates are hydrolyzed in vivo by sulfatase activity (Chapter 7, Section III), and the excretion of some sulfate conjugates may be determined by a balance between sulfotransferase and sulfatase activity (Chapter 7, Section IB). There are no data on the sulfation capacity in old animals or elderly people.

Very little is known about sex differences in conjugation. It seems that the female rat has a lower sulfation rate than the male, and therefore compensates with a higher glucuronidation as shown with paracetamol[309] and 2,6-dimethoxyphenol.[310]

Only for steroid sulfation some data are available on the effect of, e.g., hypophysectomy and hormone treatment in several animal species.[311-316] Since in most cases the effects are too complicated to allow a conclusion as to the mechanism, no further discussion of this aspect is given here. Details about development and sex differences of the sulfotransferase activities may be found in Chapter 5 (Sections IIIE, IVB5, C4, D3).

D. Dose Dependence In Vivo and in Isolated Hepatocytes

Many years ago it was observed that at increasing dose of a substrate for glucuronidation and sulfation, glucuronidation may increase relative to sulfation. Thus, phenol is conjugated with glucuronate and sulfate to about equal amounts when it is fed to rabbits at a dose level of 266 μmol/kg (25 mg/kg). However, at 4- to 10-fold higher doses this ratio changes to about 5 (Table 8).[16,59] These results were confirmed in the rat (Table 8)[265,273] and in various strains of monkeys:[317] intravenous and intramuscular injections of phenol were conjugated increasingly with glucuronic acid as the dose increased. With 1-naphthol as substrate the changes were less pronounced.[317] The data in Table 8 clearly show that the absolute amount of sulfate conjugate synthesized still increases when the percentage of the dose that is sulfated decreases. This indicates that sulfation is not yet saturated at these high doses. Depletion of sulfate plays only a minor role in this relative decrease of sulfation of phenol, because Mulder and Meerman[248] found only a small increase in the sulfation of a high dose of phenol (266 μmol/kg) in the rat by the intravenous infusion of huge amounts of sodium sulfate. Contrary to the findings in the rat and monkeys, mice did not show this shift in conjugation pattern of phenol.[250]

Only few other substrates have been tested in vivo. With 4-hydroxybenzenesulfona-mide, fed to rabbits, a similar shift from sulfate to glucuronide was observed as the dose increased.[63] The drug paracetamol, injected intraperitoneally, has been investigated in hamsters, mice, and rats in vivo.[278] When increasing the dose from 0.2 to 8 mmol/kg, a pronounced shift from sulfation to glucuronidation was observed, especially in the hamster and the rat; in mice, again the shift was only very small.

Later studies with the isolated perfused rat liver and hepatocytes have confirmed this with several substrates. In these systems a depletion of inorganic sulfate can be absolutely excluded and, therefore, the analysis of these findings in terms of mechanism involved is less ambiguous than in vivo.

One of the first studies in the isolated perfused rat liver showing a dose-dependent change in the ratio between sulfation and glucuronidation was the study by Minck et al.[318] on the metabolism of 4-nitrophenol. 4-Nitrophenol, generated in the liver from 4-nitroanisole by monooxygenase activity, is mainly sulfated. When the 4-nitroanisole concentration was increased from 25 to 100 μM (initially), in the perfusion medium especially the glucuronide conjugation of 4-nitrophenol was increased, but still sulfation was by far the most important conjugation reaction (Table 9). If, however, 4-nitrophenol itself was added directly to the perfusion medium, the increase of glucuronidation over the level obtained with 4-nitroanisole is striking: a 5- to 10-fold increase. Sulfation was slightly below the level for 4-nitroanisole. Indeed, at high 4-nitrophenol concentration in the perfusion medium, glucuronidation is the main conjugation reaction.[319] These data show that at a low rate of substrate supply, sulfation is more important than at a high rate. Since the Krebs-Ringer perfusion medium contains 1.2 mM inorganic sulfate, these results cannot be explained by depletion of sulfate. Moreover, Moldeus et al.[320] using isolated hepatocytes demonstrated that 4-nitrophenol and 4-nitroanisole behaved exactly the same in this system. Interestingly, Bray et al.[239] already in 1953 concluded that

Table 8
EFFECT OF DOSE ON SULFATION OF PHENOL IN THE RABBIT AND THE RAT

Species, dose (μmol/kg)	Phenyl sulfate (μmol/kg excreted)	Percentage of dose sulfated
Rabbit, oral dose[59]		
266	109	41[a]
530	197	37
1060	192	18
1600	303	19
2130	393	18
2660	505	19
Rat, intravenous dose[265]		
13	9	72
27	18	66
67	39	58
133	67	50
266	106	40

[a] The remainder of the dose was almost exclusively the glucuronide conjugate in all cases.

Table 9
SULFATION AND GLUCURONIDATION OF 4-NITROPHENOL IN THE ISOLATED PERFUSED RAT LIVER, WHEN 4-NITROPHENOL WAS GENERATED *IN SITU* FROM 4-NITROANISOLE, OR WAS ADDED DIRECTLY TO THE PERFUSION MEDIUM

		4-Nitrophenol conjugates in medium	
Substrate added	Initial concn., μM	Glucuronide[a]	Sulfate[a]
4-Nitroanisole	25	0.1 $\pm$ 0.01[b]	2.0 $\pm$ 0.2
	50	0.4 $\pm$ 0.1	3.5 $\pm$ 0.2
	100	0.25 $\pm$ 0.05	3.5 $\pm$ 0.6
4-Nitrophenol	25	0.7 $\pm$ 0.01	1.1 $\pm$ 0.1
	50	2.1 $\pm$ 0.2	2.5 $\pm$ 0.3
	100	5.7 $\pm$ 0.6	3.6 $\pm$ 0.3

[a] Expressed as nmol conjugate per m*l* perfusion medium per gram liver.
[b] Mean $\pm$ S.E.M., with 4 to 5 perfusions in each group.

From Minck, K., Schupp, R. R., Illing, H. P. A., Kahl, G. F., and Netter, K. J., *Naunyn-Schmiedeberg's Arch. Pharmacol.*, 279, 347, 1973. With permission of Springer-Verlag, Heidelberg.

"it is clear that the administration of a precursor (of a substrate) is equivalent to the continuous administration of its hydroxylation product at a low dose level. Thus the magnitude of the dose of an intermediate having the same metabolic fate (glucuronidation as compared to sulfation) as a given dose of its precursor (. . .) is not the equimolar dose. For instance, the dose of *p*-methoxyphenol having the same metabolic fate as anisole is only 17% of the molar dose of anisole."

Another substrate that has been tested in the isolated perfused rat liver is 4-*N*,*N*-dimethylaminophenol.[321] Increasing the prehepatic concentration of this substrate from 10 to 390 μM in the single-pass liver perfusion medium saturated both sulfation and glucuronidation of this substrate as judged by the concentrations of the conjugates in the liver effluent, which became constant above 100 μM. At low substrate supply, the sulfate conjugate predominated (ratio 4:1), but at increasing dose the glucuronide took over (ratio 1:2). The perfusion medium did not contain erythrocytes in these experiments because these bind most of the compound. When erythrocytes were included, almost only sulfation took place, presumably because only little free substrate was then available. The effect of the presence of erythrocytes is an interesting example of the pitfalls which may occur when in vivo — in vitro comparisons are made and one of the multiple factors is changed for convenience, i.e., when erythrocytes are left out. A similar major change may be observed when albumin is introduced in the incubation medium: it may keep substrates outside the hepatocyctes, and thereby prevent their sulfation.[322]

Conjugation of the phenolic substrate harmol, measured in the perfused rat liver at two-dose levels showed a similar behavior: a fivefold increase in harmol concentration in the perfusion medium (initially) resulted in a threefold increase in the amount excreted in bile as harmol sulfate, and a 11-fold increase in the glucuronide conjugate.[323] This pattern was confirmed in isolated rat hepatocytes.[324,325]

Several other substrates or precursors from which the substrate was generated usually by ring hydroxylation, have been studied in isolated hepatocytes. Biphenyl yielded predominantly the sulfate conjugate of 4-hydroxybiphenyl as metabolite.[326] The glucuronide conjugate, though present, was only 7% of the sulfate. This situation changed drastically when the supply of 4-hydroxybiphenyl was increased by using hepatocytes from phenobarbital-treated rats, and (less so) in those from 3-methylcholanthrene-treated rats: when the rate of hydroxylation of biphenyl was enhanced, glucuronidation became the predominant conjugation reaction. In order to prove that indeed the rate of supply, i.e., the concentration of 4-hydroxybiphenyl (and similarly of 2-hydroxybiphenyl) was the decisive factor, the conjugation of these hydroxylated derivatives has been determined when they were added directly to the hepatocytes in increasing concentration. In this type of experiment, the increase of glucuronidation relative to sulfation at increasing substrate concentration of 4-hydroxybiphenyl and 2-hydroxybiphenyl was confirmed. A tenfold increase in 4-hydroxybiphenyl concentration (from 7 to 70 μM) resulted, e.g., in a 20-fold increase of glucuronidation, but only a 2-fold increase in sulfation. Because sulfate availability cannot have been rate limiting in these experiments, the observed differences most likely are due to a higher K_m for glucuronidation than for sulfation for the hydroxylated biphenyls.

The concentration-dependence of conjugation for a series of substrates of decreasing polarity has been determined by Orrenius' group (Table 10)[324,325] in rat hepatocytes. Sulfation of these compounds was already saturated at 25 μM, since the rate did not increase when the substrate concentration was elevated to 200 μM. However, with the exception of 2-naphthol, the glucuronidation rate of the substrates was higher at 200 μM than at 25 μM, indicating that the K_m for glucuronidation was higher than for sulfation. 4-Nitrophenol and 4-methylumbelliferone were more rapidly sulfated than glucuronidated at 25 μM, whereas at 200 μM this was the reverse. The more water-soluble substrate paracetamol had a much higher K_m for sulfation, about 0.25 mM, but the apparent K_m for glucuronidation was still higher: 5 mM.[327]

Both sulfate and glucuronide conjugates of various hydroxylated benzo *(a)* pyrene metabolites are found in rat hepatocytes.[328-330] The sulfate conjugates are extractable into ethyl acetate, whereas the glucuronides are not, due to differences in lipid-solubility.[329,290] It has been suggested that one of the major sulfated metabolites of benzo*(a)*pyrene, the sulfate ester of 3-hydroxybenzo*(a)*pyrene, may be very persistent in mammals, because its high lipid solubility may prevent it from rapid elimination in urine.[290]

In general it seems from the above discussion that at increasing dose glucuronidation (low affinity, high capacity) takes over from sulfation (high affinity, low capacity). So

Table 10
SULFATION AND GLUCURONIDATION OF A SERIES OF SUBSTRATES OF DECREASING POLARITY BY ISOLATED RAT HEPATOCYTES[a]

Substrate	Concentration (mM)	Sulfate	Glucuronide
		(nmol/10^6 cells/min)	
Paracetamol[b]	0.25	0.77	0.40
	5.0	1.0	1.53
4-Nitrophenol	0.025	0.32	0.06
	0.20	0.31	0.63
4-Methylumbelliferone	0.025	0.65	0.10
	0.20	0.47	1.67
Harmol	0.025	0.33	0.74
	0.20	0.33	1.44
Phenolphthalein	0.025	0.07	0.28
	0.20	0.07	0.92
2-Naphthol	0.025	0.52	0.76
	0.20	0.55	0.94

[a] The polarity decreases from paracetamol to 2-naphthol.
[b] Paracetamol = Acetaminophen.

From Andersson, B., Berggren, M., and Moldeus, P., *Drug Metab. Dispos.*, 6, 611, 1978. With permission of the American Society for Pharmacology and Experimental Therapeutics.

far only very few examples of the reverse situation have been found. A simple explanation is not likely, because several factors may be involved at the same time, such as cosubstrate availability, lipid-solubility of the substrate, substrate specificity of the transferases, pharmacokinetic factors, and changes in uptake by tissues as dose increases. Briefly, this latter point means that a compound that is preferentially taken up in, for instance, the liver at low dose, may be taken up also by other tissues as the dose increases (and hepatic uptake is saturated). At low dose, therefore, the conjugation pattern of the liver may be observed, whereas at increasing dose this pattern may change because, for instance, the kidney starts contributing to the conjugation of the compound, possibly at a different ratio between sulfation and glucuronidation. At present such organ-organ competition is rather speculative, although saturation of first-pass sulfation in the gut mucosa at increasing oral dose might be cited as an example: then the liver or other organs would be presented with the unchanged drug.

One of the few examples of sulfation having a higher capacity and lower affinity than glucuronidation was observed with the substrate 7-hydroxycoumarin in isolated guinea-pig intestinal epithelial cells.[295]

E. Sulfotransferase and UDP-Glucuronosyltransferase as Determinants in the Balance Between Sulfation and Glucuronidation

Several factors will determine how much of a substrate for both sulfotransferase(s) and UDP-glucuronosyltransferase(s) will be converted to a sulfate or a glucuronide conjugate, respectively. Thus, the species differences described in Section IV A may be due to different amounts of both transferases. Dose-dependent changes in the ratio between glucuronidation and sulfation may be a result of the kinetic properties of the transferases, or a depletion of the cosubstrate. Since UDP-glucuronosyltransferase is a microsomal enzyme and sulfotransferases are cytosolic, the substrate for conjugation might show a preference for one of the enzymes, dependent on its lipid-solubility. The following factors will be briefly considered:

1. Subcellular localization of the transferases and lipid solubility of the substrate
2. Substrate specificity and enzyme kinetics of the transferases
3. Cosubstrate availability

1. Subcellular Localization of the Transferases and Lipid Solubility of the Substrate

The enzymes catalyzing glucuronidation reactions are recovered in the microsomal fraction from liver and other tissues; whether the active site is located at the inside of the microsomal vesicles (and, therefore, *in situ,* in the lumen of the endoplasmic reticulum), or at the outside is still a heatedly debated issue.[331-333] Such a localization might have an important consequence: relatively lipid-soluble substrates would have much easier access to the active site. This is suggested by in vitro data on substrate specificity of UDP-glucuronosyltransferase: there is a tendency for higher glucuronidation rates in vitro with increasing lipid solubility of the substrate.[334,335] Hänninen and Alanen[336] found increasing inhibitory potency of a series of homologue alcohols towards glucuronidation. Many more findings, extensively reviewed by Dutton in his recent monograph on glucuronidation,[274] support the contention that the active site of UDP-glucuronosyltransferase may be located in the "deeper layers of the microsomal membrane." If it is in the lumen of the endoplasmic reticulum, a "translocase" for the poorly lipid-soluble UDP-glucuronate[337] and a special mechanism for release of the formed glucuronide would be required.

Phenolsulfotransferase and most other sulfotransferases, to the contrary, are cytosolic, freely soluble enzymes (see Chapter 5, Section I). Although data on substrate specificity, especially of homologous series of substrates are scarce, nevertheless, it is clear that the active site of the sulfotransferases can easily accomodate the binding of very lipid-soluble substrates, and catalyze their sulfation.

Thus, as far as substrate specificity of the sulfotransferases properly is concerned, lipid-solubility may be of minor importance in the determination of whether a substrate is sulfated or glucuronidated. Another possibility, however, is that the phospholipid phase of the endoplasmic reticulum membranes might act as a concentrating phase for poorly water-soluble, highly lipid-soluble substances. If that is the case, glucuronidation would be the preferred conjugation reaction for those compounds in vivo, since the substrate supply for glucuronidation, (taking place in the lipid phase) would be increased as compared to that for sulfation, which would require diffusion of the substrate out of the lipid phase. Indeed, it has been shown in vitro that accumulation of poorly water-soluble substrates in the microsomal membrane takes place;[338,339] this makes it difficult to know the real substrate concentration at the active site of UDP-glucuronosyltransferase. Since most of the substrates of glucuronidation are highly lipid soluble, this may complicate the analysis of the in vitro studies on kinetic properties of the enzyme.[274,340]

Such an accumulation might be expected to occur also in vivo. Subcellular distribution studies of drugs in the liver indeed indicate that this may take place, especially at increasing dose of the compounds.[341-343] At low dose more or less selective binding proteins in the liver and other tissues, such as ligandin (Y-protein) may be able to bind the major part of many compounds, as has been shown for the cholephilic drug dibromosulphthalein (DBSP).[344] At low dose most of the drug was bound to ligandin, but at increasing dose much became bound to particulate material as isolated from the liver homogenate. Such studies on subcellular distribution have been performed for only a very limited number of drugs. This is not surprising, since the analysis and physiological relevance of the results is complicated by the unavoidable artifacts of homogenization of the tissue, and dilution of the tissue with some, usually isotonic medium. The binding at the various sites may be influenced by the ionic composition of the medium of subfractionation; further, endogenous factors, such as glutathione, which greatly enhanced the binding of bilirubin to ligandin,[345] may be required for binding. At present it can only be concluded that in vivo, drugs may be accumulated in the membrane fraction, especially at increasing dose, if they are sufficiently lipid-soluble. The question now to be considered is how would this affect the process of conjugation.

An important clue to an answer on this question comes from studies on the conjugation of substrates for both sulfation and glucuronidation that are generated by mixed function oxidase activity in the endoplasmic reticulum. The metabolism of such a compound, 4-nitroanisole, was studied by Minck et al.[318] in the perfused rat liver. It is oxidatively demethylated in the liver to 4-nitrophenol. The metabolism of 4-nitroanisole in the perfusion resulted in the appearance of almost exclusively 4-nitrophenyl sulfate. Yet, when a dose of 4-nitrophenol, equimolar to that of 4-nitroanisole, was added to the perfusion, predominantly 4-nitrophenylglucuronide was formed. One of the main differences between both experimental set-ups is that when 4-nitroanisole was added, the substrate for the subsequent conjugation is relatively slowly generated in the endoplasmic reticulum membrane by monooxygenase activity, whereas in the other case this product, 4-nitrophenol, is introduced by rapid injection at its maximum concentration in the perfusion medium. The experiment proved that at the low rate of supply of 4-nitrophenol from 4-nitroanisole, the product diffuses out of the endoplasmic reticulum membrane phase (instead of being concentrated there) into the cytosol, where the sulfotransferase is waiting for it. In isolated rat hepatocytes exactly the same was found.[320] Whether in this process the compound is freely dissolved or is bound to a binding protein in the cytosol is not known. The main conclusion, however, is that the ensuing reaction is not glucuronidation in the same phospholipid phase as oxidation, but sulfation in the cytosol. This seems a general feature, because it has been confirmed with several other products of oxidative metabolism in which a phenolic hydroxyl group had been introduced by metabolism. Both in isolated hepatocytes and the isolated perfused rat liver, preferential sulfation of the 2- and 4-hydroxylated metabolites formed from biphenyl was observed, whereas direct addition of these hydroxylated metabolites led mainly to glucuronidated conjugates.[326,346] When harmine was used as substrate for monooxygenase activity, mainly the sulfate conjugate of the product harmol was found as final product.[324,325] These examples indicate that accumulation of lipid-soluble substrates by the phospholipid phase may be of minor importance (at low doses of these substrates).

Yet, Orrenius et al.[324] suggested that increased lipophilicity of a substrate is reflected in a higher proportion of glucuronide conjugation relative to sulfate conjugation (Table 10, Section IVD). Since there is, however, no straightforward correlation between lipid solubility and glucuronidation or sulfation rate in their experiments, it is hard to draw a definite conclusion from these data. Furthermore, the conjugation processes are multistep processes, including uptake of the compounds from the medium into the cells, availability of cosubstrates, etc.

At increasing dose of the compounds to be conjugated, accumulation in the phospholipid phase of the membranes may occur. This might lead to a more rapid increase of the substrate concentration for glucuronidation than for sulfation, and, therefore, might be one explanation for the increase in glucuronidation relative to sulfation often observed at increasing dose of, for instance, phenols (see Section IVD). As yet, however, this suggestion is completely speculative. The results indicate that there is not a so-called "physiological linkage" between monooxygenase and UDP-glucuronosyltransferase, an idea proposed only because both are localized in the same membrane phase.

2. Substrate Specificity and Enzyme Kinetics of the Transferases

Obviously the kinetic properties of the transferases play an important role in the establishment of the ratio with which the glucuronide and sulfate conjugates of a certain substrate are synthesized under various conditions in the cell. Parallel in vivo and in vitro studies are required to evaluate the role of these enzymes. So far, however, comparative substrate specificity of the transferases in vitro has not been studied systematically.

One complicating factor is the choice of the enzyme preparation to be used: purified enzymes are required, but the properties of the enzyme preparation may change upon purification, especially those of UDP-glucuronosyltransferase. Microsomal UDP-glucuronosyltransferase is strongly activated in vitro by a series of manipulations which affect membrane structure of the surrounding microsomal membrane fragments. As yet it is not clear whether this transferase is completely "activated" or "latent" in vivo. Therefore, it is uncertain whether the enzyme *in situ* has to be compared with studies in vitro using the so-called "native" microsomal preparations, or the optimally activated microsomes which may have 5- to 20-fold higher activities than native microsomal preparations. A recent review discusses this problem extensively.[274] Obviously, one has to be careful with the interpretation of data obtained from studies performed under very different experimental conditions.

The physiological relevance of the in vitro-determined kinetic parameters can be tested in vivo or in cellular preparations, by administration of varying doses of the substrates: if the differences found in K_m values in vitro are also operative in vivo, the conjugation with the lowest K_m would be expected to be saturated at a lower dose than the conjugation with the higher K_m. Based on differences in enzyme kinetic factors one might expect a change of conjugation ratio as the dose is increased: if sulfation of a substrate has a very low K_m and a low V_{max} as compared to glucuronidation of the same substrate, then at low concentration the compound will be mainly sulfated, whereas at increasing concentration (= dose) glucuronidation will take over. A complication in studies on the kinetics of the transferases in vivo is that after a single dose, usually no steady state is achieved during the conjugation process because of rapid substrate consumption. In addition to that, the substrate pool from which is glucuronidated, may not be the same as that from which sulfation takes place. Part of the competition between glucuronidation and sulfation might be completely unrelated to enzyme kinetic factors, arising from preferential distribution of the substrate between the pools for sulfation and glucuronidation, respectively.

Obviously, the enzyme concentration will determine the rate of conversion (V_{max}/g of tissue; capacity). The amount of enzymic active sites may be influenced, e.g., by specific inhibition or specific induction. Genetic differences may play a role: the balance between sulfation and glucuronidation of androsterone in a certain strain of Wistar rats seemed to be dependent on the genetically determined amount of UDP-glucuronosyltransferase activity towards this substrate.[347] In rats with high activity of this enzyme much of the glucuronide was found, and in rats with a low activity, sulfation was more important.

3. Cosubstrate Availability: UDP-Glucuronate

In Section III the conclusion was reached that at high doses of a substrate for sulfation, depletion of sulfate may occur, which may lead to a decrease of sulfation rate. Clearly, any depletion of inorganic sulfate will sooner or later lead to a loss of sulfating capacity. Usually, glucuronidation has a sufficiently high capacity to take over.

UDP-glucuronate, the cosubstrate of glucuronidation, seems readily available under normal conditions: when the glucuronate group has been transferred to a substrate, uridine is "reloaded" again (through ATP, glucose-1-phosphate and NAD$^+$) with a glucuronate group.[274] However, under certain circumstances UDP-glucuronate may be decreased, as shown by the effect of ethanol on glucuronidation in isolated hepatocytes.[348] The presence of ethanol causes a shift of NAD$^+$ to NADH in the liver. This inhibits the oxidation of UDP-glucose to UDP-glucuronate and thereby decreases glucuronidation rate of harmol in the isolated rat hepatocytes. It was nicely shown that a specific inhibitor of alcohol dehydrogenase, pyrazole, prevented the effect of ethanol, indicating that it was not an effect on the glucuronyl-transfer reaction properly. Sulfation of harmol was unaffected up to at least 100 mM ethanol in the incubation medium and did not compensate for the loss of glucuronidation. In an in vivo experiment in rats that received high intravenous injections of ethanol before harmol, however, no effect whatsoever on the glucuronidation and sulfation of harmol was observed.[386]

Another way of decreasing UDP-glucuronate in the liver is by a decrease of the uridine pool. This can be brought about by galactosamine administration in the rat and other animals.[349] A decrease in glucuronidation of 1-naphthol and a compensating increase in sulfation was observed in perfused livers taken from rats that 4 hr previously had been treated with galactosamine. Similar effects of galactosamine were obtained by Meerman and Mulder.[387] They administered the same dose intraperitoneally, and observed a significant 40% decrease of glucuronidation of harmol in the rat in vivo, but for a limited period of time: only when galactosamine was administered between ½ to 2 hr before harmol (i.v.). In isolated hepatocytes, glucuronidation was much decreased by the addition of galactosamine to the incubation.[266] Unfortunately, galactosamine is rather toxic at doses that are required for a decrease of UDP-glucuronate, and, therefore, is only of limited use in vivo.

V. DRUG INTERACTIONS WITH SULFATION IN VIVO

A. Selective Inhibition In Vivo

A specific inhibitor is an important tool in the evaluation of the role of an enzymic reaction in the regulation of in vivo metabolism. In 1977, two phenolic compounds were found to selectively inhibit sulfation as compared to glucuronidation in vivo: pentachlorophenol and 2,6-dichloro-4-nitrophenol.[350] Both were very effective inhibitors of sulfation: one single dose of 26 μmol of 2,6-dichloro-4-nitrophenol per kilogram (intraperitoneally), for instance, inhibited sulfation of harmol effectively for over 48 hr in the rat. As a result of this inhibition, the percentage of harmol that became glucuronidated increased very much (Table 11). Since the biliary excretion of harmol glucuronide (which was measured in the experiments of Table 11) is much more rapid than that of harmol sulfate, the inhibition of sulfation shows much earlier as an increase in the biliary excretion of harmol glucuronide than as a decrease in that of harmol sulfate. Therefore, salicylamide which seemed to leave sulfation unaffected, but increased excretion of the glucuronide, yet also inhibited primarily sulfation, thereby caused enhanced excretion of the glucuronide conjugate. This occurred only, however, when it was injected immediately before harmol; if it was injected 45 min before harmol, it had no effect, most likely because it is rapidly eliminated.

The selectivity of inhibition of sulfation by pentachlorophenol and 2,6-dichloro-4-nitrophenol could be confirmed in vitro with harmol, phenol, and the hydroxamic acid N-hydroxyphenacetin as substrate.[350]

Further studies with 2,6-dichloro-4-nitrophenol in vivo showed that also sulfation of phenol, 4-nitrophenol, and 1-naphthol was inhibited, and a compensatory increase in the amounts of glucuronide conjugate of these substrates was found.[248,351] The

Table 11
SELECTIVE INHIBITION OF SULFATION OF PHENOLIC SUBSTRATES BY SEVERAL COMPOUNDS IN THE RAT IN VIVO

Substrate (μmol/kg) Inhibitor	Dose (μmol/kg)	Time	Route of administration	% of dose Sulfate	Glucuronide
Harmol (20 μmol/kg)[a]		0	i.v.	22	17
2,6-Dichloro-4-nitrophenol	26	−45[b]	i.p.	2	62
Pentachlorophenol	39	−45	i.p.	5	53
2,6-Dimethyl-4-nitrophenol	26	−45	i.p.	22	20
3-Methyl-2-nitrophenol	26	−45	i.p.	20	17
Salicylamide	26	−45	i.p.	22	18
Salicylamide	26	−5	i.p.	20	32
Phenol (266 μmol/kg)[c]		0	i.v.	33	39
2,6-dichloro-4-nitrophenol	104	−45	i.p.	6	59
1-Naphthol (170 μmol/kg)[d]		0	i.p.	50	49
2,6-dichloro-4-nitrophenol	125	−60	i.p.	14	81

[a] Harmol excreted in bile was collected for 2 hr in anaesthesized rats with ligated kidneys.[350]
[b] Means 45 min before harmol, the inhibitor 2,6-dichloro-4-nitrophenol was administered.
[c] Phenol conjugates were collected during 24 hr in metabolism cages.[248]
[d] Data from Dr. P. C. Hirom, St. Mary's Hospital Medical School, London.

glucuronidation of phenolphthalein, the biliary excretion of dibromosulphthalein, the acetylation of procainamide ethobromide (PAEB), and the glutathione conjugation of ethacrinic acid in the rat in vivo were unaffected by the pretreatment with 2,6-dichloro-4-nitrophenol.[351] An interesting feature of pentachlorophenol is that it is well tolerated by rats when fed for prolonged periods of time, up to 8 months.[352] A very pure preparation of this compound must be used, because even small contaminations with other polychlorinated phenols or higher molecular-weight products increase its toxicity very much.[353]

Several other phenols inhibit sulfation in vivo, most likely by competition for sulfate conjugation;[351,354] this inhibition was usually only short-lasting, probably because the compounds are rapidly eliminated. Inhibition by 4-nitrophenol is most likely the reason why the carboxylesterase inhibitor bis(4-nitrophenyl) phosphate also inhibited sulfation; this compound is hydrolyzed in vivo to 4-nitrophenol, its main metabolite.[354] Many other compounds, mostly phenols with a sterically hindered phenolic group and electron-withdrawing substituents in the phenol ring, have been tested for their potential inhibitory effect on sulfation.[354] Pentachlorophenol and 2,6-dichloro-4-nitro-phenol also effectively seem to inhibit sulfation of N-hydroxy-2-acetylaminofluorene,[355] a well-known chemical carcinogen (Chapter 8, Section II).

Neither 2,6-dichloro-4-nitrophenol nor pentachlorophenol are converted to sulfate conjugates in vivo to a measurable degree,[61,356] presumably because both are highly acidic phenols. Therefore, the inhibition must be due to either binding at the active site with an extremely low V_{max} of sulfation ("false substrate"), or another effect on the structure of the sulfotransferase.

Inhibition of sulfation by salicylamide can easily be explained by substrate competition, because salicylamide is an excellent substrate of phenolsulfotransferase[357] with a high affinity. As has been discussed in Section III, salicylamide in most experiments did not deplete sulfate because usually only a minor fraction of the sulfate pool was required for its sulfation. The effectivity of this compound in vivo is limited because it is very rapidly removed after sulfation and glucuronidation and, for instance, caused only a short-lasting inhibition of the sulfation of paracetamol in human volunteers.[243] Moreover, salicylamide also inhibits very strongly glucuronidation: in human volunteers glucuronidation of salicylate, a compound which is not conjugated with sulfate was much decreased by salicylamide.[358] Yet, the combined results[243,350,358] indicate that salicylamide is a much stronger inhibitory towards sulfation, leading to increased glucuronidation that compensates for the loss of sulfating capacity. This was confirmed in isolated rat hepatocytes with harmol or its precursor harmine as substrate.[324,325] Inclusion of salicylamide (0.5 mM) in the incubation medium decreased sulfation to about 15% of control, and increased glucuronidation, so that the total metabolism of harmol remained the same, but the ratio between sulfation and glucuronidation changed very much. Burke and Orrenius[322] found a similar inhibition of sulfation of resorufine by salicylamide in isolated rat hepatocytes; resorufine is almost completely converted into the sulfate conjugate. If salicylamide was present, reactive metabolites generated from benzo(a)pyrene in isolated rat hepatocytes were increased, and led to more covalent binding of these reactive products to DNA.[329]

Another approach to selective inhibition, namely byproduct inhibition, has been tried also. Mulder and Pilon[359] used the glucuronide and disulfate conjugates of phenolphthalein in the rat in vivo as potential inhibitors of harmol conjugation. However, the main effect was a shift of the excretory pathway of the harmol conjugates from bile to urine, without much effect on the conjugations themselves, probably because of the rapid elimination of the phenolphthalein conjugates in bile in the rat. The effect of these compounds can, therefore, much better be studied in isolated hepatocytes.[360,361] Phenolphthalein glucuronide inhibited formation of harmol glucuronide in this system (as was to be expected from the observed inhibition in vitro by this compound of glucuronidation of harmol),[359] and slightly stimulated harmol sulfation. 4-Nitrophenyl glucuronide and 2-naphthyl glucuronide were without effect. The sulfate conjugates of phenolphthalein (a disulfate) and 4-nitrophenol inhibited the sulfation of harmol. In the case of 4-nitrophenyl sulfate this inhibition, however, may have been due to free 4-nitrophenol, released by hydrolysis from the conjugate, since the sulfation of harmol is extremely sensitive to 4-nitrophenol, both in vitro[255] and in isolated hepatocytes.[360] Yet Norling et al.[360,361] showed that the conjugates may inhibit more or less selectively the respective conjugations if only they are not removed rapidly by urinary or biliary elimination.

Recently the effect of various metabolic inhibitors on sulfation and glucuronidation of 4-hydroxybiphenyl, 7-hydroxycoumarin and benzo(a)pyrene has been reported.[362] Menadione, rotenone and 2,4-dinitrophenol inhibited both conjugations. A decrease in cellular ATP and competition for conjugation may play a role.

Selective inhibition of steroid sulfation may also be possible. Brooks et al.[199] briefly mentioned that they initiated work on the specific inhibitor of estrogen sulfation 4-nitro-3-methoxyestrone in vivo; no results are available as yet.

B. Microsomal Enzyme Inducers

Pretreatment of animals with so-called microsomal enzyme inducers will affect the in vivo metabolism of drugs in many ways, and it is often impossible to pinpoint an observed effect in an unambiguous way to only one factor that was affected by the pretreatment. Thus, for instance, sulfation and glucuronidation of 1-naphthol have been measured in the isolated perfused rat liver.[363,364] After pretreatment of the donor with phenobarbital, a pronounced increase was found in glucuronidation and a reduction in sulfate formation in the subsequent perfusion. The pretreatment was shown to increase UDP-glucuronosyltransferase activity, and this may be the explanation of the decrease of sulfation. However, sulfotransferase activity has not been measured in this study. Moreover, supply rates of cofactors may have changed,[364] and liver weights were changed as a result of the pretreatment.

Similarly, the effect of a 3-methylcholanthrene pretreatment on the conjugation of 4-nitrophenol in the isolated perfused rat liver[319] does not permit a definite conclusion. It increased the rate of appearance of the sulfate conjugate in the perfusion medium, but it presumably did not change the total amount of the sulfate conjugate synthesized. Indeed, 3-methylcholanthrene did not increase sulfotransferase activity towards 4-nitrophenol in rabbit-liver homogenates in vitro.[365]

When more pathways than only glucuronidation and sulfation are possible, the analysis of the effect of microsomal enzyme inducers is even more complex. Thus, Jollow et al.[278] pretreated hamsters with 3-methylcholanthrene and phenobarbital. The 3-methylcholanthrene treatment strongly decreased the formation of the sulfate conjugate of paracetamol, whereas the excretion of the mercapturic acid of paracetamol was increased and the glucuronide unaffected. Phenobarbital pretreatment, on the other hand, increased the glucuronide, but caused only a minor decrease of the sulfate and the mercapturate. These data for phenobarbital were confirmed in isolated hepatocytes: an increase of glucuronidation of paracetamol and no effect on its sulfation was found in cells from pretreated rats.[279,327] 3-Methylcholanthrene increased glucuronidation of paracetamol in isolated rat kidney cells, and had no effect on sulfation.[289]

Nafenopin®, a hypolipidemic drug that increases liver weight and induces Z-protein when administered in vivo to rats, had no effect on the conjugation pattern of harmol in vivo, but changed the main route of elimination of harmol sulfate from urine to bile.[366]

The effect of pretreatment with various agents on the metabolism and subsequent conjugation of precursors of substrates for the conjugating enzymes is too complex to be analyzed in terms of effects of the pretreatment on the conjugation reactions.[294,322] For example, it is likely that the increase in glucuronidation of biphenyl metabolites in hepatocytes upon phenobarbital and 3-methylcholanthrene pretreatment[326,346] is due to an increase in the rate of substrate supply, and not to an inhibition of sulfation or an activation of glucuronidation (see Section IVD). Gillette[367] has given an excellent analysis of the consequences of a change in only one reaction for all the other pathways in a complex metabolic scheme, where a drug can be converted to several metabolites.

C. Other Drugs

Liver damage caused by carbon tetrachloride administration affected sulfation of 1-naphthol less severely than its glucuronidation, as measured in perfused rat liver, 24 hr after administration of 1 to 5 m*l*/kg.[349] This was confirmed for the substrate paracetamol.[368] These data indicate that even when the liver is extensively damaged by carbon tetrachloride, the sulfation reaction remains relatively intact.

In the rat and hamster, acetylsalicylic acid (aspirin) inhibited the sulfation of paracetamol, both when the latter drug was administered as such[261] or in the form of its precursor phenacetin.[369] Substrate competition is unlikely since acetylsalicylate is no substrate for sulfation. It has been suggested that acetylsalicylate inhibits the synthesis of PAPS because it also inhibited the biosynthesis of glycosaminoglycans.[370] In human volunteers no interaction between paracetamol and acetylsalicylate or salicylate was observed, possibly because lower doses were employed in these studies.[371-373] Pretreatment of rats with caffeine, codeine, ethanol, and phenobarbital did not affect phenacetin conversion into paracetamol sulfate.[369]

Several other compounds were shown not to affect sulfation in isolated rat hepatocytes: ethanol (10 m*M*), 4-methylpyrazole, lactate, and sorbitol[348] (substrate: harmol), and metyrapone and cysteamine[279,327] (substrate: paracetamol). Interestingly, the sulfation of paracetamol in the hepatocytes was considerably enhanced by the addition of cysteine (0.5 m*M*), methionine (1 m*M*), and *N*-acetylcysteine (1 m*M*) in the incubation, while there seemed to be no sulfate limitation in the incubation; the authors[327] as yet have no explanation for this effect.

VI. PHARMACOKINETICS OF SULFATION

In the in vivo studies, pharmacokinetic factors will play a role in the conjugation behavior of substrates for sulfation and glucuronidation. The route of administration (first pass effects) and the rate at which the substrate is supplied to the conjugation sites have to be considered in this respect. The first kinetic model describing rates of sulfation and glucuronidation in vivo was proposed by Bray et al.[239,374-376] They assumed first order kinetics of sulfation under their conditions, and equalled the rate of elimination of the conjugates in urine to the rate of synthesis. From the excretion data they determined the excretory deficit as a function of time; when this deficit was plotted logarithmically against time, this resulted in a straight line, and a rate of sulfation could be calculated. However, in their experiments sulfate is depleted by the substrates of sulfation, and, therefore, their assumption about first-order kinetics of sulfation cannot be valid. The problem with this kinetic model is that it is too "chemical" and does not prove whether indeed sulfation rate equals excretion rate of the product. Further it does not take into account the absorption rates of the compounds, different halflives for the various metabolites, etc.

Later kinetic models have incorporated the excretion and absorption characteristics; usually the drugs are administered intravenously to circumvent the problem of (incomplete) absorption from the gut. Enzymological parameters have been introduced in the pharmacokinetic evaluation.[377] So far, these models have not yet been extensively used to study the conjugation reactions specifically. The kinetic properties of conjugation in the liver can be determined in the isolated perfused rat liver and kinetics of sulfation of paracetamol have been investigated in this preparation.[378] The metabolism of paracetamol and its precursor, phenacetin (which is oxidatively deethylated to paracetamol by a cytochrome P_{450}-catalyzed reaction) were compared in this system in order to discriminate between two models of the liver. The "well-stirred" model describes the liver as a well-stirred compartment in which the drug in the emergent blood is in equilibrium with that in the liver.[379] The "parallel-tube" model describes the liver as a series of identical and parallel tubes with enzymes distributed evenly within the hepatocytes lining the tubes.[380] The results of Pang and Gillette[378] suggest that the liver may be viewed as an imperfectly mixed compartment with regard to the availability of the metabolite paracetamol, generated from phenacetin. A complication in this analysis is that probably the enzymes involved are not evenly distributed in the liver, but may be localized preferentially in certain zones of the liver.

The route of administration may be expected to affect the metabolic pattern. This is obvious in those cases where after oral dosage, a strong first-pass effect occurs, either at the level of the mucosa or the liver. Another factor is the fact that upon oral administration, the compound becomes available to the central compartment at a slower rate than when it is injected intravenously. This may change the conjugation pattern, because a slower rate of supply to the conjugation enzymes means a lower substrate concentration (Section IVD). An interesting observation in this respect was made by Capel et al.,[270] who administered the same dose of [^{14}C]- labeled phenol to hens by three different routes; intraperitoneally, orally, and intramuscularly. In all cases the recovery of radioactivity in urine was about the same, but there was a large difference in the ratio between sulfation and glucuronidation (Table 12). Although several explanations are possible, one of these is that the slower absorption of phenol after oral and especially intramuscular administration (tissue damage?) provides phenol at an

Table 12

SULFATION AND GLUCURONIDATION OF PHENOL AS INFLUENCED BY THE ROUTE OF ADMINISTRATION IN THE HEN[a]

Route	% of dose in 24-hr urine	Sulfate	Glucuronide
Intraperitoneal	55	56	41
Oral	57	72	28
Intramuscular (in leg muscle)	45	93	4

[a] The dose of [^{14}C]-phenol was 266 μmol/kg, and Rhode Island hens were used (2 to 2.5 kg body weight).

From Capel, I.D., Millburn, P. and Williams, R. T., *Biochem. Soc. Trans.,* 2, 875, 1974. With permission.

increasingly slower rate to the liver, the main site of sulfation, and thereby shifts the ratio towards more sulfation. Alternatively, a first pass effect at the level of the mucosa (oral administration) or the kidney (intramuscular administration in the hen leg muscle) may be involved (Section IVB).

A similar situation occurs when oral coadministration of two drugs may change the absorption rate in the gut of one of them. For example, acetylsalicylic acid was shown to slow the rate of absorption of paracetamol.[261,262]

Data on the distribution volume of phenols or other substrates of sulfation usually are not available, unless a substrate happens to be a widely used drug, such as paracetamol. This compound, however, is a relatively unusual phenol in that it is poorly lipid soluble (at pH 7), contrary to most phenols. Pharmacokinetic factors of the metabolism of paracetamol in man have been determined by several authors.[259,306,381-384]

ACKNOWLEDGMENT

I am very much indebted to Professor G. J. Dutton, Dept. of Biochemistry, University of Dundee (Scotland, U.K.) for most helpful suggestions during the preparation of this chapter.

REFERENCES

1. **Dziewiatkowski, D.,** Autoradiographic studies with [^{35}S]-sulfate, *Int. Rev. Cytol.,* 7, 159, 1958.
2. **O. D. McGee, J., Patrick, R. S., Rodger, M. C., and Luty, C. M.,** Collagen proline hydroxylase activity and [^{35}S]-sulphate uptake in human liver biopsies, *Gut,* 15, 260, 1974.
3. **Katona, E.,** Incorporation of inorganic sulfate in rat-liver Golgi, *Eur. J. Biochem.,* 63, 583, 1976.
4. **Yue, B. Y. J. T., Baum, J. L., and Sillbert, J. E.,** The synthesis of glucosaminoglycans by cultures of rabbit corneal endothelial and stromal cells, *Biochem. J.,* 158, 567, 1976.
5. **Lindahl, U., Höök, M., and Feingold, D. S.,** Structure and biosynthesis of heparin-like polysaccharides, *Fed. Proc. Fed. Am. Soc. Exp. Biol.,* 36, 19, 1976.
6. **Sobue, M., Takeuchi, J., Ito, K., Kimata, K., and Suzuki, S.,** Effect of environmental sulfate concentration on the synthesis of low and high sulfated chondroitin sulfates by chick embryo cartilage, *J. Biol. Chem.,* 253, 6190, 1978.
7. **Reggio, H. A. and Palade, G. E.,** Sulfated compounds in the zymogen granules of the guinea-pig pancreas, *J. Cell Biol.,* 77, 288, 1978.

8. **Harris, S. S. and Navia, J. M.,** Sulfate metabolism in rat calvaria cultured under vitamin A-deficient conditions, *J. Nutr.,* 108, 1777, 1978.

9. **Glimelius, B., Norling, B., Westermark, B., and Wasteson, A.,** Composition and distribution of glycosaminoglycans in cultures of human normal and malignant glial cells, *Biochem, J.,* 172, 443, 1978.

10. **Lindahl, U. and Höök, M.,** Glycosaminoglycans and their binding to biological macromolecules, *Annu. Rev. Biochem.,* 47, 385, 1978.

11. **Sjöberg, I., Carlstedt, I., Cöster, L., Malmström, A., and Fransson, L.,** Structure and metabolism of sulphated glycosaminoglycans in cultures of human fibroblasts, *Biochem. J.,* 178, 257, 1979.

12. **Ward, J. W. and Packham, M. A.,** Characterization of the sulfated glycosaminoglycan on the surface and in the storage granules of rabbit platelets, *Biochim. Biophys. Acta,* 583, 196, 1979.

13. **Blaschke, E.,** Studies on sulphomucopolysaccharides and ATP in adrenergic neurons, *Acta Physiol. Scand. Suppl.,* 466, 1, 1979.

14. **Farooqui, A. A.,** Metabolism of sulfolipids in mammalian tissues: a review, *Int. J. Biochem.,* 9, 709, 1978.

15. **Brunngraber, E. G.,** *Neurochemistry of Aminosugars,* Charles C Thomas, Springfield, Ill., 1979.

16. **Porteous, J. W. and Williams, R. T.,** Studies in detoxication. 19. The metabolism of benzene. I (a) The determination of phenol in urine with 2,6-dichloro-quinonechloroimide. (b) the excretion of phenol, glucuronic acid and ethereal sulphate by rabbits receiving benzene and phenol. (c) observations on the determination of catechol, quinol and muconic acid in urine, *Biochem. J.,* 44, 46, 1949.

17. **Bray, H. G., Humphris, B. G., Thorpe, W. V., White, K., and Wood, P. B.,** Kinetic studies of the metabolism of foreign organic compounds. 2. The formation of phenols from certain precursors, *Biochem. J.,* 52, 412, 1952.

18. **Laidlaw, J. C. and Young, L.,** Biochemical studies of toxic agents. 4. A study of etheral sulphate formation *in vivo* using radioactive sulphur, *Biochem. J.,* 54, 142, 1953.

19. **Robinson, D., Smith, J. N., Spencer, B., and William, R. T.,** Studies in detoxication. 43. A study of the arylsulphatease activity of takadiastase towards some phenolic ethereal sulphates, *Biochem. J.,* 51, 202, 1952.

20. **Abrams, L. S. and Elliott, H. W.,** Morphine metabolism *in vivo* and *in vitro* by homozygous Gunn rats, *J. Pharmacol. Exp. Ther.,* 189, 285, 1974.

21. **Coburn, S. P., Mahuren, J. D., and Schaltenbrand, W. E.,** Identification of 5'-deoxypyridoxine-3-sulfate as the major urinary metabolite of 5'-deoxypyridoxine in rats with comments on the inhibition of arylsulfatase activity and manganese dioxide oxidation at neighboring groups, *Anal. Biochem.,* 80, 942, 1978.

22. **Ahlborg, U. G., Mansoor, E., and Thumberg, T.,** Inhibition of β-glucuronidase by chlorinated hydroquinones and benzoquinone, *Arch. Toxicol.,* 37, 81, 1977.

23. **Roy, A. B.,** Enzymological aspects of steroid conjugation, in *Chemical and Biological Aspects of Steroid Conjugation,* Bernstein, S. and Solomon, S., Eds., Springer Verlag, Berlin, 1970, 74.

24. **McKenna, J. and Norymberski, J. K.,** Steroid sulfates. 1. Some solvolytic reactions of the salts of steroid sulfates, *J. Chem. Soc.,* 3889, 1957.

25. **Burstein, S. and Lieberman, S.,** Kinetic and mechanisms of solvolysis of steroid hydrogen sulfates, *J. Am. Chem. Soc.,* 80, 5235, 1958.

26. **Kornel, L.,** Studies on steroid conjugates. 4. Demonstration and identification of solvolyzable corticosteroids in human urine and plasma, *Biochemistry,* 4, 444, 1965.

27. **Bradlow, H. L.,** The hydrolysis of steroid conjugates, in *Chemical and Biological Aspects of Steroid Conjugation,* Burnstein, S. and Solomon, S., Eds., Springer Verlag, New York, 1970, 143.

28. **Goren, M. B. and Kochansky, M. E.,** The stringent requirement for electrophiles in the facile solvolytic hydrolysis of neutral sulfate ester salts, *J. Org. Chem.,* 38, 3510, 1973.

29. **Aso, T., Aedo, A. R., and Cekan, S. Z.,** Simultaneous determination of the sulphates of dehydroepiandrosterone and pregnenolone in plasma by radioimmuno-assay following a rapid solvolysis, *J. Steroid Biochem.,* 8, 1105, 1977.

30. **Paulson, G., Simpson, M., Giddings, J., Bakke, J., and Stolzenberg, K.,** The convertion of arysulfate ester salts to alkylaryl derivatives suitable for analysis by electron impact mass spectrometry, *Biomed. Mass Spectrom.,* 5, 413, 1978.

31. **Murray, S. and Baillie, T. A.,** Direct derivatization of sulphate esters for analysis by gaschromatography mass spectrometry, *Biomed. Mass Spectr.,* 6, 82, 1979.

32. **Palmer, R. H. and Bolt, M.,** Bile salt sulfates. 1. Synthesis of lithocholic acid sulfates and their identification in human bile, *J. Lipid Res.,* 12, 671, 1971.

33. **Campbell, C. B., McGuffie, C., and Powell, L. W.,** The measurement of sulphated and non-sulphated bile acids in serum using gas-liquid chromatography, *Clin. Chim. Acta,* 63, 249, 1975.

34. **Van Berge-Henegouwen, G. P., Allan, R. N., Hofmann, A. F., and Yu, P. Y. S.,** A facile hydrolysis-solvolysis procedure for conjugated bile acid sulfates, *J. Lipid Res.,* 18, 118, 1977.

35. **Cantafora, A., Angelico, M., Attili, A. F., Ercoli, L., and Capocaccia, L.,** An improved gas-chromatographic method for the determination of sulfated and unsulfated bile acids in serum, *Clin. Chim. Acta,* 95, 501, 1979.

36. **Nair, P. P., Gordon. M., and Reback, J.,** The enzymatic cleavage of the carbon-nitrogen bond in 3α, 7α, 12α-trihydroxy-5β-cholan-24-oylglycine, *J. Biol. Chem.,* 242, 7, 1967.

37. **Sjövall, J. and Vihko, R.,** Determination of androsterone and dehydroepiandrosterone sulfates in human serum by gas-liquid chromatography, *Steroids,* 6, 597, 1965.

38. **Sjövall, J. and Vihko, R.,** Chromatography of conjugated steroids on lipophilic Sephadex, *Acta Chem. Scand.,* 20, 1419, 1966.

39. **Jänne, O., Vihko, R., Sjövall, J., and Sjövall, K.,** Determination of steroid mono- and di-sulfates in human plasma, *Clin. Chim. Acta,* 23, 405, 1969.

40. **Makino, I., Shinozaki, K., Nakagawa, S., and Mashino, K.,** Measurement of sulfated and non-sulfated bile acids in human serum and urine, *J. Lipid Res.,* 15, 132, 1974.

41. **Coertz, G. R., Crepy, O. C., Judas, O. E., Longchampt, J. E., and Jayle, M.,** Séparation des fractions sulfo- et glucurono-conjugées des steroids urinaires: mise au point d'une méthode analitique, *Clin. Chim. Acta,* 51, 277, 1974.

42. **Bradlow, H. L.,** Modified technique for the elution of polar steroid conjugates from Amberlite®-XAD-2, *Steroids,* 30, 581, 1977.

43. **Musey, P. I., Collins, D. C., and Preedy, J. R. K.,** Isocratic separation of estrogen conjugates on DEAE-Sephadex, *Steroids,* 29, 657, 1977.

44. **Parmentier, G. and Eyssen, H.,** Thin layer chromatography of bile salt sulphates, *J. Chromatogr.,* 152, 285, 1978.

45. **Eriksson, H., Taylor, W., and Sjövall, J.,** Occurrence of sulfated 5α-cholanoates in rat bile, *J. Lipid Res.,* 19, 177, 1978.

46. **Pageaux, J. F., Duperray, B., Anker, D., and Dubois, M.,** Bile acid sulfates in serum bile acids determination, *Steroids,* 34, 73, 1979.

47. **Kohno, Y., Matsuo, K., Tanaka, M., Furukawa, T., and Nagasaki, N.,** Simultaneous determination of noradrenaline and 3-methoxy-4-hydroxyphenylethylene glycol sulfate in discrete brain regions of the rat, *Anal. Biochem.,* 97, 352, 1979.

48. **Summerfield, J. A., Billing, B. H., and Shackleton, C. H. L.,** Identification of bile acids in the serum and urine in cholestasis. Evidence for 6α-hydroxylation of bile acids in man, *Biochem. J.,* 154, 507, 1976.

49. **Van Berge-Henegouwen, G. P., Hofmann, A. F., and Ruben, A. T.,** A simple batch adsorption procedure for the isolation of sulfated and nonsulfated bile acids from serum, *Clin. Chim. Acta,* 73, 469, 1976.

50. **Peltonen, J. I., Laatikainen, T. J., and Hesso, A.,** Determination of conjugated steroids in amniotic fluid, *J. Steroid Biochem.,* 10, 499, 1979.

51. **Cowen, A. E., Korman, M. G., Hofmann, A. F., Turcotte, J., and Carter, J. A.,** Radioimmunoassay of sulfated lithocholates, *J. Lipid Res.,* 18, 698, 1977.

52. **Demers, L. M. and Hepner, G. W.,** Radioimmunoassay of serum bile acids, *Clin. Chem.,* 22, 602, 1976.

53. **Sanyaolu, A. A., Eccles, S. S., and Oakley, R. E.,** An antiserum for oestrone sulphate, *J. Endocrinol.,* 69, 11P, 1976.

54. **Cass, O. W., Cowen, A. E., Hofmann, A. F., and Coffin, S. B.,** Thin-layer chromatographic separation of sulfated and non-sulfated lithocholic acids and their glycine and taurine conjugates, *J. Lipid Res.,* 16, 159, 1975.

55. **Raedsch, R., Hofmann, A. F., and Tserng, K. Y.,** Separation of individual sulfated bile acid conjugates as calcium complexes using reversed-phase partition thin-layer chromatography, *J. Lipid Res.,* 20, 796, 1979.

56. **Musey, P. I., Collins, D. C., and Preedy, J. R. K.,** Separation of estrogen conjugates by high pressure liquid chromatography, *Steroids,* 31, 583, 1978.

57. **Goto, J., Kato, H., and Nambara, T.,** Separation of sulfated bile acids by high performance liquid chromatography, *Lipids,* 13, 908, 1978.

58. **Ragan, M. A. and MacKinnon, M. D.,** Paired-ion reversed phase high performance liquid chromatography of phenol sulfates in synthetic mixtures, algal extracts and urine, *J. Chromatogr.,* 178, 505, 1979.

59. **Williams, R. T.,** Studies in detoxication. 1. The influence of (a) dose and (b) *o-*, *m-* and *p-*substitution on the sulphate detoxication of phenol in the rabbit, *Biochem. J.,* 32, 878, 1938.

60. **Williams, R. T.,** Metabolism of phenolics in animals, in *Biochemistry of Phenolic Compounds,* Harborne, J. B., Ed., Academic Press, New York, 1964, chap. 6

61. **Dodgson, K. S., Smith, J. N., and Williams, R. T.,** Studies in detoxication. 29. The orientation of glucuronic acid conjugation in chloroquinol, *Biochem. J.,* 46, 124, 1950.

62. **Ahlborg, U. G.,** Metabolism of Chlorophenols: Studies on Dechlorination in Mammals, Ph.D. thesis, University of Stockholm, 1977.

63. **Sammons, H. G., Shelswell, J., and Williams, R. T.,** Studies in detoxication. 10. The conjugation and oxidation of *p*-hydroxybenzenesulphonamide in the rabbit. The characterization of *p*-sulphonamido-phenylglucuronide, *Biochem. J.,* 35, 557, 1941.

64. **Miller, J. J., Powell, G. M., Olavesen, A. H., and Curtiss, C. G.,** The fate of 2,6-dimethoxy [U-^{14}C]-phenol in the rat, *Xenobiotica,* 4, 285, 1974.

65. **Dacre, J. C.,** The metabolism of 3,5-di-*tert.*-butyl-4-hydroxytoluene and 3,5-di-*tert.*-butyl-4-hydroxy-benzoic acid in the rabbit, *Biochem. J.,* 78, 758, 1961.

66. **Dacre, J. C., Denz, F. A., and Kennedy, T. H.,** The metabolism of butylated hydroxyanisol in the rabbit, *Biochem. J.,* 64, 777, 1956.

67. **Levy, G., Tsuchiya, T., and Amsel, L. P.,** Limited capacity for salicylic phenolic glucuronide formation and its effect on the kinetics of salicylate elimination in man, *Clin. Pharmacol. Ther.,* 13, 258, 1972.

68. **Van Ginneken, C. A. M., Van Rossum, J. M., and Fleuren, H. L. J. M.,** Linear and non-linear kinetics of drug elimination, *J. Pharmacokinet. Biopharm.,* 2, 395, 1974.

69. **Buhler, D. R.,** Characterization of the glucuronide conjugate of chlorphenesin carbamate from the rat and from man, *Biochem. Pharmacol.,* 14, 371, 1965.

70. **Boström, H. and Vestermark, A.,** Studies on sulphates. 7. On the excretion of sulphate conjugates of primary aliphatic alcohols in the urine of rats, *Acta Physiol. Scand.,* 48, 88, 1960.

71. **Boyland, E. and Manson, R.,** The metabolism of 2-naphthylamine and 2-naphthylhydroxylamine derivatives, *Biochem. J.,* 101, 84, 1966.

72. **Hathway, D. E.,** *Foreign Compound Metabolism in Mammals,* Vol. 1-5, Chemical Society London, 1970-1979.

73. **Hearse, D. J., Powell, G. M., Olavesen, A. H., and Dodgson, K. S.,** The influence of some physico-chemical factors on the biliary excretion of a series of structurally related aryl sulphate esters, *Biochem. Pharmacol.,* 18, 181, 1969.

74. **Curtis, C. G., Hearse, D. J., and Powell, G. M.,** Renal excretion of some aryl sulphate esters in the rat, *Xenobiotica,* 4, 595, 1974.

75. **Kinoshita, N. and Gelboin, H. V.,** β-glucuronidase-catalyzed hydrolysis of benzo[*a*]pyrene-3-glu-curonide and binding to DNA, *Science,* 199, 307, 1978.

76. **Mead, C. J. and Finamore, F. J.,** The occurrence of ascorbic acid sulfate in the brine shrimp, *Artemia Salina, Biochemistry,* 8, 2652, 1969.

77. **Baker, E. M., Hammer, D. C., March, S. C., Tolbert, B. M., and Canham, J. E.,** Ascorbate sulfate: a urinary metabolite of ascorbic acid in man, *Science,* 173, 826, 1971.

78. **Lillard, P. W. and Seib, P. A.** Monosulfate esters of L-ascorbic acid, in *ACS Symposium Series,* American Chemical Society, Washington, D.C., 77, 1, 1978.

79. **Bond, A. D., McClelland, B. W., Einstein, J. R., and Finamore, F. J.,** Ascorbic acid 2-sulfate of the brine shrimp, *Artemia salina, Arch. Biochem. Biophys.,* 153, 207, 1972.

80. **Hornig, D., Gallo-Torres, H. E., and Weiser, H.,** A biliary metabolite of ascorbic acid in normal and hypophysectomized rats, *Biochim. Biophys. Acta,* 320, 549, 1973.

81. **March, S. C.,** Some Aspects of the Synthesis, Analysis and Occurrence of Ascorbate-2-sulfate and its Metabolism in Rats, Ph.D. thesis, University of Colorado, Boulder; *Diss. Abstr. B,* 34, 1411, 1973.

82. **Manowitz, P., Shapiro, S. S., and Goldstein, L.,** Ascorbate 2-sulfate levels in metachromatic leucodystrophy patients, *Biochem. Med.,* 18, 274, 1977.

83. **Quadri, S. F., Seib, P. A., and Deyoe, C. W.,** Improved method of preparing L-ascorbic acid 2-sulfate, *Carbohydr. Res.,* 29, 259, 1973.

84. **Hatanaka, H., Ogawa, Y., and Egami, F.,** L-Ascorbic acid sulfate esters with special reference to enzymic hydrolysis, *J. Biochem (Tokyo),* 75, 861, 1974.

85. **Verlangieri, A. J.,** Possible biological and pharmacological significance of L-ascorbic acid and L-ascorbic acid 2-sulfate on cholesterol metabolism, metabolic sulfation and atherogenesis, Ph.D. thesis, University of Pennsylvania, Philadelphia; *Diss. Abstr. B,* 34, 3635, 1974.

86. **Muccino, R. R., Markezich, P., Vernice, G. G., Perry, C. W., Cupano, J., and Liebman, A. A.,** The preparation of L-Ascorbic acid [^{35}S] 2-sulfate having a high specific activity, *Methods Enzymol.,* 62, 39, 1979.

87. **Mumma, R. O. and Verlangieri, A. J.,** Isolation of ascorbic acid 2-sulfate from selected rat organs, *Biochim. Biophys. Acta,* 273, 249, 1972.

88. **Bigler, W. N. and Kelly, D. M.** Liquid chromatographic analysis of ascorbate and ascorbate-2-sulfate, *Ann. N. Y. Acad. Sci.,* 258, 70, 1975.

89. **Tsujimura, M., Yoshikawa, H., Hasegawa, T., and Suzuki, T.,** Studies on the determination of ascorbic acid 2-sulfate by high speed liquid chromatography and column chromatography, *Vitamins,* 51, 207, 1977.

90. **Baker, F. M., Hammer, D. C., Kennedy, J. E., and Tolbert, B. M.,** Interference by ascorbate 2-sulfate in the dinitrophenylhydrazine assay of ascorbic acid, *Anal. Biochem.,* 55, 641, 1973.

91. **Tsujimura, M., Yoshikawa, H., Kasai, T., Hasegawa, T., and Suzuki, T.,** Studies on the determination of ascorbic acid-2-sulfate by bromidehydrazine, *Method Vitamin,* 52, 541, 1978.

92. **Terada, M., Watanabe, Y., Kunitomo, M., and Hayashi, E.,** Differential rapid analysis of ascorbic acid and ascorbic acid 2-sulfate by dinitrophenylhydrazine method, *Anal. Biochem.,* 84, 604, 1978.

93. **Mohamran, M., Rucker, R. B., and Hodges, R. E.,** Formation *in vitro* of ascorbic acid 2-sulfate, *Biochim. Biophys. Acta,* 437, 305, 1976.

94. **Tolbert, B. M., Downing, M., Carlson, R. W., Knight, M. K., and Baker, E. M.,** Chemistry and metabolism of ascorbic acid and ascorbate sulfate, *Ann. N. Y. Acad. Sci.,* 258, 48, 1975.

95. **Baker, E. M., Halven, J. E., Johnson, D. O., Joyce, B. E., Knight, M. K., and Tolbert, B. M.,** Metabolism of ascorbic acid and ascorbic-2-sulfate in man and the subhuman primate, *Ann. N. Y. Acad. Sci.,* 258, 72, 1975.

96. **Atkins, G. L., Dean, B. M., Griffin, W. J., and Watts, R. W. E.,** Quantitative aspects of ascorbic acid metabolism in man, *J. Biol. Chem.,* 239, 2975, 1964.

97. **Chatterjee, J. B.,** Ascorbic acid metabolism, *World Rev. Nutr. Diet,* 30, 69, 1978.

98. **Hornig, D.** Metabolism of ascorbic acid, in *Vitamin C,* Birch, C. G. and Parker, K. J., Eds., John Wiley & Sons, New York, 1974, 91.

99. **Powell, G. M., Parry, T. J., and Curtis, C. G.,** An entrogastric circulation, *Biochem. Soc. Trans.,* 6, 141, 1978.

100. **Quadri, S. F.,** Improved method of synthesis of L-ascorbate 2-sulfate and its recovery from some cereal products, Ph.D. thesis, Kansas State University, Manhattan; *Diss. Abstr. B,* 34, 4431, 1974.

101. **Mumma, R. O., McKee, E. E., Verlangieri, A. J., and Barron, P. G.,** Antiscorbutic effect of ascorbic acid 2-sulfate in the guinea-pig, *Nutr. Rep. Int.,* 6, 133, 1972.

102. **Kueniz, W., Avenia, R., and Kamm, J. J.,** Studies on the antiscorbutic activity of ascorbate-2-sulfate in the guinea-pig, *J. Nutr.,* 104, 952, 1974.

103. **Machlin, L. J., Garcia, F., Kuenzing, W., Richter, C. B., Spiegel, H. E., and Brin, M.,** Lack of anti-scorbutic activity of ascorbate 2-sulfate in the rhesus monkey, *Am. J. Clin. Nutr.,* 29, 825, 1976.

104. **Verlangieri, A. J. and Mumma, R. O.,** *In vivo* sulfation of cholesterol by ascorbic acid 2-sulfate, *Atherosclerosis,* 17, 37, 1973.

105. **Hornig, D., Weber, F., and Wiss, O.,** Effect of ascorbic acid 2-sulfate on the faecal excretion of exogenous cholesterol in the rat, *Z. Klin. Chem. Klin. Biochem.,* 2, 62, 1974.

106. **Finamore, F. J., Feldman, R. P., and Cosgrove, G. E.,** L-ascorbic acid, L-ascorbate 2-sulfate, and atherogenesis, *Int. J. Vitam. Nutr. Res.,* 46, 275, 1976.

107. **Hayashi, E., Yamada, J., Kunitomo, M., Terada, M., Tomita, T., and Kinoshita, J.,** Fundamental studies on physiological and pharmacological actions of L-ascorbate 2-sulfate. 1. On the hypolipidemic effects. *J. Nutr. Sci. Vitaminol.,* 22, 201, 1976.

108. **Finamore, F. J., Feldman, R. P., Serrano, L. J., and Cosgrove, G. E.,** L-Ascorbate-2-sulfate and mobiliation of cholesterol from plaque deposition in rabbit aortas, *Int. J. Vitam. Nutr. Res.,* 47, 62, 1977.

109. **Hayashi, E., Yamada, J., Kunimoto, M., Terada, M., and Watanabe, Y.,** Fundamental studies on physiological and pharmacological actions of L-ascorbate 2-sulfate. 6. Effects of L-ascorbate 2-sulfate on lipid metabolism in guinea-pig, *Jpn. J. Pharmacol.,* 28, 133, 1978.

110. **Shapiro, S. S. and Poon, J. P.,** Apparent sulfation of glycosaminoglycans by ascorbic acid 2-[^{35}S] sulfate: an explanation, *Biochim. Biophys. Acta,* 385, 221, 1975.

111. **Hatanaka, H. and Egami, F.,** Sulfate incorporation from ascorbate 2-sulfate into chondroitin sulfate by embryo chick cartilage epiphyses, *J. Biochem. (Tokyo),* 80, 1215, 1976.

112. **Hatanaka, H., Egami, F., Kato, T., and Nagatsu, T.,** Ascorbate 2-sulfate inhibits dopamine β-hydroxylase reaction, but not ascorbate oxidase reaction, *J. Biochem. (Tokyo),* 78, 821, 1975.

113. **Roy, A. B.,** L-Ascorbic acid 2-sulphate A substrate for mammalian arylsulphatases, *Biochim. Biophys. Acta,* 377, 356, 1975.

114. **Helwig, J. J., Farooqui, A. A., Bollack, C., and Mandel, P.,** Purification and some properties of arylsulphatases A and B from rabbit kidney cortex, *Biochem. J.,* 165, 127, 1977.

115. **Fluharty, A. L., Stevens, R. L., Miller, R. T., Shapiro, S. S., and Kihara, H.,** Ascorbic acid-2-sulfate sulfohydrolase activity of human arylsulfatase A, *Biochim. Biophys. Acta,* 429, 508, 1976.

116. **Stevens, R. L., Fluharty, A. L., Shapiro, S. S., Miller, R. T., Davis, L. L., and Kihara, H.,** Assay procedures for ascorbic acid-2-sulfate sulfohydrolase, *Anal. Biochem.,* 79, 23, 1977.

117. **Palmer, R. H.,** The formation of bile acid sulfates: a new pathway of bile acid metabolism in humans, *Proc. Natl. Acad. Sci. U.S.A.,* 58, 1047, 1967.

118. **Palmer, R. H.,** Bile acid sulfates. 2. Formation, metabolism and excretion of lithocholic acid sulfates in the rat, *J. Lipid Res.,* 12, 680, 1971.

119. **Small, D. M. and Admirand, W.,** Solubility of bile salts, *Nature (London),* 221, 265, 1969.
120. **Carey, M. C., Wu, S. J., and Watkins, J. B.,** Solution properties of sulfated monohydroxy bile salts. Relative insolubility of the disodium salt of glycolithocholate sulfate, *Biochim. Biophys. Acta,* 575, 16, 1979.
121. **Matern, S. and Gerok, W.,** Pathophysiology of the enterohepatic circulation of bile acids, *Rev. Physiol. Biochem. Pharmacol.,* 85, 135, 1979.
122. **Low-Beer, T. S., Tyor, M. P. and Lack, W.,** Effects of sulfation of taurolithocholic and glycolithocholic acids on their intestinal transport, *Gastroenterology,* 56, 721, 1969.
123. **Admirand, W. H., Stiehl, A., and Thaler, M. M.,** Sulfation of bile salts: an important metabolic pathway in cholestasis, *Gastroenterology,* 62, 190, 1972.
124. **Makino, I., Nakagawa, S., and Shinozaki, K.,** Sulfated bile acids in urine of patients with hepatobiliary diseases, *Lipids,* 8, 47, 1973.
125. **Stiehl, A., Earnest, D. L., and Admirand, W. H.,** Sulfation and renal excretion of bile salts in patients with cirrhosis of the liver, *Gastroenterology,* 68, 534, 1975.
126. **Makino, I., Hashimoto, H., Shinozaki, K., Yoshino, K., and Nakagawa, S.,** Sulfated and nonsulfated bile acids in urine, serum and bile of patients with hepatobiliary diseases, *Gastroenterology,* 68, 545, 1975.
127. **Summerfield, J. A., Cullen, J., Barnes, S., and Billing, B. H.,** Evidence for renal control of urinary excretion of bile acids and bile acid sulphates in the cholestatic syndrome, *Clin. Sci. Mol. Med.,* 52, 51, 1977.
128. **Van Berge Henegouwen, G. P., Brandt, K. H., Eyssen, H., and Parmentier, G.,** Sulphated and unsulphated bile acids in serum, bile and urine of patients with cholestasis, *Gut,* 17, 861, 1976.
129. **Gadacz, T. R., Allan, R. N., Mack, E., and Hofmann, A. F.,** Impaired lithocholate sulfation in the rhesus monkey: a possible mechanism for chenodeoxycholate toxicity, *Gastroenterology,* 70, 1125, 1976.
129a. **Yousef, I. M., Vonk, R. J., Massé, D, Tuchweber, B., and Roy, C. C.,** Glycolithocholic acid sulfate disodium salt-induced intrahepatic cholestasis in rats, *Gastroenterology,* 76, 1302, 1979.
130. **Cowen, A. E., Korman, M. G., Hofmann, A. F., and Cass, O. W.,** Metabolism of lithocholate in healthy man. 1. Biotransformation and biliary excretion of intravenously administered lithocholate, litholcholylglycine and their sulfates, *Gastroenterology,* 69, 59, 1975.
131. **Cowen, A. E., Korman, M. G., Hofmann, A. F., and Cass, O. W.,** Metabolism of lithocholate in healthy man. 2. Enterohepatic circulation, *Gastroenterology,* 69, 67, 1975.
132. **Cowen, A. E., Korman, M. G., Hofmann, A. F., and Cass, O. W.,** Metabolism of lithocholate in healthy man. 3. Plasma disappearance of radioactivity after intravenous injection of labeled lithocholate and its derivatives, *Gastroenterology,* 69, 77, 1975.
133. **Stiehl, A., Ast, E., Czygan, P., Fröhling, W., Raedsch, R., and Kommerall, B.,** Poolsize, synthesis and turn-over of sulfated and non-sulfated cholic acid and chenodeoxycholic acid in patients with cirrhosis of the liver, *Gastroenterology,* 74, 572, 1978.
134. **Czygan, P., Ast, E., Fröhling, W., Stiehl, A., and Kommerell, B.,** Synthesis and excretion of bile acid sulfate esters in the isolated perfused rat kidney, in *Bile Acid Metabolism in Health and Disease,* Paumgartner, G. and Stiehl, A., Eds., MTP Press, Baltimore, 1977, 83.
135. **Summerfield, J. A. Gollan, J. L., and Billing, B. H.,** Synthesis of bile acid monosulphates by the isolated perfused rat kidney, *Biochem, J.,* 156, 339, 1976.
136. **Parmentier, G., Mertens, J., and Eyssen, H.,** in *Advances in Bile Acid Research,* Matern, S., Hackenschmidt, J., Back, P., and Gerok, W., Eds., F. K. Schattauer Verlag, Stuttgart, 1975, 139.
137. **Taylor, W.,** The bile acid composition of rabbit and cat gall-bladder bile, *J. Steroid Biochem.,* 8, 1077, 1977.
138. **Hammerman, K. J., Chen, L. J., Fernandez-Corugedo, A., and Earnest, D. L.,** Sex differences in hepatic sulfation of taurolithocholate in the rat, *Gastroenterology,* 75, 1021, 1978.
139. **Watkins, J. B. and Brown, E. R.,** Conjugation and sulfation of lithocholic acid in fetal liver, in *Bile Acid Metabolism in Health and Disease,* Paumgartner, G. and Stiehl, A. Eds., MTP Press, Baltimore, 1977, 65.
140. **Laatikainen, T. J., Lehtonen, P. J., and Hesso, A. E.,** Fetal sulfated and nonsulfated bile acids in intrahepatic cholestasis of pregnancy, *J. Lab. Clin. Invest.,* 92, 185, 1978.
141. **Chen. L., Thaler, M. M., Bolt, R. J., and Golbus, M. S.,** Enzymatic sulfation of bile salts. 3. Enzymatic sulfation of tauro-lithocholate in human and guinea-pig fetuses and adults, *Life Sci.,* 22, 1817, 1978.
142. **Stiehl, A.,** Bile acid sulphates in cholestasis, *Eur. J. Clin. Invest.,* 4, 59, 1974.
143. **Van Berge Henegouwen, G. P., Brandt, K. H., Ruben, A. T., and Van Leusen, R.,** Sulphation of bile acids: liver or kidney?, *Lancet,* 1, 374, 1977.
144. **Barnes, S., Summerfield, J. A., Gollan, J. L., and Billing, B. H.,** Renal mechanisms influencing the bile acid composition of cholestatic urine, in *Bile Acid Metabolism in Health and Disease,* Paumgartner, G. and Stiehl, A., Eds., MTP Press, Baltimore, 1977, 89.

145. **Jensen, R. T., Davis, R. A., and Kern, F.,** Increased sulfation and decreased 7α-hydroxylation of deoxycholic acid in ethinylestradiol-induced cholestasis in rats, *Gastroenterology,* 73, 314, 1977.

146. **Fröhling, W. and Stiehl, A.,** Bile salt glucuronides: identification and quantitative analysis in the urine of patients with cholestasis, *Eur. J. Clin. Invest.,* 6, 67, 1976.

147. **Back, P. and Gerok, W.,** Differences in renal excretion between glyco-, tauro-conjugates, sulfoconjugates and glucuronoconjugates of bile acids in cholestasis, in *Bile Acid Metabolism in Health and Disease,* Paumgartner, G. and Stiehl, A., Eds., MTP Press, Baltimore, 1977, 93.

148. **Fröhling, W., Stiehl, A., Czygan, P., Liersch, M., Kommerell, B., Rotthauwe, H. W., and Becker, M.,** Induction of bile acid glucuronide formation in children with intrahepatic cholestasis, in *Bile Acid Metabolism in Health and Disease,* Paumgartner, G. and Stiehl, A., Eds., MTP Press, Baltimore, 1977, 101.

149. **Haslewood, E. S. and Haslewood, G. A. D.,** Preparation of the 3-monosulphates of cholic acid, chenodeoxycholic acid and deoxycholic acid, *Biochem. J.,* 155, 401, 1976.

150. **Parmentier, G. and Eyssen, H.,** Synthesis of the specific monosulphates of cholic acid, *Steroids,* 26, 721, 1975.

151. **Tserng, K. Y. and Klein, P. D.,** Synthesis of sulfate esters of lithocholic acid, glycolithocholic acid, and taurolithocholic acid with sulfur trioxide triethylamine, *J. Lipid Res.,* 18, 491, 1977.

152. **Tserng, K. Y. and Klein, P. D.,** Bile acid sulfates. 2. Synthesis of 3-mono-sulfates of bile acids and their conjugates, *Lipids,* 13, 479, 1978.

153. **Tserng, K. Y. and Klein, P. D.,** Bile acid sulfates. 3. Synthesis of 7- and 12-monosulfates of bile acids and their conjugates using a sulfur trioxide-triethylamine complex, *Steroids,* 33, 167, 1979.

154. **Fried, A. A., Petrow, V., and Lack, L.,** The synthesis of diazo, halo and sulfoxy bile acid derivatives: potential affinity labels, *Steroids,* 34, 171, 1979.

155. **Bernstein, S. and Solomon, S.,** Eds., *Chemical and Biological Aspects of Steroid Conjugation,* Springer Verlag, Berlin, 1970.

156. **Gauthier, R., Vigneault, N., Bleau, G., Chapdelaine, A., and Roberts, D. K.,** Solubilization and partial purification of steroid sulfatase of human placenta, *Steroids,* 31, 783, 1978.

157. **Cronholm, T.,** Position of the sulfate group in steroid sulfates from human plasma, *Steroids,* 14, 285, 1969.

158. **Ruokonen, A. and Vihko, R.,** Steroid metabolism in human and boar testis tissue. Steroid concentrations and the position of the sulfate group in steroid sulfates, *Steroids,* 23, 1, 1974.

159. **Laatikainen, T. and Vihko, R.,** Quantitation of $C_{19}O_2$ and $C_{21}O_2$ steroid mono- and disulfates in human bile, *Steroids,* 14, 119, 1969.

160. **Huhtaniemi, I. and Vihko, R.,** Identification and measurement of sulphate-conjugated neutral steroids in the intestinal contents of early and midterm foetuses, *J. Endocrinol.,* 57, 143, 1973.

161. **Kornel, L. and Miyabo, S.,** Studies on steroid conjugates. 9. Urinary excretion of sulfate conjugated metabolites of cortisol in man, *Steroids,* 25, 697, 1975.

162. **Miyabo, S. and Kornel, L.,** Corticosteroids in human blood. 6. Isolation, characterization and quantitation of sulfate conjugated metabolites of cortisol in human plasma, *J. Steroid Biochem.,* 5, 233, 1974.

163. **Yamamoto, Y., Manyon, A. T., Osawa, Y., Kirdani, R. Y., and Sandberg, A. A.,** Androgen metabolism in the baboon: a comparison with the human, *J. Steroid Biochem.,* 9, 751, 1978.

164. **Barford, P. A., Olavesen, A. H., Curtis, C. G., and Powell, G. M.,** Metabolic fates of diethylstilboestrol sulphates in the rat, *Biochem. J.,* 164, 423, 1977.

165. **Frey, M. J., Jirku, H., and Levitz, M.,** Levels of *N*-acetylglucosaminides and sulfo-*N*-acetylglucosaminides of 15α-hydroxyestrone and 15α-hydroxyestradiol in human late pregnancy urine, *J. Clin. Endocrinol. Metab.,* 32, 532, 1971.

166. **Yamamoto, Y., Ishihara, M., Kirdani, R. Y., Osawa, Y., and Sandberg, A. A.,** Studies of phenolic steroids in human subjects. 19. Renal conjugation of 15α-hydroxyestradiol-3-sulfate, *J. Clin. Endocrinol. Metab.,* 43, 144, 1976.

167. **Pasqualini, J. R.,** Metabolic conjugation and hydrolysis of steroid hormones in the fetoplacental unit, in *Metabolic Conjugation and Metabolic Hydrolysis,* Vol. 2, Fishman, W. H., Ed., Academic Press, New York, 1970, 154.

168. **Layne, D. S., Labow, R. S., and Williamson, D. G.,** The formation and metabolism by animal tissues of glycosides of steroid hormones, in *Advances in Sex Hormone Research,* Vol. 1, Thomas, J. A. and Singhal, R. L., Eds., University Park Press, Baltimore, 1975, 1.

169. **Harvey, P. R. C. and Hobkirk, R.,** The metabolism of estrone and estradiol-17β and their 3-sulfates by female guinea-pig liver microsomes, *Steroids,* 30, 115, 1977.

170. **Ingelman-Sundberg, M., Rane, A., and Gustafsson, J.,** Properties of hydroxylase systems in the human fetal liver active on free and sulfoconjugated steroids, *Biochemistry,* 14, 429, 1975.

171. **Gustafsson, J. and Ingelman-Sundberg, M.,** Multiple forms of cytochrome P-450 in rat liver microsomes. Separation and some properties of different hydroxylases active on free and sulphoconjugated steroids, *Eur. J. Biochem.,* 64, 35, 1976.

172. **Ingelman-Sundberg, M.,** Specific reductive metabolism of steroid sulphates in rat liver, *Biochim. Biophys. Acta,* 431, 592, 1976.

173. **Montelius, J., Gustafsson, J., Ingelman-Sundberg, M., and Rydström, J.,** Binding and hydroxylation of sulfoconjugated steroids in adrenal cortex mitochondria, *Biochim. Biophys. Acta,* 488, 502, 1977.

174. **Lebeau, M. and Baulieu, E.,** On the significance of the metabolism of steroid hormone conjugates, in *Metabolic Conjugation and Metabolic Hydrolysis,* Vol. 3, Fishman, W. H., Ed., Academic Press, New York, 1973, 151.

175. **Ruokonen, A., Laatikainen, T., Laitinen, E. A., and Vihko, R.,** Free and sulfate-conjugated neutral steroids in human testis tissue, *Biochemistry,* 11, 1411, 1972.

176. **Ruokonen, A.,** Steroid metabolism in testis tissue: the metabolism of pregnenolone, pregnenolone sulfate, dehydroepiandrosterone, and dehydroepiandrosteone sulfate in human and boar testis in vitro, *J. Steroid Biochem.,* 9, 939, 1978.

177. **Dessypris, A. G.,** Testosterone sulfate, its biosynthesis, metabolism, measurement, function and properties, *J. Steroid Biochem.,* 6, 1287, 1975.

178. **Matsui, M. and Hakozaki, M.,** Comparison of biliary metabolites of androsterone glucuronide and androsterone sulphate in female rats, *J. Steroid Biochem.,* 8, 1243, 1977.

179. **Matsui, M. and Kinwyama, Y.,** Comparative fate of testosterone and testosterone sulphate in female rats: $C_{19}O_2$ and $C_{19}O_3$ steroid metabolites in the bile, *J. Steroid Biochem.,* 8, 323, 1977.

180. **Gustafsson, J., Pousette, Å., Stenberg, Å. and Wrange, Ö.,** High-affinity binding of 4-androstene-3,-17-dione in rat liver, *Biochemistry,* 14, 3942, 1975.

181. **Carlestedt-Duke, J., Gustafsson, J., and Gustafsson, S. A.,** Sexual differences in hepatic metabolism and intracellular distribution of corticosterone studied by pulse labeling with [1,2,6,7-³H] corticosterone, *Biochemistry,* 14, 639, 1975.

182. **Laatikainen, T., Laitinen, E. A., and Vihko, R.,** Secretion of free and sulfate-conjugated neutral steroids by the human testis. Effect of administration of human chorionic gonadotropin, *J. Clin. Endocrinol. Metab.,* 32, 59, 1971.

183. **Legault, Y., Bleau, G., Chapdelaine, A., and Roberts, K. D.,** The binding of sterol sulfates to hamster spermatozoa, *Steroids,* 34, 89, 1979.

184. **Höller, M., Grochtmann, W., Napp, M., and Breuer, H.,** Studies on the metabolism of oestrone sulphate. Comparative perfusions of oestrone and oestrone sulphate through isolated rat livers, *Biochem. J.,* 166, 363, 1977.

185. **Oertel, G. W., Groot, K. and Brühl, P.,** Über Steroid-Konjugate in Plasma. 14. Zur Bindung von sulfokonjugierten Steroiden an Plasmaproteine, *Biochem. Z.,* 341, 10, 1965.

186. **Watanabe, H.,** Some factors in the biliary excretion of estrogens, *Adv. Steroid Biochem. Pharmacol.,* 5, 239, 1976.

187. **Mason, M.,** Effects of conjugated steroids on enzymes, in *Metabolic Conjugation and Metabolic Hydrolysis,* Vol. 1, Fishman, W. H., Ed., Academic Press, New York, 1970, 121.

188. **Tipping, E., Ketterer, B., and Christodoulides, L.,** Interaction of small molecules with phospholipid bilayers. Binding to egg phosphatidylcholine of some organic anions that bind to ligandin and amino azo-dye-binding protein A, *Biochem. J.,* 180, 327, 1979.

189. **Tipping, E., Ketterer, B., Christodoulides, L., and Enderby, G.,** The non-covalent binding of small molecules by ligandin. Interactions with steroids and their conjugates, fatty acids, bromosulphophthalein, carcinogens, glutathione and related compounds, *Eur. J. Biochem.,* 67, 583, 1976.

190. **Miyazaki, T., Mizukoshi, H., and Araki, Y.,** Biliary and urinary metabolites of estrone in the guinea-pig, *J. Steroid Biochem.,* 9, 115, 1978.

191. **Matsui, M. and Hakozaki, M.,** Disulphates of 16-oxygenated ketonic C_{19} steroids as biliary metabolites of androsterone sulphate in female rats, *Steroids,* 31, 219, 1978.

192. **Matsui, M. and Hakozaki, M.,** Variations in biliary metabolites of androsterone in female rats, *J. Steroid Biochem.,* 8, 319, 1977.

193. **Yamamoto, Y., Osawa, Y., Kirdani, R. Y., and Sandberg, A. A.,** Testosterone metabolites in dog bile, *Steroids,* 31, 233, 1978.

194. **Robinson, A. R., Henneberry, G. O., and Common, R. H.,** Steroid estrogen conjugates of hens' urine: identification of radioactive estrone-β-glucuronide, estrone sulphate, estradiol-17β-3-sulphate and estradiol-17α-3-sulphate as metabolites of injected [¹⁴C]estrone, *Biochim. Biophys. Acta,* 326, 93, 1973.

195. **Ikegami, S., Kamiya, Y., and Tamura, S.,** Studies on astrosaponins. 5. A novel steroid conjugate, 5α-pregn-9(11)-ene-3β,6α-dio-20-one-3-sulfate, from a starfish saponin asterosaponin, A, *Tetrahedron,* 29, 1807, 1973.

196. **Creange, J. E. and Szego, C. M.,** Sulphation as a metabolic pathway for oestradiol in the sea urchin *Strongylocentrotus fransiscanus, Biochem. J.,* 102, 898, 1967.

197. **Mulder, E., Lamers-Stahlhofen, G. J. M., and Van der Molen, H. J.,** Interaction between steroids and membranes. Uptake of steroids and steroid sulphates by resealed erythrocyte ghosts, *J. Steroid Biochem.,* 4, 369, 1973.

198. **Kurtenbach, P., Benes, P., and Oertel, G. W.,** On steroid conjugates in plasma. Biosynthesis of lipophile steroid sulfoconjugates from steroid sulfate, *Eur. J. Biochem.,* 39, 541, 1973.

199. **Brooks, S. C., Rozhin, J., Pack, B. A., Horn, L., Godefroi, V. C., Locke, E. R., Zemlicka, J., and Singh, D. V.,** Role of sulfate conjugation in estrogen metabolism and activity, *J. Toxicol. Environmental Health,* 4, 283, 1978.

200. **Aso, T., Aedo, A. R., and Cekan, S. Z.,** Simultaneous determination of the sulphates of dehydroepiandrosterone and pregnenolone in plasma by radioimmunoassay following a rapid solvolysis, *J. Steroid Biochem.,* 8, 1105, 1977.

201. **Baillie, T. A., Anderson, R. A., Sjövall, K., and Sjövall, J.,** Identification and quantification of 16α-hydroxy C_{21} steroid sulphates in plasma from pregnant women, *J. Steroid Biochem.,* 7, 203, 1976.

202. **Taylor, N. F. and Shackleton, C. H. L.,** Gaschromatographic steroid analysis for diagnosis of placental sulfatase deficiency: a study of nine patients, *J. Clin. Endocrin. Metab.,* 49, 78, 1979.

203. **Viinikka, L., Jänne, O., Perheentupa, J., and Vihko, R.,** Congenital adrenal hyperplasia. Plasma and urinary steroid conjugates in seven children with steroid 21-hydroxylase deficiency, *Clin. Chim. Acta,* 48, 359, 1973.

204. **Grose, J. H., Nowaczynski, W., Kuchel, O., and Genest, J.,** Isolation of aldosterone urinary metabolites, glucuronides and sulfate, *J. Steroid Biochem.,* 4, 551, 1973.

205. **Adams, J. B., Archibald, L., and Clarke, C.,** Adrenal dehydroepiandrosterone and human mammary cancer, *Cancer Res.,* 38, 4036, 1978.

206. **Fahl, W. E. and Rose, D. P.,** Effect of estrogen-containing oral contraceptives on urinary corticosteroid sulfate excretion, *Clin. Chim. Acta,* 63, 189, 1975.

207. **Martin, F., Adlercreutz, H., Lindström, B., Dencker, H., Rimer, U., and Sjöberg, N.,** Mass fragmentographic determination of conjugated neutral 7-ketosteroids in peripheral and portal venous blood: effect of ampicillin administration, *J. Steroid Biochem.,* 6, 1371, 1975.

208. **Reed, M. J., Fotherby, K., and Steele, S. J.,** Metabolism of ethynyloestradiol in man, *J. Endocrinol.,* 55, 351, 1972.

209. **Gustafsson, J. and Sjövall, J.,** Identification of 22-, 24- and 26-hydroxycholesterol in the steroid sulphate fraction of faeces from infants, *Eur. J. Biochem.,* 8, 467, 1969.

210. **Sorgue, Y. and Miravet, L.,** Chromatographic separation of vitamin D_3 sulfate and vitamin D_3, *Steroids,* 31, 653, 1978.

211. **Le Boulch, N. and Marnay-Gulat, C.,** Elimination urinaire de cholecalciférol sous forme d'ester sulfurique chez le rat, *Biochimie,* 53, 1219, 1971.

212. **Spencer, B.,** Endogenous sulphate acceptors in rat liver, *Biochem. J.,* 77, 294, 1960.

213. **Parke, D. V.,** *The Biochemistry of Foreign Compounds,* Pergamon Press, Oxford, 1968.

214. **Scheline, R. R.,** *Mammalian Metabolism of Plant Xenobiotics,* Academic Press, New York, 1978.

215. **Davis, V. E., Huff, J. A., and Brown, H.,** Free and conjugated serotonin excretion in carcinoid syndrome, *J. Lab. Clin. Med.,* 66, 390, 1965.

216. **Martin-Gal, E.,** 5-Hydroxytryptamine-*O*-sulfate: an alternative route of serotonin inactivation in brain, *Brain Res.,* 44, 309, 1972.

217. **Axelrod, J., Kopin, I. J., and Mann, J. D.,** 3-Methoxy-4-hydroxyphenyl glycol sulfate, a new metabolite of epinephrine and norepinephrine, *Biochim. Biophys. Acta,* 36, 576, 1959.

218. **Karoum, F., Lefèvre, H., Bigelow, L. B., and Costa, E.,** Urinary excretion of 4-hydroxy-3-methoxy-phenylglycol and 4-hydroxy-3- methoxyphenylethanol in man and rat, *Clin. Chim. Acta,* 43, 127, 1973.

219. **Demet, E. M. and Halaris, A. E.,** Origin and distribution of 3-methoxy-4-hydroxyphenylglycol in body fluids, *Biochem. Pharmacol.,* 28, 3043, 1979.

220. **Meek, J. L. and Neff, N. H.,** Acidic and neutral metabolites of norepinephrine: their metabolism and transport from brain, *J. Pharmacol. Exp. Ther.,* 181, 457, 1972.

221. **Braestrup, C.,** Gaschromatographic evidence for the presence of 3-methoxy-4-hydroxyphenylethanol in rat brain, *Biochem. Pharmacol.,* 21, 1775, 1972.

222. **Bronaugh, R. L., Hattox, S. E., Hoehn, M. M., Murphy, R. C., and Rutledge, C. O.,** The separation and identification of dopamine 3-*O*-sulfate and dopamine 4-*O*-sulfate in urine of Parkinsonism patients, *J. Pharmacol. Exp. Ther.,* 195, 441, 1975.

223. **Buu, N. T. and Kuchel, O.,** The direct conversion of dopamine-3-*O*-sulfate to norepinephrine by dopamine-β-hydroxylase, *Life Sci.,* 24, 783, 1979.

224. **Buu, N. T. and Kuchel, O.,** Dopamine-4-*O*-sulfate: a possible precursor of free norepinephrine, *Can. J. Biochem.,* 57, 1159, 1979.

225. **Tallan, H. H., Bella, S. T., Stein, W. H. and Moore, S.,** Tyrosine-*O*-sulfate as a constituent of normal human urine, *J. Biol. Chem.,* 217, 703, 1955.

226. **John, R. A., Rose, F. A., Westeman, F. S., and Dodgson, K. S.,** The detection and determination of L-tyrosine *o*-sulphate in rabbit and other mammalian urine, *Biochem. J.,* 100, 278, 1966.

227. **Fluharty, A. L., Stevens, R. L., Goldstein, E. B., and Kihara, H.,** The activity of arylsulfatase A and B on tyrosine *O*-sulfates, *Biochim. Biophys. Acta,* 566, 321, 1979.

228. **Dodgson, K. S. and Rose, F. A.,** Sulfohydrolases, in *Metabolism of Sulfur Compounds,* Greenberg, D.M., Ed., Academic Press, New York, 1975, 359.

229. **Heirwegh, K. P. M., Meuwissen, J. A. T. P., and Fevery, J.,** Critique of the assay and significance of bilirubin conjugation, *Adv. Clin. Chem.,* 16, 239, 1973.

230. **Isselbacher, K. J. and McCarthy, E. A.,** Identification of a sulfate conjugate of bilirubin in bile, *Biochim. Biophys. Acta,* 29, 658, 1958.

231. **Noir, B. A. and Nanet, H.,** A study of the ethyl anthranilate azo derivatives of bilirubin sulfate. Confirmation of the existence of bilirubin sulphate conjugates in bile, *Biochim. Biophys. Acta,* 372, 230, 1974.

232. **Kawai, T. and Okayama, P.,** Direct bilirubin. 2. Bilirubin sulfate fraction, *Igakkai Zasshi,* 84, 330, 1972; *Chem. Abstr.,* 80, 67937f.

233. **Huxtable, R. and Barbeau, A.,** Eds., *Taurine,* Raven Press, New York, 1976.

234. **Robeson, B. L. and Martin, W. G.,** Taurine synthesis from sulfate in the rat induced by dietary zinc, *Fed. Proc.,* 37, 537, 1978.

235. **Flynn, T. J., Desmukh, D. S., Subba Rao, G., and Pieringer, R. A.,** Sulfogalactosyl diacylglycerol: occurrence and biosynthesis of a novel lipid in rat brain, *Biochem. Biophys. Res. Commun.,* 65, 122, 1975.

236. **Fleischer, B. and Smigel, M.,** Solubilization and properties of galactosyltransterase and sulfotransferase activities of Golgi membranes in Triton X-100, *J. Biol. Chem.,* 253, 1623, 1978.

237. **Tennekoon, G. and McKhann, G. M.,** Galactocerebroside sulfotransferase: further characterization of the enzyme from rat brain, *J. Neurochem.,* 31, 329, 1978.

238. **Jutzi, H., Siegrist, H. P., Burkart, T., Wiesmann, U., and Herschkowitz, N. N.,** Diminished cerebroside-sulfotransferase activity in the Jimpy mouse mutant due to altered lipid composition in microsomal membranes, *Biochim. Biophys. Acta,* 552, 413, 1979.

239. **Bray, H. G., Humphris, B. G., Thorpe, W. V., White, K., and Wood, P. B.,** Kinetic studies of the metabolism of foreign compounds. 4. The conjugation of phenols with sulphuric acid, *Biochem. J.,* 52, 419, 1952.

240. **Krijgsheld, K. R., Scholtens, E., and Mulder, G. J.,** Concentration of inorganic sulfate in serum of mammals, species difference and circadian rhythm, *Comp. Biochem. Physiol.,* 67A, 683, 1980.

241. **Levy, G. and Matsuzawa, T.,** Pharmacokinetics of salicylamide elimination in man, *J. Pharmacol. Exp. Ther.,* 156, 285, 1967.

242. **Büch, H., Rummel, W., Pfleger, K., Eschrich, C., and Texter, N.,** Ausscheidung freien und kunjugierten Sulfates bei Ratte und Menschen nach Verabreichung von *N*-Acetyl-*p*-Aminophenol, *Naunyn-Schmiedebergs Arch. Pharmacol.,* 259, 276, 1968.

243. **Levy, G. and Yamada, H.,** Drug biotransformation interactions in man. 3. Acetaminophen and salicylamide, *J. Pharm. Sci.,* 60, 215, 1971.

244. **Roe, D.,** Effects of methionine and inorganic sulfate on indole toxicity and indican excretion in rats, *J. Nutr.,* 101, 645, 1971.

245. **Smith, I. and Mitchell, P. D.,** The effect of oral inorganic sulphate on the metabolism of 4-hydroxyphenethylamine (Tyramine) in man: tyramine *O*-sulphate measurement in human urine, *Biochem. J.,* 142, 189, 1974.

246. **Bennett, P. N., Blackwell, E., and Davies, D. S.,** Competition for sulphate during detoxification in the gut wall, *Nature (London),* 258, 247, 1975.

247. **Houston, J. B. and Levy, G.,** Drug biotransformation interactions in man. 6. Acetaminophen and ascorbic acid, *J. Pharm. Sci.,* 65, 1218, 1976.

248. **Mulder, G. J. and Meerman, J. H. N.,** Glucuronidation and sulphation *in vivo* and *in vitro:* selective inhibition of sulphation by drugs and deficiency of inorganic sulphate, in *Conjugation Reactions in Drug Biotransformation,* Aitio, A., Ed., Elsevier/North Holland Publishing, Amsterdam, 1978, 389.

249. **Galinsky, R. E., Slattery, J. T., and Levy, G.,** Effect of sodium sulfate on acetaminophen elimination by rats, *J. Pharm. Sci.,* 68, 803, 1979.

250. **Herbai, G.,** A double insotope method for determination of the miscible inorganic sulfate pool of the mouse applied in *in vivo* studies of sulfate incorporation into costal cartilage, *Acta Physiol. Scand.,* 80, 470, 1970.

251. **Mulder, G. J. and Scholtens, E.,** The availability of inorganic sulphate in blood for sulphate conjugation of drugs in rat liver *in vivo.* [^{35}S]– sulphate incorporation into harmol sulphate, *Biochem. J.,* 172, 247, 1978.

252. **Mulder, G. J. and Keulemans, K.,** Metabolism of inorganic sulphate in the isolated perfused rat liver. Effect of sulphate concentration on the rate of sulphation by phenol sulphotransferase, *Biochem. J.,* 176, 959, 1978.

253. **Slotkin, T. A., Di Stefano, V., and Au, W. Y. W.,** Blood levels and urinary excretion of harmine and its metabolites in man and rats, *J. Pharmacol. Exp. Ther.,* 173, 26, 1970.

254. **Mulder, G. J. and Hagedoorn, A. H.,** UDP glucuronyltransferase and phenol sulphotransferase *in vivo* and *in vitro.* Conjugation of harmol and harmalol, *Biochem. Pharmacol.,* 23, 2101, 1974.

255. **Mulder, G. J.,** A method for comparison of the properties of UDP glucuronyltransferase and phenolsulfotransferase from rat liver, with a joint substrate, *Anal. Biochem.,* 64, 350, 1975.

256. **Krijgsheld, K. R., Scholtens, E., and Mulder G. J.,** Sulfation of phenols in relation to the serum sulfate concentration in the rat, submitted.

257. **Houston, J. B. and Levy, G.,** Modification of drug biotransformation by vitamin C in man, *Nature (London),* 255, 78, 1975.

258. **Slattery, J. T. and Levy, G.,** Reduction of acetaminophen toxicity by sodium sulfate in mice, *Res. Commun. Chem. Pathol. Pharmacol.,* 18, 167, 1977.

259. **Levy, G.,** Pharmacokinetics and toxicological implications of glucuronide and sulfate conjugation of certain nonnarcotic analgesics in man, in *Conjugation Reactions in Drug Biotransformation,* Aitio, A., Ed., Elsevier/North Holland Publishing, Amsterdam, 1978, 469.

260. **Greiling, H. and Schulder, B.,** Zur Wirkungsweise der Salizylsäure, Azetylsalicylsäure and des Salizylamids, *Z. Rheumaforsch.,* 22, 47, 1963.

261. **Wong, L. T., Solomonrai, G., and Thomas, B. H.,** Metabolism of [14C] paracetamol and its interactions with aspirin in hamsters, *Xenobiotica,* 6, 575, 1976.

262. **Heading, R. C., Ninmo, J., Prescott, L. F., and Tothill, P.,** The dependence of paracetamol absorption on the rate of gastric emptying, *Br. J. Pharmacol.,* 47, 415, 1973.

263. **Galinsky, R. E. and Levy, G.,** Effect of *N*-acetylcysteine on the pharmacokinetics of acetaminophen in rats, *Life Sci.,* 25, 693, 1979.

264. **Thor, H., Moldeus, P., and Orrenius, S.,** Metabolic activation and hepatotoxicity. Effect of cysteine, *N*-acetylcysteine and methionine on glutathione biosynthesis and bromobenzene toxicity in isolated rat hepatocytes, *Arch. Biochem. Biophys.,* 192, 405, 1979.

265. **Weitering, J. G., Krijgsheld, K. R., and Mulder, G. J.,** The availability of inorganic sulphate as a rate limiting factor in the sulphate conjugation of xenobiotics in the rat. Sulphation and glucuronidation of phenol, *Biochem. Pharmacol.,* 27, 757, 1979.

266. **Moldeus, P., Andersson, B., and Gergely, V.,** Regulation of glucuronidation and sulfate conjugation in isolated hepatocytes, *Drug Metab. Dispos.,* 7, 416, 1979.

267. **Kobayashi, K., Kimura, S., and Akitake, H.,** Studies on the metabolism of chlorophenols in fish. 7. Sulfate conjugation of phenol and PCP by fish liver, *Bull. Jpn. Soc. Sci. Fish.,* 42, 171, 1976.

268. **Capel, I. D., French, M. R., Millburn, P., Smith, R. L., and Williams, R. T.,** The fate of [14C] phenol in various species, *Xenobiotica,* 2, 25, 1972.

269. **French, M. R., Babbunmi, E. A., Golding, R. R., Bassir, O., Caldwell, J., Smith, R. L., and Williams, R. T.,** The conjugation of phenol, benzoic acid, 1-naphthylacetic acid and sulphadimethoxine in the lion, civet and genet, *FEBS Lett.,* 46, 134, 1974.

270. **Capel, I. D., Millburn, P., and Williams, R. T.,** Route of administration and the conjugation of phenol in hens, *Biochem. Soc. Trans.,* 2, 875, 1974.

271. **Caldwell, J., French, M. R., Idle, J. R., Renwick, A. G., Bassir, O., and Williams, R. T.,** Conjugation of foreign compounds in the elephant and hyena, *FEBS Lett.,* 60, 391, 1975.

272. **Kao, J., Bridges, J. W., and Faulkner, J. K.,** Metabolism of [14C] phenol by sheep, pig and rat, *Xenobiotica,* 9, 141, 1979.

273. **Oehme, F. W. and Davis, L. E.,** The comparative toxicity and biotransformation of phenol, *Toxicol. Appl. Pharmacol.,* 17, 283, 1970.

274. **Dutton, G. J.,** *Glucuronidation of Drugs and Other Compounds,* CRC Press, Boca Raton, Fla., 1980.

275. **Mulder, G. J. and Bleeker, B.,** UDP glucuronyltransferase and phenolsulfotransferase from rat liver *in vivo* and *in vitro.* 4. Species differences in harmol conjugation and elimination in bile and urine *in vivo,* *Biochem. Pharmacol.,* 24, 1481, 1975.

276. **Capel, I. D., Millburn, P., and Williams, R. T.,** The conjugation of 1- and 2-naphthols and other phenols in the cat and pig, *Xenobiotica,* 4, 601, 1974.

277. **Miller, J. J., Powell, G. M., Olavesen, A. H., and Curtis, C. G.,** The metabolism and toxicity of phenols in cats, *Biochem. Soc. Trans.,* 1, 1163, 1973.

278. **Jollow, D. J., Thorgeirsson, S. S., Potter, W. Z., Hashimoto, M., and Mitchell, J. R.,** Acetaminophen-induced hepatic necrosis. 6. Metabolic disposition of toxic and non-toxic doses of acetaminophen, *Pharmacology,* 12, 251, 1974.

279. **Moldeus, P.,** Paracetamol metabolism and toxicity in isolated hepatocytes from rat and mouse, *Biochem. Pharmacol.,* 27, 2859, 1978.

280. **Smith, R. L. and Timbrell, J. A.,** Factors affecting the metabolism of phencetin.1. Influence of dose, chronic dosage, route of administration and species on the metabolism of 1-[^{14}C]-acetyl phenacetin, *Xenobiotica,* 4, 489, 1974.

281. **Miller, R. P. and Fischer, L. J.,** Urinary excretion of acetaminophen by the rat, *J. Pharm. Sci.,* 63, 969, 1974.

282. **Kao, J., Faulkner, J., and Bridges, J. W.,** Metabolism of aniline in rats, pigs and sheep, *Drug Metab. Dispos.,* 6, 549, 1978.

283. **Merits, I.,** Formation and metabolism of [^{14}C] dopamine 3-*O*-sulfate in dog, rat and guinea-pig, *Biochem. Pharmacol.,* 25, 829, 1976.

284. **Williams, R. T.,** Inter-species variations in the metabolism of xenobiotics, *Biochem. Soc. Trans.,* 2, 13, 1974.

285. **Smith, R. L.,** Species differences in drug metabolism, in *Drug Metabolism from Microbe to Man,* Parke, D. V. and Smith, R. L., Eds. Taylor & Francis, London, 1977.

286. **Quebbeman, A. J. and Rennick, B. R.,** Catechol transport by the renal tubule in the chicken, *Am. J. Physiol.,* 214, 1201, 1968.

287. **Watrous, W. M. and Fujimoto, J. M.,** Inhibition of morphine metabolism by catechol in the chicken kidney, *Biochem. Pharmacol.,* 20, 1479, 1971.

288. **Quebbeman, A. J. and Anders, M. W.,** Renal tubular conjugation and excretion of phenol and *p*-nitrophenol in the chicken: differing mechanisms of renal transfer, *J. Pharmacol. Exp. Ther.,* 184, 695, 1973.

289. **Jones, D. P., Sundby, G. B., Ormstad, K., and Orrenius, K.,** Use of isolated kidney cells for study of drug metabolism, *Biochem. Pharmacol.,* 28, 929, 1979.

290. **Cohen, G. M., Haws, S. M., Moore, B. P., and Bridges, J. W.,** Benzo*(a)*pyren-3-yl hydrogen sulphate, a major ethyl acetate-extractable metabolite of benzo*(a)*pyrene in human, hamster and rat lung cultures, *Biochem. Pharmacol.,* 25, 2561, 1976.

291. **Cohen, G. M. and Moore, B. P.,** The metabolism of benzo*(a)*pyrene, 7,8-dihydro-7,8-dihydroxyben-zo*(a)*pyrene and 9,10-dihydro-9,10-dihydroxybenzo*(a)*-pyrene by short-term organ cultures of hamster lung, *Biochem. Pharmacol.,* 26, 1481, 1977.

292. **Mehta, R. and Cohen, G. M.,** Major differences in the extent of conjugation with glucuronic acid and sulphate in human peripheral lung, *Biochem. Pharmacol.,* 28, 2479, 1979.

293. **Hartiala, K.,** Metabolism of hormones, drugs and other substances by the gut, *Physiol. Rev.,* 53, 496, 1973.

294. **Shirkey, R. J., Kao, J., Fry, J. R., and Bridges, J. W.,** A comparison of xenobiotic metabolism in cells isolated from rat liver and small intestinal mucosa, *Biochem. Pharmacol.,* 28, 1461, 1979.

295. **Dawson, J. R. and Bridges, J. W.,** Xenobiotic metabolism by isolated intestinal epithelial cells from guinea pig, *Biochem. Pharmacol.,* 28, 3299, 1979.

296. **Dawson, J. R. and Bridges, J. W.,** Conjugation and excretion of metabolites of 7-hydroxycoumarin in the small intestine of rats and guinea pigs, *Biochem. Pharmacol.,* 28, 3291, 1979.

297. **Josting, D., Winne, D., and Bock, K. W.,** Glucuronidation of paracetamol, morphine and 1-naphthol in the rat intestinal loop, *Biochem. Pharmacol.,* 25, 613, 1976.

298. **Conolly, M. E., Davies, D. S., Dollery, C. T., Morgan, C. D., Paterson, J. W., and Sandler, M.,** Metabolism of isoprenaline in dog and man, *Br. J. Pharmacol.,* 46, 458, 1972.

299. **Powell, G. M., Miller, J. J., Olavesen, A. H., and Curtis, C. G.,** Liver as major organ of phenol detoxication?, *Nature,* 252, 234, 1974.

300. **George, C. F., Blackwell, E. W., and Davies, D. S.,** Metabolism of isoprenaline in the intestine, *J. Pharm. Pharmacol.,* 26, 265, 1974.

301. **Gram, T. E.,** Ed., *Extrahepatic Drug Metabolism,* Spectrum Publishing, Holliswood, N. Y., 1980.

302. **Hänninen, O.,** Age and exposure factors in drug metabolism, *Acta Pharmacol. Toxicol.,* 36(Suppl. 2), 3, 1975.

303. **Percy, A. K. and Yaffe, S. J.,** Sulfate metabolism during mammalian development, *Pediatrics,* 33, 975, 1964.

304. **Pulkkinen, M. O.,** Sulphate conjugation during development in human, rat and guinea-pig, *Acta Physiol. Scand.,* 66, 115, 1966.

305. **Hiles, R. A., Caudill, D., Birch, C. G., and Eichhold, T.,** The metabolism and disposition of 3,4,4′-trichlorocarbanilide in the intact and bile duct-cannulated adult and in the newborn Rhesus monkey *(M. mulatta), Toxicol. Appl. Pharmacol.,* 46, 593, 1978.

306. **Miller, R. P., Roberts, R. J., and Fischer, L. J.,** Acetaminophen elimination kinetics in neonates, children and adults, *Clin. Pharmacol. Ther.,* 19, 284, 1976.

307. **Rollins, D. E., Von Bahr, C., Glaumann, H., Moldeus, P., and Rane, A.,** Acetaminophen: potentially toxic metabolite formed by human fetal and adult liver microsomes and isolated fetal liver cells, *Science,* 205, 1414, 1979.

308. **Rane, A., Sjöqvist, F., and Orrenius, S.,** Drugs and fetal metabolism, *Clin. Pharmacol. Ther.*, 14, 666, 1973.

309. **Smith, G. E. and Griffuths, L. A.,** Comparative metabolic studies of phenacetin and structurally-related compounds in the rat, *Xenobiotica*, 6, 217, 1976.

310. **Miller, J. J., Powell, G. M., Olavesen, A. H., and Curtiss, C. G.,** The fate of 2,6-dimethyl [U-^{14}C] phenol in the rat, *Xenobiotica*, 4, 285, 1974.

311. **Carlstedt-Duke, J. and Gustafsson, J. A.,** Sexual differences in hepatic sulphurylation of deoxycorticosterone in rats, *Eur. J. Biochem.*, 36, 177, 1973.

312. **Anderson, C. H. and Chatterton, R. T.,** Effect of hypophysectomy on estrogen conjugation and on plasma and tissue concentrations of tritium after administration of [^{3}H]-estradiol-17, *Steroids*, 28, 785, 1976.

313. **Djøseland, O.,** Androgen metabolism by rat epididymis. 4. The formation of conjugates, *Steroids*, 27, 617, 1976.

314. **Hart, G. W.,** Glycosaminoglycan sulfotransferases of the developing chick cornea, *J. Biol. Chem.*, 253, 347, 1978.

315. **Singer, S. S., Kutzer, T., and Lee, A.,** Enzymatic sulfation of steroids. 8. Control of hepatic cortisol sulfation and glucucorticoid sulfotransferases of rats by the pituitary gland, *Endocrinology*, 104, 571, 1979.

316. **Lambiotte, M. and Sjövall, J.,** Hydroxylation and sulfation of bile acids in rat hepatoma cultures under the influence of a glucucorticoid, *Biochem. Biophys. Res. Commun.*, 86, 1089, 1979.

317. **Mehta, R., Hirom, P. C., and Millburn, P.,** The influence of dose on the pattern of conjugation of phenol and 1-naphthol in non-human primates, *Xenobiotica*, 8, 445, 1978.

318. **Minck, K., Schupp, R. R., Illing, H. P. A., Kahl, G. F., and Netter, K. J.,** Interrelationship between demethylation of *p*-nitroanisole and conjugation of *p*-nitrophenol in rat liver, *Naunyn-Schmiedebergs Arch. Pharmacol.*, 279, 347, 1973.

319. **Hamada, N. and Gessner, T.** Effect of 3-methylcholanthrene pretreatment on glucuronidation and sulfation in perfused rat liver, *Drug Metab. Dispos.*, 3, 407, 1975.

320. **Moldeus, P., Vadi, H., and Berggren, M.,** Oxidative and conjugative metabolism of *p*-nitroanisole and *p*-nitrophenol in isolated rat liver cells, *Acta Pharmacol. Toxicol.*, 39, 17, 1976.

321. **Eyer, P. and Kampffmeyer, H. G.** Biotransformation of 4-dimethylaminophenol in the isolated perfused rat liver and in the rat, *Biochem. Pharmacol.*, 27 2223, 1978.

322. **Burke, M. D. and Orrenius, S.,** The effect of albumin on the metabolism of ethoxyresorufin through *O*-deethylation and sulphate conjugation using isolated rat hepatocytes, *Biochem. Pharmacol.*, 27, 1533, 1978.

323. **Mulder, G. J., Hayen-Keulemans, K., and Sluiter, N. E.,** UDP glucuronyltransferase and phenolsulphotransferase from rat liver *in vivo* and *in vitro*. Characterization of conjugation and biliary excretion of harmol *in vivo* and in the perfused liver, *Biochem. Pharmacol.*, 24, 103, 1975.

324. **Orrenius, S., Andersson, B., Jernström, B., and Moldeus, P.,** Isolated hepatocytes as an experimental tool in the study of drug conjugation reactions, in *Conjugation Reactions in Drug Biotransformation*, Aitio, A., Ed., Elsevier/North Holland Publishing, Amsterdam, 1978, 273.

325. **Andersson, B., Berggren, M., and Moldeus, P.,** Conjugation of various drugs in isolated hepatocytes, *Drug Metab. Dispos.*, 6, 611, 1978.

326. **Wiebkin, P., Fry, J. R., Jones, C. A., Lowing, R. K., and Bridges, J. W.,** Biphenyl metabolism in isolated rat hepatocytes: effect of induction and nature of the conjugates, *Biochem. Pharmacol.*, 27, 1899, 1978.

327. **Moldeus, P.,** Paracetamol metabolism and toxicity studied in isolated hepatocytes from mouse, in *Conjugation Reactions in Drug Biotransformation*, Aitio, A., Ed., Elsevier/North Holland Publishing, Amsterdam, 1978, 293.

328. **Vadi, H., Moldeus, P., Capdevilla, J., and Orrenius, S.,** The metabolism of benzo(α)pyrene in isolated rat liver cells, *Cancer Res.*, 35, 2083, 1975.

329. **Burke, M. D., Vadi, H., Jernström, B., and Orrenius, S.,** Metabolism of benzo(α)pyrene with isolated hepatocytes and the formation and degradation of DNA-binding derivatives, *J. Biol. Chem.*, 252, 6424, 1977.

330. **Jones, C. A., Moore, B. P., Cohen, G. M., Fry, J. R., and Bridges, J. W.,** Studies on the metabolism and excretion of benzo(α)pyrene in isolated adult rat hepatocytes, *Biochem. Pharmacol.*, 27, 693, 1978.

331. **Berry, C. S.,** Critical evaluation of UDP-*N*-acetylglucosamine and product glucuronides as allosteric effectors of UDP-glucuronyltransferase, in *Conjugation Reactions in Drug Biotransformation*, Aitio, A., Ed., Elsevier/North Holland Publishing, Amsterdam, 1978, 233.

332. **Vessey, D. A. and Zakim, D.,** Are glucuronidation reactions compartmented?, in *Conjugation Reactions in Drug Biotransformation*, Aitio, A., Ed., Elsevier/North Holland Publishing, Amsterdam, 1978, 247.

333. **Hallinan, T.**, Comparison of compartmented and of conformational phospholipid constraint models for the intramembranous arrangement of UDP-glucuronyltransferase, in *Conjugation Reactions in Drug Biotransformation,* Atio, A., Ed., Elsevier/North Holland Publishing, Amsterdam, 1978, 257.

334. **Mulder, G. J. and Van Doorn, A. B. D.**, A rapid NAD⁺-linked assay for microsomal uridine diphosphate glucuronyltransferase of rat liver and some observations on substrate specificity of the enzyme, *Biochem. J.,* 151, 131, 1975.

335. **Illing, H. P. A.**, Effects of activating agents on UDP glucuronosyltransferase activity towards acceptor substrates of different octanol/buffer partition coefficients, *Biochem. Soc. Trans.,* 6, 1211, 1978.

336. **Hänninen, O. and Alanen, K.**, The competitive inhibition of *p*-nitrophenyl-β-D-glucopyranosiduronic acid synthesis by aliphatic alcohols *in vitro, Biochem. Pharmacol.,* 15, 1465, 1966.

337. **Berry, C. and Hallinan, T.**, Summary of a novel, three component regulatory model for uridine diphosphate glucuronyltransferase, *Biochem. Soc. Trans.,* 4, 650, 1976.

338. **Vessey, D. A. and Zakim, D.**, The binding of non-polar molecules by microsomal membranes and its relation to the enzymology of UDP-glucuronyltransferase, in *Metabolism and Chemistry of Bilirubin and related Tetrapyrrols,* Bakken, A. F. and Fog, J., Eds., Rikshospitalet, Oslo, 1975, 83.

339. **Zakim, D. and Vessey, D. A.**, Membrane-bound estrone as substrate for microsomal UDP-glucuronyltransferase, *J. Biol. Chem.,* 252, 7534, 1977.

340. **Mulder, G. J.**, Heterogeneity of hepatic microsomal uridine diphosphate glucuronyltransferase: a critical evaluation, *Biochem. Soc. Trans.,* 2, 1172, 1974.

341. **Miller, H. H. and Jondorf, W. R.**, The subcellular distribution of *(±)* 2,3-dehydroemetine and (-) emetine in rat liver and changes in hepatic lipid content after treatment of rats with *(±)* dehydroemetine, *J. Pharm. Pharmacol.,* 22, 659, 1970.

342. **Levine, W. G. and Singer, R. W.**, Hepatic intracellular distribution of foreign compounds in relation to their biliary excretion, *J. Pharmacol. Exp. Ther.,* 183, 411, 1972.

343. **Bickel, M. H. and Steele, J. W.**, Binding of basic and acidic drugs to rat tissue subcellular fractions, *Chem. Biol. Interact.,* 8, 151, 1974.

344. **Blom, A., Weitering, J. G., and Meijer, D. K. F.**, Subcellular distribution of DBSP in relation to its transport in the liver. Influence of Y and Z protein, submitted.

345. **Meuwissen, J. A. T. P., Zeegers, M., Srai, K. S., and Ketterer, B.**, Effect of glutathione on the activity of bilirubin-binding proteins from rat liver cytosol, *Biochem. Soc. Trans.,* 5, 1404, 1977.

346. **Kahl, G. F., Müller, W., Kahl, R., Jonen, H. G., and Netter, K. J.**, Differential inhibition of biphenyl hydroxylation in perfused rat liver, *Naunyn-Schmiedebergs Arch. Pharmacol.,* 304, 297, 1978.

347. **Matsui, M. and Aoyagi, S.**, Variability of androsterone metabolism in male Wistar rats, *Biochem. Pharmacol.,* 28, 1023, 1979.

348. **Moldeus, P., Andersson, B., and Norling, A.**, Interaction of ethanol oxidation in isolated hepatocytes, *Biochem. Pharmacol.* 27, 2583, 1978.

349. **Otani, G., Abou-El-Makarem, M. M., and Bock, K. W.**, UDP-glucuronyltransferase in perfused rat liver and in microsomes. 3. Effects of galactosamine and carbontetrachloride on the glucuronidation of 1-naphthol and bilirubin, *Biochem. Pharmacol.,* 25, 1293, 1976.

350. **Mulder, G. J. and Scholtens, E.**, Phenolsulphotransferase and uridine diphosphate glucuronyltransferase from rat liver in vivo and in vitro. 2,6-dichloro-4-nitrophenol as selective inhibitor of sulphation, *Biochem. J.,* 165, 553, 1977.

351. **Koster, H., Scholtens, E., and Mulder, G. J.**, Inhibition of sulfation of phenols *in vivo* by 2,6-dichloro-4-nitrophenol: selectivity of its action in relation to other conjugations in the rat *in vivo, Med. Biol.,* 57, 340, 1979.

352. **Kimbrough, R. D. and Linder, R. E.**, The effect of technical and purified pentachlorophenol in the rat liver, *Toxicol. Appl. Pharmacol.,* 46, 151, 1978.

353. **Goldstein, J. A., Friesen, M., Linder, R. E., Hickman, P., Hass, J. R., and Bergman, H.**, Effects of pentachlorophenol on hepatic drug metabolizing enzymes and porphyria related to contamination with chlorinated dibenzo-*p*-dioxins and dibenzofuran, *Biochem. Pharmacol.,* 26, 1549, 1977.

354. **Koster, H., Scholtens, E., and Mulder, G. J.**, Inhibition of sulphation of phenolic substances by the carboxylesterase inhibitor bis-(*p*-nitrophenyl)-phosphate in the rat *in vivo, Biochem. Pharmacol.,* 28, 2685, 1979.

355. **Meerman, J. H. N., Van Doorn, A. B. D., and Mulder, G. J.**, Inhibition of sulfate conjugation of *N*-hydroxy-2-acetylaminofluorene in the isolated perfused rat liver and in the rat *in vivo* by pentachlorophenol and low-sulfate, *Cancer Res.,* 40, 3772, 1980.

356. **Hultmark, D., Sundh, K., Wachtmeister, C. A., and Arrhenius, E.**, Dichloro-*p*-nitroanisole *O*-demethylase. A convenient assay for microsomal mixed function oxidase in isolated rat hepatocytes, *Biochem. Pharmacol.,* 27, 1129, 1978.

357. **Davis, D. C.**, Radioisotopic assay for rat liver sulfotransferase activity, *Biochem. Pharmacol.,* 24, 975, 1975.

358. **Levy, G.,** Drug biotransformation interactions in man: non-narcotic analgesics, *Ann. N. Y. Acad. Sci.,* 179, 38, 1971.

359. **Mulder, G. J. and Pilon, A. H. E.,** UDP glucuronyltransferase and phenolsulfotransferase from rat liver in vivo and in vitro. 3. The effect of phenolphthalein and its sulfate and glucuronide conjugate on conjugation and biliary excretion of harmol, *Biochem. Pharmacol.,* 24, 517, 1975.

360. **Norling, A., Moldeus, P., Andersson, B., and Hänninen, O.,** Passage of glucuronides and sulphates into isolated hepatocytes and action on conjugation reactions, in *Conjugation Reactions in Drug Biotransformation,* Aitio, A., Ed., Elsevier/North Holland Publishing, Amsterdam, 1978, 303.

361. **Norling, A., Andersson, B., Berggren, M., and Moldeus, P.,** Uptake of glucuronides into isolated hepatocytes and their effects on glucuronide and sulphate conjugation, *Acta Pharmacol. Toxicol.,* 43, 311, 1978.

362. **Wiebkin, P., Parker, G. L., Fry, J. R., and Bridges, J. W.,** Effect of various metabolic inhibitors on biphenyl metabolism in isolated rat hepatocytes, *Biochem. Pharmacol.,* 28, 3315, 1979.

363. **Bock, K. W. and Fröhling, W.,** UDP glucuronyltransferase activity in isolated perfused rat liver, *Naunyn-Schmiedebergs Arch. Pharmacol.,* 277, 103, 1973.

364. **Bock, K. W. and White,** I. N. H., UDP-glucuronyltransferase in perfused rat liver and in microsomes: influence of phenobarbital and 3-methylcholanthrene, *Eur. J. Biochem.,* 46, 451, 1974.

365. **Gram, T. E., Litterst, C. L., and Mimnaugh, E. G.,** Enzymatic conjugation of foreign chemical compounds by rabbit lung and liver, *Drug Metab. Dispos.,* 2, 254, 1974.

366. **Jorritsma, J., Meerman, J. H. N., Vonk, R. J., and Mulder, G. J.,** Biliary and urinary excretion of drug conjugates: effect of diuresis and choleresis on excretion of harmol suphate and glucuronide in the rat, *Xenobiotica,* 9, 247, 1979.

367. **Gillette, J R. and Mitchell, J. R.,** Drug actions and interactions: theoretical considerations, in *Handbook of Pharmacology,* Vol. 28 (Part 3.), Academic Press, New York, 1975, 359.

368. **Siegers, C. P. and Schütt, A.,** Dose dependent biliary and renal excretion of paracetamol in the rat, *Pharmacology,* 18, 175, 1979.

369. **Smith, R. L. and Timbrell, J. A.,** Factors affecting the metabolism of phenacetin. 2. Effect of aspirin, caffeine, codeine, ethanol and phenobarbital on the metabolism of [acetyl-^{14}C] phenacetin in the rat, *Xenobiotica,* 4, 503, 1974.

370. **Bostrom, H., Bernstein, K., and Whitehouse, M. W.,** Biochemical properties of anti-inflammatory drugs. II. Effects on sulfate [^{35}S] metabolism *in vitro, Biochem. Pharmacol.,* 13, 413, 1964.

371. **Amsel, L. P. and Davison, C.,** Simultaneous metabolism of aspirin and acetaminophen in man, *J. Pharm. Sci.,* 61, 1474, 1972.

372. **Levy, G. and Regardh, C. G.,** Drug biotransformation interactions in man. 5. Acetaminophen and salicylic acid, *J. Pharm. Sci.,* 60, 608, 1971.

373. **Ramachander, G., Williams, F. D., and Emele, J. F.,** Effect of concurrent administration of choline salicylate and acetaminophen on their mutual biotransformation in the rat, *J. Pharm. Sci.,* 62, 1498, 1973.

374. **Bray, H. G., Thorpe, W. V., and White, K.,** Kinetic studies of the metabolism of foreign organic compounds. 1. The formation of benzoic acid from benzamide, toluene, benzylalcohol and benzaldehyde and its conjugation with glycine and glucuronic acid in the rabbit, *Biochem. J.,* 48, 88, 1951.

375. **Bray, H. G., Humphris, B. G., Thorpe, W. V., White, K., and Wood, P. B.,** Kinetic studies of the metabolism of foreign organic compounds. 3. The conjugation of phenols with glucuronic acid, *Biochem. J.,* 52, 416, 1952.

376. **Bray, H. G., Thorpe, W. V., and White, K.,** Kinetic studies of the metabolism of foreign organic compounds. 5. A mathematical model expressing the metabolic fate of phenols, benzoic acid and their precursors, *Biochem. J.,* 52, 423, 1952.

377. **Pang, K. S., Rowland, M., and Tozer, T. N.,** *In vivo* evaluation of Michaelis-Menten constants of drug eliminating systems, *Drug Metab. Dispos.,* 6, 197, 1978.

378. **Pang, K. S. and Gillette, J. R.,** Kinetics of metabolite formation and elimination in the perfused rat liver preparation: differences between the elimination of preformed acetaminophen and acetaminophen formed from phenacetin, *J. Pharmacol. Exp. Ther.,* 207, 178, 1978.

379. **Rowland, M., Benet, L. Z., and Graham, G. G.,** Clearance concepts in pharmacokinetics, *J. Pharmacokinet. Biopharm.,* 1, 123, 1973.

380. **Winkler, K., Keiding, S., and Tygstrup, N.,** Clearance as a quantitative measure of liver function, in *The Liver: Quantitative Aspects of Structure and Function,* Paumgartner, G. and Preisig, R., Eds., S. Karger, Basel, 1973, 144.

381. **Cummings, A. J., Martin, B. K., and Park, G. S.,** Kinetic considerations relating to the accrual and elimination of drug metabolites, *Br. J. Pharmacol.,* 29, 136, 1967.

382. **Cummings, A. J., King, M. L., and Martin, B. K.,** A kinetic study of drug elimination: the excretion of paracetamol and its metabolites in man, *Br. J. Pharmacol.,* 29, 150, 1967.

383. **Mrochek, J. E., Katz, S., Christie, W. H., and Dinsmore, S. R.,** Acetaminophen metabolism in man, as determined by high-resolution liquid chromatography, *Clin. Chem.,* 20, 1086, 1974.
384. **Slattery, J. T. and Levy, G.,** Acetaminophen kinetics in acutely poisoned patients, *Clin. Pharmacol. Ther.,* 25, 184, 1979.
385. **Levy, G. L., Khanna, N. N., Soda, D. M., Tsuzuki, O., and Stern, L.,** Pharmacokinetics of acetaminophen in the human neonate: formation of acetaminophen glucuronide and sulfate in relation to plasma bilirubin concentration and D-glucaric excretion, *Pediatrics,* 55, 818, 1975.
386. **Koster, H. and Mulder, G. J.,** unpublished data, 1978.
387. **Meerman, J. H. N. and Mulder, G. J.,** unpublished data, 1977.

Chapter 7

THE FATE OF SULFATE ESTERS IN VIVO

G. M. Powell and A. H. Olavesen

TABLE OF CONTENTS

I. THE BIOLOGICAL STATUS OF SULFOCONJUGATES— HYDROLYSIS IN RELATION TO SULFATION

Within the animal world there are many sulfate esters and related sulfoconjugates. The sulfate moiety is bound to a wide variety of molecules, and thus the far-reaching effects of sulfate esterification are manifest in many diverse compounds. Such common usage of sulfoconjugation in the body can be rationalized in terms of the physico-chemical characteristics of sulfate esters. Due emphasis must be placed on their ionization properties because the sulfate group is highly acidic and is fully ionized under all pH conditions existing in the body. In macromolecules having many sulfate groups, polyanions are formed which bind cations and, in addition, the highly ionic nature of the molecule results in water being held in a structured manner.

A. The Effects of Sulfoconjugation on Biological Activity

In chemical terms, the sulfate moiety creates a similar environment in all molecules. Nevertheless, even a cursory consideration of the sulfate esters in the body reveals that the introduction of sulfate groups equips the various molecules for diverse biological functions. For example, the importance of the sulfate moiety in connective tissues is clearly related to its water-holding ability and to the cation-binding affinity in relation to ion-exchange and ion balance in vivo.[1] Further, the introduction of a sulfate moiety into smaller molecules clearly alters the overall solubility properties of those molecules. This is particularly well demonstrated in the hydrophobic steroids like cholesterol and the bile acids where the introduction of the sulfate group converts the molecule into one having amphipathic properties. These properties may be very important for the function of a molecule as illustrated in the bile salts of many primitive animals where the sulfate moiety, in association with a suitable hydrophobic moiety provides the necessary physical properties for a surface-active agent.[2] In this connection, cholesterol sulfate has been implicated as an amphipathic lipid which stabilizes the erythrocyte membrane.[3,4] The sterol conjugate decreases significantly the osmotic fragility of erythrocytes exposed to hypotonic saline solutions.[5] This effect involves some degree of specificity, and both the sterol side chain and the sulfate moiety are essential for the effect.[3] In another context, the introduction of sulfate into cholesterol fits it for the quite different role of biosynthetic intermediate. This is a recurring theme when considering steroid sulfate esters in general, for it is well known that many act as important biosynthetic intermediates.[6,7] The question arises as to why the sulfate conjugates of steroids are the intermediates of choice, rather than the free steroids, in certain biosynthetic pathways. The answer may well lie in the amphipathic nature of the steroid sulfates and the intracellular location of the enzymes involved in their metabolism. One of the most striking differences between the metabolism of unconjugated and sulfoconjugated steroids is the sulfate-specific 20β-reduction of the 21-sulfates of corticosterone and deoxycorticosterone in male rat-liver microsomal preparations.[8] It is interesting that the reduction occurs in the immediate neighborhood of the sulfate group perhaps indicating that the polar, highly nucleophilic sulfate group interacts with the enzyme surface and that this interaction is a prerequisite for enzyme catalysis. A similar mechanism seems to be involved in hydroxylations catalyzed by the steroid sulfate-specific hydroxylase system present in female rat-liver microsomes.[9,10] In this case also, hydroxylation occurs in the vicinity of the sulfate group, and a special type of cytochrome P_{450} molecule with an electrophilic substrate-binding site has been suggested to participate in the catalysis. In general, it has been shown that the steroid sulfates are good substrates for hepatic reducing enzymes and in many cases they are even better substrates than their unconjugated analogues.

The question also arises as to what effect the introduction of sulfate into proteins might have on their biological activity. Currently, only one amino acid sulfate, L-tyrosine sulfate, is known to occur as an integral part of proteins. L-Tyrosine sulfate is a component of mammalian fibrinogen[11-14] and gastrin II,[15] and although this has been known for some time, the physiological contribution which this modified amino acid makes to the functions of these proteins is still open to question.

Some of the consequences of introducing a sulfate group into small molecules arise from changes in properties associated with increased water solubility and decreased lipid solubility. This is reflected in the importance of biological sulfation in the excretion of phenolic and steroidal end-products of metabolism. Thus, it is hardly surprising that sulfation is an aid to excretion since the introduction of sulfate satisfies the classic detoxication criteria: increase in polarity and thus water solubility and concomitant decrease in hydrophobicity, all combining to limit cellular uptake and favor excretion. For example, it is known that steroid sulfates penetrate slowly into reconstituted cells compared with the free steroids,[16] and arylsulfate esters, in general, seem to enjoy a limited distribution in vivo and are rapidly excreted.[17,18]

In addition to affecting the water solubility of hydrophobic molecules, the introduction of the sulfate moiety also affects the biological activity of such molecules by blocking those groups which normally have physiological consequences (for example, phenolic groups). This general rule for naturally occurring anutrients, generally referred to as foreign compounds, is not necessarily applicable to endogenous molecules. For example, information is available on some hormonal sulfates which suggests that the sulfated form of the hormone retains its biological activity. It has been claimed that sulfation of estrone is a prerequisite for the hormonal effect on protein biosynthesis[19] and dehydroepiandrosterone sulfate has estrogenic properties[20] affecting the development of chick embryo frontal bones in vitro.[21] By contrast, testosterone sulfate has only slight androgenic activity,[22] and serotonin sulfate does not stimulate aortic contraction.[23] What emerges is that with respect to the hormone sulfates there is no general rule as to whether the sulfoconjugate has biological activity or not. The situation is equally confused with regard to two vitamins, C and D, both of which are known to occur as sulfates in vivo. The antirachitic property of vitamin D sulfate in human milk was reported some time ago,[24] but no further information either on the extent of the formation of the sulfate or on its relative potency has been forthcoming. As might be expected, considerable attention has been paid to L-ascorbic acid 2-sulfate, but the situation with respect to this vitamin has been confused by conflicting reports on its possible antiscorbutic properties.[25,26] It has been suggested that ascorbic acid 2-sulfate may be involved in the sulfation of cholesterol.[27,28] Another suggested role is that of sulfate donor to glycosaminoglycans although some research does not support this idea.[29] (See Chapter 6, Section IIC.)

Uncertainties about the effects of sulfoconjugation on the activity of naturally occurring molecules are also apparent when one considers drugs and xenobiotic compounds in general. Although in many instances, sulfoconjugation is compatible with detoxication and inactivation, in other cases this may not be so, and pharmacological activity is not necessarily lost on sulfation. Thus, morphine 3-sulfate has some analgesic properties and reduces the intensity of morphine withdrawal symptoms.[30-32] Similarly, diethylstilbestrol sulfate shows estrogenic activity,[33] but it is not entirely certain whether this activity is due to the ester sulfate or its hydrolyzed product since it is known that inorganic sulfate is liberated from the ester in vivo.[34,35] By contrast, lithocholic acid sulfate is less toxic than the parent acid, and sulfoconjugation is an important protective mechanism in patients receiving chenodeoxycholate therapy for cholesterol gallstones.[36] (See further Chapter 6, Section IID.)

Yet another consequence of sulfation must be considered because various studies have revealed that sulfoconjugation may confer biological properties not possessed by the parent molecule. For example, serine sulfate reacts with and inactivates aspartate aminotransferase.[37] Further, ethanolamine sulfate is an irreversible, active-site-directed inhibitor both in vivo and in vitro of rat-brain 4-aminobutyrate aminotransferase,[38] and estrogen sulfates are powerful inhibitors of glutathione *S*-tranferase.[39] In short, the sulfation of some molecules may be regarded as a process of intoxication rather than detoxication, a concept that has been explored by Mulder.[40] Sulfation of *N*-hydroxy-*N*-acetyl-2-aminofluorene in vivo[41] certainly produces an intoxicating effect and the sulfoconjugate has been identified as a possible ultimate hepatocarcinogen in the rat.[42] Collectively, the data available illustrate that the situation is complex. The simplistic view that sulfation automatically leads to the loss of pharmacological activity of naturally occurring and xenobiotic molecules is quite clearly untenable.

B. Sulfation in Relation to Desulfation

That there are many uncertainties about the roles of some sulfoconjugates should not obscure the fact that the importance of sulfoconjugation is not in doubt. It is quite clear that the enzymes responsible for the biosynthesis of sulfate esters, the sulfotransferases, fulfill well-defined and undeniably essential biological roles. Sulfotransferases are instrumental in producing such important molecules as the glycosaminoglycans and the steroid sulfates and also provide a detoxication facility. All these are essential for the maintenance and well-being of the body. Of equal importance to the enzymes responsible for the formation of sulfate esters are those responsible for their desulfation — the sulfatases. These enzymes were accorded their rightful status when it was realized that they are concerned with degrading some physiologically important esters formed by the sulfotransferase system. Thus, the body possesses a vital sulfation/desulfation cycle concerned with the biosynthesis and turnover of the sulfate esters. Paradoxically, the importance of that balance is best demonstrated when it is disrupted, and a considerable body of information has accumulated from studies in which the levels of naturally occurring sulfoconjugates in urine, bile, and plasma have been monitored in normal and disease states. In addition, it has been shown that defects in sulfatase activity are associated with rare metabolic diseases. Elucidation of the biochemistry of metachromatic leucodystrophy showed that the tissues were low in arylsulfatase activity.[43] There are a number of connective tissue related disorders which are associated with sulfatase deficiencies of one kind or another.[44,45] All lead to defects in the degradation of one or other of the connective tissue polysaccharides coupled with severe skeletal deformities. A multiple sulfatase deficiency[46] has also been described in which there is general sulfatase deficiency affecting not only polysaccharide sulfates but also cereboside sulfate and some steroid sulfates. Placental sulfatase deficiency[47] has also been reported. This condition differs from the other sulfatase deficiencies in being sex-linked and only male fetuses are affected.

It is now important to consider, to assess, and also to speculate on how the various factors discussed in this section may be related to the fate of sulfoconjugates, their distribution, transport, pharmacological activity, biological halflives, and modes of excretion. This contribution seeks to explore these areas, dealing first of all with the sulfatase enzymes, their substrate requirements and their biological roles, and secondly, with what is known of the metabolism of sulfate esters. Finally, the distribution of sulfate esters in vivo together with their sites of formation and metabolism will be considered, and the consequences of these parameters will be assessed.

II. THE SULFATASES

The sulfatases catalyze the hydrolysis of sulfate esters according to Equation 1 where ROH may be a phenol, simple alcohol, or carbohydrate or indeed almost any hydroxyl-containing compound.

$$ROSO_3^- + H_2O \rightarrow ROH + H^+ + SO_4^{2-} \tag{1}$$

The ability of mammals to desulfate sulfate esters has been appreciated for a very long time, and a number of reviews[48-51] describe the early history and development of this field. As information has accumulated over the years, it has become abundantly clear that the capacity for desulfation in mammals is far from simple and cannot be ascribed to a single hydrolytic enzyme. It is now known that a whole variety of compounds containing the sulfate moiety, in a variety of chemical environments are suitable substrates for desulfation in vivo. This implies and indeed reflects the multiplicity of enzymes which are available to achieve sulfate removal from diverse molecules. Difficulties arise when one considers the multiplicity of the sulfatases and their contribution to the whole organism in acting as a desulfating system. Although the specificities of some of the enzymes have been clarified a good deal in recent years, and their roles are better understood, much more information is required before a complete picture can be presented. Much of the confusion which has arisen, in relation to specificity, function, and distribution, has been due to the use of synthetic substrates in the early years of sulfatase research. Nevertheless, synthetic substrates have been important in providing the initial classification of sulfatase activity, which is still used. The convenience of these unphysiological substrates, particularly the chromogenic ones, was instrumental in amassing information on the wisespread distribution of the enzymes in nature, delineating their distribution intracellularly and also in pinpointing disease states where the absence of certain sulfatases suggested possible roles for their activity in vivo.

A. The Classification of Sulfatases

The synthetic substrates which have been used extensively to measure sulfatase activity are 4-hydroxyacetophenone sulfate (4-acetylphenyl sulfate), 4-nitrophenyl sulfate, and 2-hydroxy-5-nitrophenyl sulfate (nitrocatechol sulfate) illustrated in Figure 1. By using these compounds, it became apparent that sulfatase enzymes could be conveniently classified into two main groups on the basis of their activities and specificities towards these substrates. One group of enzymes was more active towards the simpler arylsulfates (4-acetylphenyl sulfate and 4-nitrophenyl sulfate) while members of the other group were more active towards nitrocatechol sulfate than towards the simpler esters.[50] Activity towards 4-acetylphenyl sulfate is localized in the microsomal fraction, whereas the activity towards nitrocatechol sulfate is associated with the lysosomes. The microsomal enzyme (named arylsulfatase C) was characterized by its alkaline optimum pH and its greater activity towards 4-acetylphenyl sulfate and 4-nitrophenyl sulfate than towards nitrocatechol sulfate. Activity is inhibited by cyanide but not by sulfate or phosphate ions. Lysosomal enzyme activity on the other hand, was characterized by an acid pH optimum and high activity towards nitrocatechol sulfate. Further, activity is inhibited by phosphate ions but not by cyanide, the converse of the situation with arylsulfatase C. Two arylsulfatase enzymes with these properties are present in the lysosomes. They have been designated arylsulfatases A and B and were distinguished initially on the basis of their different kinetic properties.[52,53] Thus, it has

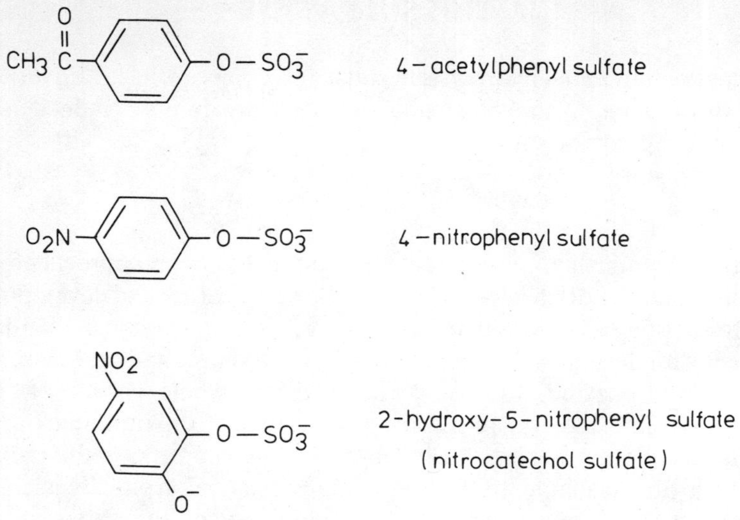

FIGURE 1. Chemical structure of some nonphysiological substrates for arylsulfatase S.

become clear that mammalian tissues contain at least three distinct arylsulfatases which have been classified as either Type I or Type II according to whether their properties resemble those of arylsulfatase C or arylsulfatases A and B.[54] This classification has proven useful, but Dodgson and Rose[55] have warned against misusing it by carrying the analogy too far and by applying the definition too rigidly.

1. Arylsulfatase C

As previously discussed, arylsulfatase C activity, as assayed using nonphysiological substances, is located in the microsomal fraction. Dodgson and Rose[56] are firmly of the opinion that the natural substrate for arylsulfatase C is estrone sulfate and that the estrogen sulfatase activity is concerned with regulating estrogen levels in vivo. The 3β-sulfates of the 5α and Δ^5 series of steroids are also hydrolyzed by the microsomal fraction.[57] Thus, the sulfate esters of epiandrosterone, pregnenolone, and androstene-diol can serve as substrates for microsomal sulfatase activity. The question arises as to whether this activity is due to a separate enzyme or whether it is identical with arylsulfatase C. This question is unresolved mainly because sulfatase activity is tightly bound to the microsomal membrane and consequently difficult to solubilize. One theoretical argument in favor of two distinct enzyme activities can be made on the basis of the structures of the substrates hydrolyzed by microsomes (see Figure 2). Those with the estrogen skeleton (estrone sulfate) may be considered to be arylsulfate esters, whereas those in which ring A is not aromatic (e.g., dehydroepiandrosterone sulfate) are steroid sulfates. Hence, it would not be surprising if more than one enzyme were necessary to remove sulfate in these very different chemical environments.

2. Arylsulfatases A and B

Type II arylsulfatase activity is located in the lysosomes. It is now clear that arylsulfatases A and B are not true arylsulfatases, but by chance are active towards nitrocatechol sulfate. In fact, both enzymes attack sulfate groups attached to carbohydrate residues, and in vivo arylsulfatase A is certainly concerned with the turnover of cerebroside sulfate[45,58] and arylsulfatase B with the desulfation of *N*-acetyl galactosamine 4-sulfate residues during glycosaminoglycan turnover[59] (see Figure 3).

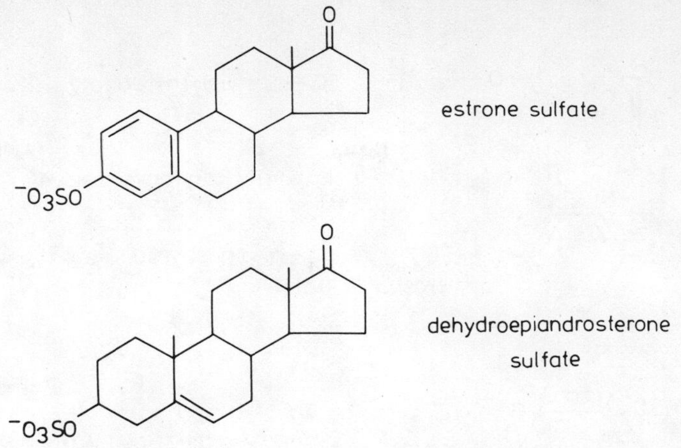

estrone sulfate

dehydroepiandrosterone sulfate

^-O_3SO

FIGURE 2. Chemical structure of substrates for microsomal sulfatase activity.

3. Other Carbohydrate Sulfatases

A number of other mammalian lysosomal sulfatases have been discovered, all of which appear to be concerned with glycosaminoglycan turnover.[44,45] Their discovery has stemmed from the studies of inherited metabolic diseases of connective tissue. Thus in the lysosomes there is a complex set of sulfatase enzymes acting on the closely related substrates shown in Figure 3.

4. Sulfamatases

Mammals also possess enzymes which hydrolyze $N-SO_3^-$ linkages.[55]

$$R.NH.SO_3^- + H_2O \rightarrow R.NH_3^+ + SO_4^{2-} \tag{2}$$

These are the sulfamatases also found in the lysosomes. They are involved in the turnover of connective tissue polysaccharide containing the sulfamate group, for example, heparin and heparan sulfate whose structures are shown in Figure 4.

5. Sulfatophosphate Sulfatases

Two further distinct sulfatases are present in the mammalian liver cells.[55,56] They hydrolyze the sulfatophosphate linkage according to the following equation:

$$R-O-\overset{\overset{O}{\parallel}}{\underset{\underset{O^-}{|}}{P}}-O-SO_3^- + H_2O \rightarrow R-O-\overset{\overset{O}{\parallel}}{\underset{\underset{O^-}{|}}{P}}-O^- + SO_4^{2-} + 2H^+ \tag{3}$$

where R represents adenosine or its 3′-phosphate derivative. The substrates are thus adenosine 5′-sulfatophosphate (APS) and adenosine 3′-phosphate 5′-sulfatophosphate (PAPS). The APS-sulfatase has a bimodal distribution in the liver cell with distinct forms of the enzyme in the cytosol and the lysosomes.[60] Much less information is available on PAPS-sulfatase,[55] but PAPS is certainly degraded by the lysosomes, cytosol, and endoplasmic reticulum of mammalian liver (see Chapter 4, Section V for further information).

B. Sulfatase Activity in Relation to Drug Metabolism

It is quite clear that mammals are capable of desulfating, enzymically, a wide variety of compounds containing sulfate moieties covalently bound to widely differing chemical

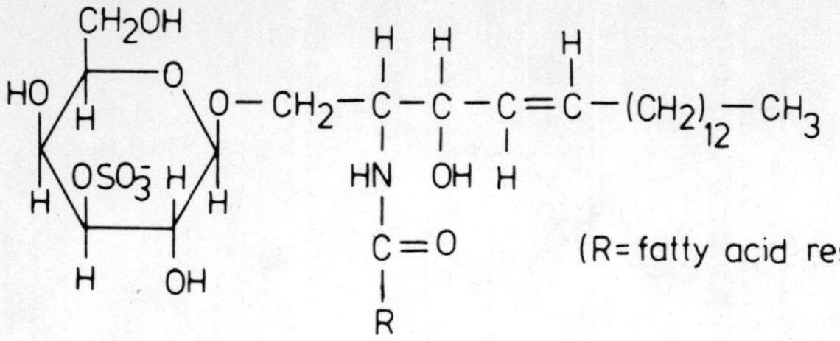

cerebroside sulfate

(R= fatty acid residue)

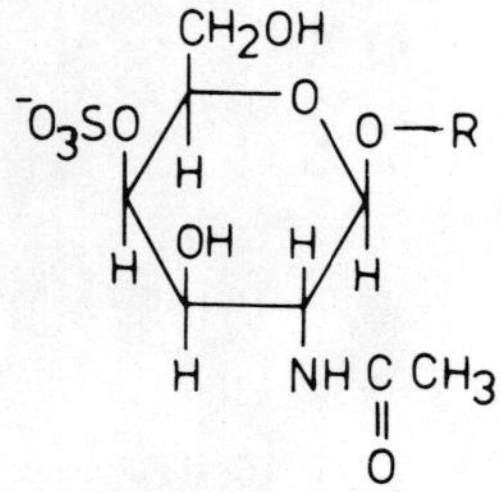

(R = polysaccharide)

N-Acetylgalactosamine 4-sulfate

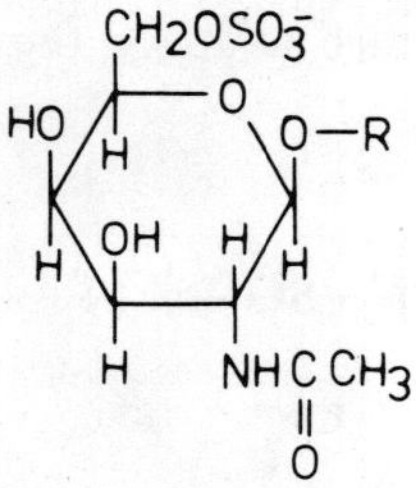

(R=polysaccharide)

N-Acetylgalactosamine 6-sulfate

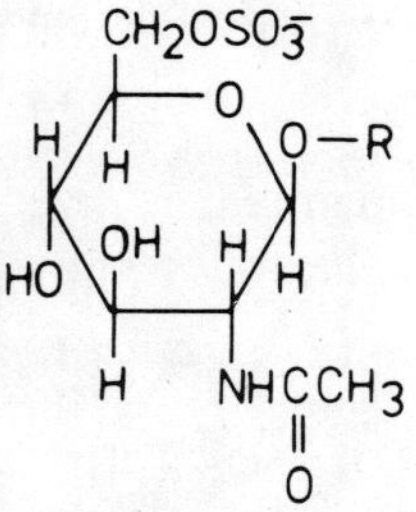

(R=polysaccharide)

N-Acetylglucosamine 6-sulfate

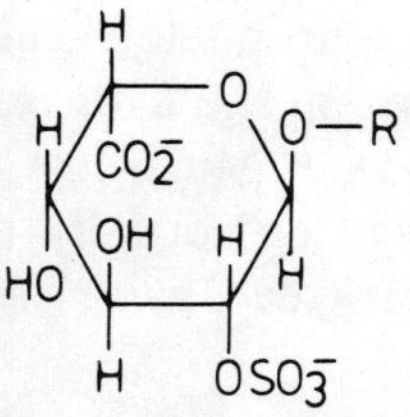

(R=polysaccharide)

∝-L-Iduronic-acid 2-sulfate

FIGURE 3. Chemical structure of some physiological substrates for lysosomal sulfatases.

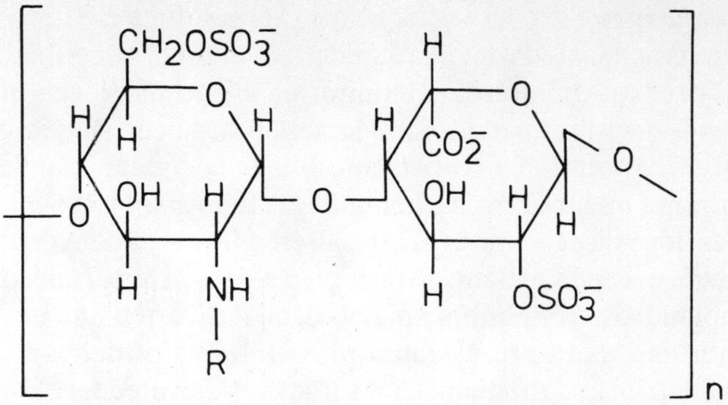

Heparin ;   R = predominantly SO_3^-

Heparan sulfate ;   R = predominantly Acetyl

FIGURE 4. Structures of heparin and heparan sulfate.

structures. Thus, the body possesses an arsenal of enzymes which can attack chemically disparate sulfate esters. An understanding of their physiological roles has been reached only very slowly, but from the data accumulated over a number of years, it now seems that the enzymes present in insoluble form in the smooth endoplasmic reticulum are concerned with the regulation of estrogen levels, while the lysosomal enzymes are concerned with the turnover of macromolecules containing carbohydrate sulfates. The roles which the enzymes might play in relation to drug metabolism are even more difficult to assess mainly because it is only recently that the definitive substrates have been identified for the enzymes in vivo. Nevertheless, many investigations using nonphysiological substrates have revealed that the enzymes may attack compounds other than those for which they were evolved. This is well illustrated by the fact that nonphysiological substrates like 4-nitrophenyl sulfate can be hydrolyzed in vivo. Studies such as these are particularly relevant in assessing the status of sulfatases with respect to the fates of drugs. It cannot be emphasized too strongly that if suitable substrates are presented to the sulfatase enzymes, then hydrolysis will occur and that sulfate esters formed from foreign compounds, such as drugs, or sulfate esters exogenously supplied may undergo desulfation by one or more of the sulfatase enzymes. The point must also be made that although various drugs, sulfated in vivo, may be relatively poor substrates for the sulfatase enzymes, even limited desulfation may give rise to native drug or its metabolic derivatives with subsequent prolongation of its halflife which may result in toxic effects.

III. SULFATASES AND THE FATE OF SULFATE ESTERS IN VIVO

A. Sulfate Esters in Urine

In view of the ubiquitous distribution of the sulfatase enzymes and the wide variety of substrates which they hydrolyze, it is perhaps surprising that so many sulfate esters of diverse structure are excreted in the urines of mammals. Mammalian urines contain many steroid sulfates and a large number derived from C_{18}-, C_{19}-, and C_{21}-steroids have been identified in human urine.[21,61] Disulfate derivatives of some steroids are also present in human urine.[62] The concentrations of urinary steroid sulfates are potentially of much clinical interest as indicators of hormonal metabolism. For example, it is known that the level of urinary estrogen sulfates increases during pregnancy,[63] that dehydroepiandrosterone sulfate levels alter during labor[64] and are affected by diet and obesity.[65] In pregnancy, there is also elevated urinary excretion of corticosteroid conjugates and large increases in plasma testosterone sulfate.[21] There are indications[66] that increasing age is associated with increased production of steroid sulfates by gonadal tissue. There has been much interest in monitoring the urinary levels of steroid sulfates both in normal and in various pathological states. It has been suggested, for example, that the levels of urinary sulfated corticosteroid may be valuable indicators of normal and abnormal adrenal metabolism. Other changes in urinary steroid sulfate levels are associated with various disease states. Thus, altered levels of dehydroepiandrosterone sulfate have been recorded in patients with benign essential hypertension.[67] In operative stress, dehydroepiandrosterone sulfate metabolism is diverted and urinary levels fall.[68] In Cushings syndrome there are elevated plasma levels of dehydroepiandrosterone sulfate, and pregenetriol and pregnanetriol sulfates.[69] Elevated levels of corticosterone sulfate are associated with breast cancer,[70] and urines of women taking estrogen contraceptives contain higher-than-normal levels of steroid sulfates.[71]

Normal urine also contains a variety of nonsteroidal sulfate esters, and a substantial proportion of these represent inactivation products of anutrients of exogenous origin. They are the detoxication products of naturally occurring phenolic anutrients presented to the body via the gastrointestinal tract either in the food supply or as a result of bacterial metabolism in the gut. Thus, depletion of the intestinal flora markedly influences the urinary phenol excretion pattern,[72,73] and certain sulfates (phenyl sulfate and indoxyl sulfate) are lacking completely from the urines of germ-free animals.[74] However, in such animals there is a well-differentiated pattern of sulfate conjugates (20 to 45 in number) which is independent of the bacterial flora in the gut.[74]

Not all the nonsteroidal sulfate esters present in urine can be classified as detoxication products of exogenous anutrients. It is well known that sulfoconjugates of compounds of endogenous origin are normal urinary constituents. Some of these were identified and recorded many years ago, but it is noteworthy that there are interesting recent additions to the list. Those sulfate esters present include L-tyrosine sulfate and 4-hydroxyphenylpyruvate sulfate which arise from the degradation of polypeptides containing L-tyrosine sulfate residues.[75-77] Other urinary sulfate esters derived from endogenous phenols include estrone sulfate,[78,79] serotonin sulfate,[80] 2-amino-3-hydroxyacetophenone sulfate,[81] 5-hydroxyindolylacetic acid sulfate,[82] and dopamine sulfate.[83] Ascorbic acid 2-sulfate is also present in urine,[84] but its origin is not known.

B. Sulfate Esters Inert In Vivo

Attempts have been made to assess the importance and the definitive roles of the sulfatases by studying the fates in vivo of various sulfate esters of diverse structure. Early work established that a number of compounds, both naturally occurring and foreign, were excreted unchanged in the urine following their administration to experimental animals. For example, it was shown that the sulfates of phenol,[85] 1-naphthol, and 2-naphthol[86] were excreted largely unchanged with 10% hydrolysis at the most. Subsequent work has established that a range of sulfate esters (both naturally occurring and synthetic) are excreted in the urines of experimental animals receiving them. They include naphthyl 2-sulfate,[16] 5,6,7,8-tetrahydronaphthyl 2-sulfate,[16] D-glucose 6-sulfate,[87] D-galactose 6-sulfate,[87] N-acetyl glucosamine 6-sulfate,[88] N-acetyl galactosamine 6-sulfate,[89] 5-hydroxytryptamine sulfate,[90] ethyl sulfate, and ethanolamine sulfate.[91] There is also some evidence that ascorbic acid 2-sulfate is not desulfated in vivo,[27] but all studies involving the [^{35}S]-labeled molecule should perhaps be treated with caution in view of the finding that the radiolabeled ester undergoes modification when stored in the solid state.[92] Mention should also be made of phenolphthalein disulfate, another sulfate ester which is excreted unchanged, but in this case the route of elimination is biliary in both rats[93,94] and guinea pigs.[34] Collectively, these findings have established that the excretion of administered sulfate esters is a common phenomenon, and that many sulfate esters (both synthetic and of endogenous origin) are not attacked by the sulfatases in vivo. There is also abundant evidence that sulfation is a device commonly employed for the detoxication of drugs and that the sulfoconjugates once formed are not subject to attack by the sulfatases since they appear in the urine. This view is substantiated by studies with such drugs as salicylamide,[95] isoprenaline[96] and anthranilamide,[97] and others.[98-103]

C. Sulfate Esters Desulfated In Vivo

It is hardly surprising that research reports amassed throughout a number of years, on the excretion of nonmetabolized sulfate esters led to the popular belief that sulfate esters are inert in vivo. Gradually this view has been abandoned because there is now overwhelming evidence that this is not so. It has been established that sulfate esters are not necessarily inert and may undergo a variety of metabolic transformations. For example, many sulfate esters are extensively desulfated, viz. 4-nitrophenyl sulfate,[50] triiodothyronine sulfate,[104] biphenyl 4-sulfate,[105] cyclohexylphenyl 2-sulfate,[105] cyclohexylphenyl 4-sulfate,[105] and estrone sulfate.[106-108] All these studies have been carried out with [^{35}S]-labeled sulfate esters, and the extent of sulfohydrolysis has been determined by measuring the amounts of $^{35}SO_4^{2-}$ released in vivo. The extent of desulfation may vary from one species to another, and this can be rationalized in terms of species differences in enzyme levels. Thus, the extensive desulfation of estrone sulfate in the rat[107] would be forecast since the ester is a substrate for estrogen sulfate sulfohydrolase which is probably identical with arylsulfatase C. The guinea pig has low levels of this enzyme, and desulfation of administered estrone sulfate is accordingly much less.[109,110] Similar arguments, in terms of enzyme complement have been applied to the very different metabolic fates of diethylstilbestrol sulfate esters in the rat[34] and guinea pig.[35]

It is hardly surprising that substances such as 4-nitrophenyl sulfate which have been used to assay sulfohydrolase activity in vitro should be readily desulfated in vivo. However, the fate in vivo of compounds like nitrocatechol sulfate does not lend itself to such rationalization since although it has long been the substrate of choice for assaying mammalian lysosomal sulfatase activity, and substantial hydrolysis in vivo might be expected, this does not occur. The explanation for the discrepancy between the experimental findings and theoretical prediction lies in the rapid urinary excretion of the ester.[111]

IV. THE ELIMINATION OF SULFATE ESTERS

A. Urinary Excretion

The presence of diverse sulfoconjugates in substantial concentrations in urine and bile is entirely predictable if conjugation with sulfuric acid is viewed solely as a detoxication device. Sulfoconjugation has long been viewed as an aid to urinary excretion, and certainly the addition of sulfate to an unionized functional group, converting it into a fully ionized group, substantially changes the physical properties of the molecule. Generally, it becomes more polar, less lipid soluble, and thus more readily excreted in the urine. The efficacy of the device is borne out by the fact that many phenolic compounds appear in the urine as ester sulfates. Nevertheless, the actual mechanisms by which the kidney handles sulfoconjugates are still largely obscure. Many sulfate esters, both of steroids[112] and of simple phenols[17,105,113] are firmly bound to plasma proteins, and this may well be an important influence in the movement of compounds between blood and urine. There may be further complications because there are indications that at least one sulfate ester (tyrosine sulfate) may undergo tubular reabsorption.[114] Studies on the mode of excretion of sulfate esters by the kidney have been hampered by the lack of suitable methods for their estimation in the plasma. However, Sperber,[115] taking advantage of the renal portal system in birds, showed that a number of phenolic sulfate esters are secreted by the renal cells. More recently, sulfate ester excretion in mammals was studied,[113] and the findings limit the widely held view that sulfation of phenols is solely concerned with the introduction of a highly polar group which hinders tubular reabsorption since it was established that phenyl sulfate, 2-naphthyl sulfate, and nitrocatechol sulfate are secreted into the renal tubular fluid. Similar results were obtained with dehydroepiandrosterone sulfate and showed that this ester competes with phenyl sulfate for renal excretion.[116] Thus, it seems vey likely that the detoxication effect produced by sulfation of phenols is coupled with a secretory process in the kidney, which aids the rapid elimination of potentially toxic compounds. The secretory mechanism has not been elucidated, but there is evidence that uptake at the peritubular membrane is an active process. Thus, it has been shown that the renal excretion of extrarenally formed morphine sulfate and catechol sulfate is blocked by probenecid, but that excretion of the same conjugates formed within the cells is not.[117,118] From studies on the renal handling of phenol and 4-nitrophenol it has been suggested[119] that the process of excreting sulfoconjugates does not necessarily involve active transport, the high tubular excretion ratios simply reflecting the trapping, in urine, of conjugates to which the peritubular membrane is relatively impermeable. What emerges from the limited number of studies on the renal handling of sulfoconjugates is that the addition of sulfate does not necessarily signal direct and simple transport into urine.

B. Biliary Excretion

Biliary excretion of sulfoconjugates is a common phenomenon, but an understanding of the process and its implication in many ways parallels that of our understanding of urinary excretion. Thus, although the excretion of various sulfate esters in the bile is well documented, little is known about the mechanisms involved. Among the sulfoconjugates of endogenous compounds which appear in the bile are triiodothyronine sulfate,[104] estrogen sulfates,[120] various steroid sulfates[61,121-124] and steroid disulfates,[125,126] bilirubin sulfate,[127] the sulfates of glycolithocholate and taurolithocholate,[128] and bile acid sulfates.[129] There are also many examples of the biliary elimination of the sulfoconjugates of xenobiotics. The drug morphine is eliminated via the bile as the sulfate conjugate although only in some species.[130-132] Other examples include Terbutaline,[99] Topanol,[102] iodinated phenoxybenzoic acid—a hypocholesterolaemic agent,[133] the analgaesic 1-*n*-butyryl-4-cinnamylpiperazine,[134] and carbenoxolone.[135]

It has been proposed[136,137] that the prerequisites for biliary elimination are a suitable balance of hydrophilic and lipophilic properties, the presence of a strongly polar anionic group, and a minimum molecular weight which is species dependent. The significance of the presence of the sulfate moiety in relation to these criteria has not been evaluated, but some studies have been designed to investigate this particular point. The biliary excretion of exogenously supplied [^{35}S]-labeled sulfate esters has shown that, although significant percentages of the [^{35}S] dose appeared in the bile after the administration of [^{35}S]-labeled biphenyl 4-sulfate, cyclohexylphenyl 4-sulfate, and cyclohexylphenyl 2-sulfate, in all cases the esters were further metabolized by hydroxylation and conjugation with glucuronic acid before biliary excretion occurred.[105] Other sulfate esters are known to be conjugated with glucuronic acid before biliary elimination, for example, nitrocatechol sulfate.[111] In the case of cortisone 21-sulfate, reduction is followed by glucuronic acid conjugation.[138] Rationalization for the formation of these double conjugates on the grounds of molecular weight was suggested since some sulfate esters would reach and exceed the molecular weight threshold by the addition of a glucuronic acid moiety.[139] This view gains support from data obtained with phenolphthalein disulfate which does meet the molecular weight requirement and which appears in the bile unchanged.[139] However, studies in the rat on the sulfate esters of diethylstilbestrol strongly suggest the involvement of other factors.[34] Although both the monosulfate and the disulfate of diethylstilbestrol are eliminated via the bile as diethylstilbestrol monosulfate monoglucuronide, it has been suggested that factors other than molecular weight are the determinants of the extent of biliary elimination. Thus, the results obtained with both esters have been explained on the basis of transport and location of the esters in the liver cell, the activity of arylsulfatase C of rat liver—and the affinity of a UDP-glucuronosyltransferase for diethylstilbestrol monosulfate. These claims have been supported by subsequent work with several compounds in the guinea pig.[35,140] Further, the differences in the nature of the biliary compounds in rats and guinea pigs is apparently explicable in terms of the relative activities of hepatic sulfatase, sulfotransferase, and UDP-glucuronosyltransferase systems. However, it is clear that the full significance of the sulfate moiety on choleophiles will not emerge until it is possible to describe, in detail, the molecular mechanisms by which compounds, in general, appear in the bile. It has been shown that some sulfate and glucuronide conjugates compete at some stage for biliary elimination[94] and Powell et al.[141] have put forward a model system which describes the elimination of phenolphthalein disulfate. However, the relationship between sulfate conjugation and biliary elimination is still very poorly understood. A number of reports[142,143] in the literature suggest that the urinary and biliary pathways of excretion may be complementary to each other. Hirom et al.[142] have illustrated that complementation is dependent upon the molecular weight of the compounds being excreted. Thus, compounds of molecular weight less than 350, whose major route of elimination is urinary, are not excreted in bile to any significant extent even when urinary excretion is prevented by kidney ligation. Similarly, compounds in the molecular weight range 450 to 850, which are excreted predominantly in bile are not excreted in urine even when the biliary route is obstructed. It is only for compounds in the molecular weight range 350 to 450 that there is a compensatory interrelationship between the urinary and biliary routes. Other studies[143] designed to investigate urinary and biliary compensatory characteristics using physiological means (diuresis and choleresis) have shown that, for harmol sulfate, urine and bile are compensatory pathways of elimination that can be influenced by urine and bile flow. However, the precise factors governing these effects are still unclear.

V. METABOLIC MODIFICATION OF SULFATE ESTERS
OTHER THAN AT THE C-O-S BOND

A. Hydroxylation and Further Conjugation

Some sulfate esters, although not substrates for the mammalian sulfatases, are metabolized to yield intermediates which, in turn, give rise to urinary inorganic sulfate. For example, cortisone 21-[^{35}S]-sulfate is reduced to the corresponding 3α-hydroxy-5α-pregnane derivative which is excreted in bile after conjugation with glucuronic acid.[138] The [^{35}S] eventually appears, in part, as $^{35}SO_4^{2-}$ in the urine: the route by which this occurs is unknown. No sulfatase capable of hydrolyzing corticosteroid 21-sulfates is known in mammalian tissues, and it may be that the double conjugate, or the aglycone formed from it through the action of intestinal β-glucuronidase, is absorbed from the gastrointestinal tract, and a metabolite of this yields inorganic sulfate. Similar arguments have been proposed to explain the appearance of inorganic sulfate in urines of animals receiving either cyclohexylphenyl 4-sulfate or the 2-sulfate derivative[105] since neither is a substrate for the microsomal sulfatase[91] and both appear in the bile as glucuronic acid derivatives following hydroxylation in the liver.

B. Indirect Sulfate Loss

It is well known that hydrolytic attack by sulfatases is not the only means by which inorganic sulfate may be liberated from sulfate esters in vivo. In the case of serine sulfate, extensive release of inorganic sulfate occurs,[144] but experiments in vitro[145] have shown that the products of enzymic degradation are pyruvate and ammonia in addition to inorganic sulfate, implying that the enzyme is not a simple sulfatase. Because of this, it has been suggested[146,147] that the inorganic sulfate produced in vivo following injection of dipeptides containing serine sulfate originates from the free ester liberated by dipeptidase action. This must certainly be true for glycyl-L-serine sulfate which cannot act as a substrate for a desulfating enzyme. L-Threonine sulfate is another amino acid sulfate yielding inorganic sulfate in experimental animals, but in this instance direct enzymic desulfation is also unlikely although the mechanism of sulfate release is not known.[148]

C. ω,β-Oxidation

Further examples of sulfate release not involving sulfatase action are furnished by a number of simple primary and secondary alkyl sulfates. They give rise to some inorganic sulfate following their administration to experimental animals, but this is not due to alkyl sulfatase activity which is absent from mammalian tissues. Explanation is afforded by the nature of the metabolism of the esters and the instability of the metabolites. The esters are subjected to ω,β-oxidation with the production of short chain sulfated carboxylic acids, the precise nature of which depends on the structure of the hydrophobic chains of the parent molecules. Dodecyl sulfate,[149] decyl sulfate, octadecyl sulfate,[150] undecyl sulfate,[151] and hexadecyl sulfate[152] yield three-, four-, or five-carbon carboxylic acid sulfates. In particular, it has been established that butyric acid 4-sulfate, the product of ω,β-oxidation of even-numbered carbon alkyl sulfates undergoes nonenzymic desulfation at physiological pH.[153] The metabolism of 2-ethylhexyl sulfate[154] in rat and rabbit may also be rationalized in terms of modification of the hydrophobic chain prior to loss of the sulfate moiety. Recent studies with octyl 2-sulfate[155] indicate that secondary sulfates, in general, undergo sulfate loss in vivo following ω,β-oxidation. These results illustrate the importance of attack on the carbon skeleton remote from the sulfate moiety leading to unstable products which undergo spontaneous loss of sulfate. They also underline the pitfall of interpreting the appearance of inorganic sulfate as an indication of sulfatase attack. In this connection, it should be noted that inorganic sulfate is released from dopamine 3-sulfate during its conversion to norepinephrine by dopamine β-hydroxylase in the presence of ascorbic acid.[156] It is interesting that ascorbic acid 2-sulfate competitively inhibits dopamine-β-hydroxylase activity, and it has been suggested that ascorbic acid 2-sulfate may play a regulatory role in the biosynthesis of norepinephrine.[157] Loss of sulfate from dopamine 3-sulfate has been reported,[83] but other studies[158] indicate that the ester is metabolically inert. It seems almost certain that the disparity in results is due to the different dose levels used. Dopamine 4-sulfate is not metabolically inert but undergoes desulfation and deamination.[159]

D. Conjugation with Glutathione

Yet another example of sulfate release unrelated to sulfatase activity is given by the metabolism of aralkyl sulfate esters in the rat. It has been concluded that the aralkylation of glutathione is an early step in the formation of aralkylmercapturic acids from aralkyl esters.[160,161] Rat-liver supernatant preparations catalyze the reactions of some arylalkyl sulfate esters to yield S-aralkylglutathione derivatives.[162] Sulfate ions are released from benzyl sulfate, 2-menaphthyl (naphth-1-yl methyl) sulfate, phenanthr-9-ylmethyl sulfate but not from prop-1-yl sulfate, L-serine sulfate, phenyl sulfate, or estrone sulfate. Mercapturic acid formation can also occur as a conjugation device for the metabolism of short-chain alkyl sulfates. Thus, n-butyl, n-pentyl and n-hexyl mercapturic acids,[163,164] were detected as urinary metabolites of the corresponding alkyl sulfate esters after their administration to rats. Very little of the corresponding alkyl mercapturic acid was detected after administration of alkyl sulfates of chain length longer than six carbons. Thus, the mechanism operates for short-chain alkyl sulfates only and may not represent a significant pathway in the metabolism of the longer-chain analogues. The disubstituted sulfate esters, diethyl sulfate and di-n-propyl sulfate yield ethyl and n-propyl mercapturic acids, respectively, in the rat.[164]

E. General Comments

A number of references have already been made to sulfate esters which are metabolized in vivo without initial loss of the sulfate moiety. To these must be added the sulfate ester of the amino acid tyrosine which is metabolized by the rat to yield two major products, the sulfate esters of 4-hydroxyphenylpyruvic acid[165] and 4-hydroxy-phenylacetic acid.[166] What has emerged over a number of years is that sulfate esters cannot be treated as a homogenous group but that each sulfate ester must be considered as an individual case. Its desulfation or further metabolism may not be simply predicted. The most potent illustrations of this fact, still not fully appreciated, come from studies with the steroid sulfates which exploded the erstwhile popular view that all sulfate esters are the endproducts of metabolism and are thus inert in vivo. Drastic revision of this view was necessary when it was recognized that steroid sulfates may play important roles in metabolic interconversions. Recognition of the roles which steroid sulfates may play in these conversions began with observations on cholesterol sulfate metabolism[167] and were fruitfully extended to other sulfated steroids such as dehydroepiandrosterone sulfate.[125] Subsequent studies evaluated by Pasqualini[168] unequivocally established the involvement of steroid sulfates in metabolic processes where they fulfill roles as biosynthetic intermediates and also in transport. The functions of steroid sulfates in hormone biosynthesis have been appraised by Dominguez et al.[169]

VI. THE DISTRIBUTION OF SULFATE ESTERS IN RELATION TO THEIR METABOLISM

The metabolism of exogenously supplied sulfate esters should be considered in terms of site of entry into the animal, transport to various organs, and the metabolic capabilities of those organs. Particular attention should be directed towards the distribution of sulfate esters both at the organ and subcellular level because their ultimate fate depends upon their interaction with the appropriate enzymes. The classical view sees the presence of the sulfate moiety as a severely limiting factor in the entry of sulfate esters into cells and indeed this view is substantiated in a number of studies on estrone and its sulfate. Uptake of the sulfate into isolated liver cells is much slower,[170] and studies with the isolated perfused liver system suggest a slower uptake of estrone sulfate than estrone.[171,172] However, a sulfate ester is not necessarily precluded from extensive cellular penetration. Indeed, their penetration to seemingly unlikely sites no longer occasions surprise. For instance, it is now accepted that sulfate esters like dehydroepiandrosterone sulfate[173] and estrone sulfate[174] are able to enter the brain. Thus, sulfate esters do not comprise a homogenous group with respect to distribution, but each ester must be separately considered.

Further factors having far-reaching influences on the metabolic fates of sulfate esters are the routes and rates of elimination. With respect to urinary excretion, the rate of elimination may well limit the extent of desulfation. Nitrocatechol sulfate is a case in point, and the insignificant extent of desulfation is explained by its rapid urinary excretion, an argument supported by the fact that appreciable hydrolysis of the ester occurs in the isolated perfused liver system.[111] Thus, although the capacity of the liver for metabolizing sulfate esters can be usefully assessed in the isolated perfused system, quantitatively the results may be different from those in the whole animal, a point further illustrated by studies using octan-2-sulfate.[91]

When ester sulfates are eliminated in the bile, they may appear unchanged or as double conjugates (glucuronide sulfates) depending on the species.[34,35,105] Usually, an enterohepatic circulation is established with subsequent prolongation of biological halflife.[175] The possible complexities attendant on an enterohepatic circulation with successive modifications of the molecule with each cycle are illustrated by studies with cortisone 21-sulfate.[138] It has already been noted that the sulfate is eventually released and appears in the urine. Inorganic sulfate also appears in urines of guinea pigs receiving estrone sulfate, but the ester is excreted unchanged in guinea-pig bile, and there are indications that it may be desulfated in the gut lumen.[109]

Contrary to popular belief, the sulfate group appears not to restrict absorption from the gastrointestinal tract. A variety of substances including simple phenolic sulfates,[105] primary[149] and secondary alkyl sulfates,[91] and alkylethoxy sulfates[176] are readily absorbed from the gut.

A. The Distribution of Sulfate Esters In Vivo
1. The Distribution of Sulfate Esters in Relation to Desulfation
In order to obtain a comprehensive picture of the metabolism of sulfate esters, experiments should be designed to investigate distributions in vivo and the capacities of individual organs to bring about metabolic transformations. The technique of whole-body radioautography used to study the distribution of a series of administered sulfate esters[177] showed that, in general, they were not widely distributed in vivo. However, with certain compounds there was a dramatic uptake and concentration by various tissues. Hepatic tissues were most commonly involved, but with some esters accumulation was noted in other tissues. For example, following the administration of [^{35}S]-labeled L-threonine sulfate, L-serine sulfate, and L-serylglycine sulfate to immature rats there was a marked accumulation of radioactivity in brown fat, although the physiological significance of this is still obscure.[177] From inspecting the distribution patterns obtained with a whole range of sulfate esters, a general rule emerged: metabolism could be correlated with tissue accumulation. Thus, sulfuric acid esters such as D-glucose 6-sulfate, which are excreted largely unchanged, show little or no cellular accumulation.[178] By contrast, other esters known to undergo substantial metabolic conversion yielded quite different distribution patterns, and although the precise nature of the pattern varied from one ester to another, they all showed cellular uptake and accumulation.[18] For example, [^{35}S]-labeled esters such as cortisone sulfate and the alkyl sulfates gave distribution patterns dominated by accumulation of radioactivity in the liver and subsequent experiments using isolated perfused liver confirmed the metabolic capacity of that organ with respect to these compounds.[138,149] By using whole-body radioautography it is sometimes possible to gain insight into the nature of the metabolic conversions. Thus, the localization of radioactivity in cartilaginous tissue and gastric mucosa is characteristic of the distribution of inorganic [^{35}S]-sulfate and provides evidence of the release of inorganic sulfate from administered esters.[18]

Every mammalian tissue that has been examined contains at least one of the sulfatases,[55] but the extent of sulfate release from administered sulfate esters will be dictated by the extent of uptake into various tissues and the suitability of the esters as substrates for the enzymes. In this context, the results obtained following the administration of naturally occurring sulfate esters may be misleading. For example, little desulfation occurs of cerebroside sulfate or its monosaccharide constituent, D-galactose 6-sulfate,[87] in spite of the fact that it is now recognized that the sulfatide is a substrate for arylsulfatase A. In retrospect, the small amount of desulfation with respect to D-galactose 6-sulfate is hardly surprising in view of its rapid urinary excretion and the known limited ability of at least one sugar sulfate (D-glucose 6-sulfate)[178] to penetrate liver tissue. Although the [^{35}S]-labeled sulfatide readily enters the liver, as evidenced by the appearance of radiolabel in the bile, it may be that there is restriction on its penetration to the enzyme site. Thus, the physiological significance of small amounts of desulfation may be underestimated, particularly when the desulfation is expressed as a percentage of administered radioactivity, and seemingly small amounts of desulfation should not be ignored. Such arguments are applicable to studies with the polymeric substrates chondroitin 4-sulfate[179] and heparan sulfate.[180] When either material was administered to experimental animals, the major urinary component in early urine collections was unchanged polymer, but in later urine samples, although the amounts were small, the levels of inorganic sulfate were of the same order as those of sulfated polymeric material. The evidence suggests the cellular uptake of both polymers is followed by total removal of sulfate groups in the lysosomes. Thus, the liberation of seemingly insignificant amounts of inorganic sulfate becomes an observation of considerable importance. Extreme caution should be exercised when interpreting data obtained when endogenous sulfate esters are administered exogenously.

2. The Distribution of Sulfate Esters in Relation to Other Metabolic Modifications

The influence which the distribution of a molecule may have on its metabolic fate is well illustrated by studies with the sulfate ester of L-tyrosine.[181] The ester is not metabolized in the mouse[182] but in the rat undergoes extensive transamination,[166] and this species difference is reflected in differences in distribution patterns.[177] In mice there is no cellular accumulation and although mouse tissues are rich in the transaminase, metabolism does not occur because the substrate does not penetrate to the enzyme sites. In rats, tissue accumulation was recorded but only in the renal subcortex,[183] a region where the transaminase is particularly concentrated. Although rat liver is also rich in transaminase activity, the substrate does not enter the liver. It is, however, able to penetrate as the peptide L-tyrosylglycine sulfate.[184]

B. The Significance of the Site of Sulfation

Thus far, this section has been concerned with the fate of sulfate esters of exogenous origin. However, sulfate esters are commonly formed in vivo, and some of these may be pharmacologically active. With regard to the fates of sulfate esters formed in vivo, the factors to be considered are largely the same as those already discussed for sulfates of exogenous origin. In addition, their formation sites are also of paramount importance. Because of the wide distribution of the sulfotransferases, sulfate esters could, in theory, be formed at many sites in the body. However, with respect to the sulfation of foreign compounds, most studies have concentrated on the liver and more recently on the gastrointestinal tract.[185] Whether an orally administered drug is sulfated either in the liver or the gut may have important consequences for pharmacological activity and clearance rates. For example, the effects of milligram doses of isoprenaline, a sympathomimetic amine by the oral route are relatively slight compared with the profound effects of microgram quantities administered intravenously.[96] Although isoprenaline is an excellent substrate for catechol *O*-methyl transferase, this enzyme appears to have a relatively minor role in the inactivation of the orally administered drug which is largely metabolized to a sulfoconjugate in the gut wall.[186-188] The capacity of the normal gastrointestinal tract for sulfation is of considerable import particularly since it is saturable.[95] Clearly, whether a drug enters the portal system either as native drug or as the sulfoconjugate may have far-reaching implications. Similar considerations may be applied to compounds entering the body via the lung. Pulmonary tissues represent the first line of defense of the body to inhaled foreign compounds, and there seems little doubt that sulfoconjugation may be quantitatively highly significant in the metabolism of xenobiotics by the lung. The formation has been demonstrated of benzo(*a*)pyrene-3-yl sulfate by cultures of pulmonary cells from a number of species including the human,[189] and it is known that some phenols presented intratracheally enter the systemic circulation in sulfated form.[190] However, pulmonary phenol sulfotransferase activity is apparently not available to all xenobiotics, as indicated in studies with isoprenaline. This compound is sulfated only to a minor extent by the lung,[191] although the major metabolite was isoprenaline sulfate following inhalation[192] by whole animals. It was concluded that inhaled isoprenaline is subsequently swallowed and sulfated by the gastrointestinal tract.

Once in the systemic circulation, the movement of sulfate esters into various organs may be affected by the extent of binding to plasma proteins. It is well known that sulfate esters in general are extensively bound to plasma protein,[17,105,113,149,150] a factor which may also affect their clearance rates by the kidney.[40,193]

The influences of the site of sulfation on the movement of molecules in vivo may be more complex. Many sulfate esters formed in the liver are eliminated via the bile while others are passed into the blood. The liver also directs different conjugates of the same compound into different body fluids. Thus the sulfoconjugates of harmol[194] and dibenzoxapine[195] enter the blood while their corresponding glucuronides are eliminated in the bile. How these distinctions are made is not known but clearly they are important in controlling the subsequent fate and half-life of a compound in vivo. The role of the liver in the synthesis and distribution of sulfate esters is best illustrated, perhaps, paradoxically, when hepatic function is abnormal. In patients with hepatobiliary diseases there is a marked increase in the urinary excretion of cholate and chenodeoxycholate and further, these bile acids are present, to a major extent, as their sulfate esters.[196-198] It may well be that the kidney contributes substantially to the sulfation of bile acids under these conditions since it has been shown that bile acids are sulfated by the isolated perfused kidney.[199]

VII. CONCLUDING REMARKS

It is now abundantly clear that the behavior and metabolic fates of sulfate esters vary considerably. The diversity depends upon a number of factors including the chemical nature of the compound, its concentration, site of formation, and the species of animal. Despite the complexity imposed by these variables, certain generalizations can be made. It is now generally accepted that naturally occurring sulfate esters fall into two groups: first, those destined for excretion and second, those which are essential biosynthetic intermediates, important structural compounds, or molecules essential to control systems or transport.

In recent times much progress has been made in clarifying the significance of the balance between sulfation and desulfation. The roles of sulfotransferases and the sulfatases have been rationalized, to some extent, in terms of the synthesis and degradation of connective tissue components and the interconversion of estrone and its sulfoconjugate. However, many difficulties still arise when attempting to assess the importance of sulfation and desulfation in relation to drugs, their metabolism, pharmacological activity, and excretion. In spite of increasing knowledge of the metabolic fates of sulfate esters it is not possible to predict, with any degree of certainty, whether a particular sulfate ester will be excreted or retained and be biologically active.

Another aspect of drug sulfoconjugation which has far-reaching implications, but about which very little is known, is how sulfoconjugates may interact with enzymes. Many enzyme systems are known which normally metabolize anionic substrates and one may speculate as to how these enzymes may interact with, or be affected by, sulfoconjugates. Little information is available but it may be significant that D-fructose 1-phosphate-6-sulfate is an alternative substrate for both aldolase and fructose, 1,6-diphosphatase.[200] In addition, dihydroxyacetone sulfate is known to act as a substrate analogue for α-glycerol phosphate dehydrogenase,[201] and phosphofructokinase can use D-fructose 6-sulfate as an alternative substrate.[202] Although this area is largely unexplored, these examples illustrate how sulfate esters could integrate into metabolic pathways possibly modifying their effectiveness with the sequelae of disturbing energy balance in the cell.

There is no doubt that the addition of the sulfate moiety has a dramatic effect on the physico-chemical properties of molecules covalently bound to the group. These changes in property should be regarded in the light of current knowledge which provides plenty of evidence that not all sulfate esters can be considered solely as endproducts of metabolism and whose only fate is elimination.

REFERENCES

1. **Comper, W. D. and Laurent, T. C.,** Physiological function of connective tissue polysaccharides, *Physiol. Rev.,* 58, 255, 1978.
2. **Haslewood, G. A. D.,** Comparative biochemistry of bile salts, in *The Biliary System,* Taylor, W., Ed., Blackwell Scientific Publications, Oxford, 1965, 107.
3. **Bleau, G., Bodley, F. H., Longpré, J., Chapdelaine, A., and Roberts, K. D.,** Cholesterol sulfate. 1. Occurrence and possible biological function as an amphipathic lipid in the membrane of the human erythrocyte, *Biochim. Biophys. Acta,* 352, 1, 1974.
4. **Bleau, G., Lalumière, G., Chapdelaine, A., and Roberts, K. D.,** Red cell surface structure: stabilization by cholesterol sulfate as evidenced by scanning electron microscopy, *Biochim. Biophys. Acta,* 375, 220, 1975.
5. **Lalumière, G., Longpré, J., Trudel, J., Chapdelaine, A., and Roberts, K. D.,** Cholesterol sulfate. II. Studies on its metabolism and possible function in canine blood, *Biochim. Biophys. Acta,* 394, 120, 1975.
6. **Roberts, K. D., Vandewiele, R. L., and Lieberman, S.,** The conversion *in vivo* of dehydroisoandrosterone sulfate to androsterone and etiocholanolone glucuronidates, *J. Biol. Chem.,* 236, 2213, 1961.
7. **Roberts, K. D., Bandi, L., Calvin, H. I., Drucker, W. D., and Lieberman, S.,** Evidence that steroid sulfates serve as biosynthetic intermediates. IV. Conversion of cholesterol sulfate *in vivo* to urinary C_{19} and C_{21} steroidal sulfates, *Biochemistry,* 3, 1983, 1964.
8. **Ingelman-Sundberg, M.,** Specific reductive metabolism of steroid sulfates in rat liver, *Biochim. Biophys. Acta,* 431, 592, 1976.
9. **Gustafsson, J.-Å. and Ingelman-Sundberg, M.,** Regulation and properties of a sex-specific hydroxylase system in female rat liver microsomes active on steroid sulfates, *J. Biol. Chem.,* 249, 1940, 1974.
10. **Gustafsson, J.-Å. and Ingelman-Sundberg, M.,** Regulation and substrate specificity of a steroid sulfate-specific hydroxylase system in female rat liver microsomes, *J. Biol. Chem.,* 250, 3451, 1975.

11. **Jevons, F. R.,** Tyrosine O-sulfate in fibrinogen and fibrin, *Biochem. J.,* 89, 621, 1963.

12. **Blombäck, B. and Doolittle, R. F.,** Amino acid sequence studies on fibrinopeptides from several species, *Acta Chem. Scand.,* 17, 1819, 1963.

13. **Blombäck, B., Blombäck, M., and Gröndahl, N.J.,** Studies on fibrinopeptides from mammals, *Acta Chem. Scand.,* 19, 1789, 1965.

14. **Krajewski, T. and Blombäck, B.,** The location of tyrosine-*O*-sulfate in fibrinopeptides, *Acta Chem. Scand.,* 22, 1339, 1968.

15. **Gregory, H., Hardy, P. M., Jones, D. S., Kenner, G. W., and Sheppard, R. C.,** The antral hormone, gastrin, *Nature (London),* 204, 931, 1964.

16. **Mulder, E., Lamers-Stahlhofen, G. J. M., and van der Molen, H. J.,** Interaction between steroids and membranes. Uptake of steroids and steroid sulfates by resealed erythrocyte ghosts, *J. Steroid Biochem.,* 4, 369, 1973.

17. **Hearse, D. J., Powell, G. M., and Olavesen, A. H,.,** The mode of excretion and metabolic fate of potassium naphthyl 2-^{35}S-sulfate and potassium 5,6,7,8-tetrahydronaphthyl 2-^{35}S-sulfate, *Biochem. Pharmacol.,* 18, 197, 1969.

18. **Hearse, D. J., Powell, G. M., Olavesen, A. H., and Dodgson, K. S.,** The application of whole-body autoradiography to a study of the distribution, metabolism and mode of excretion of ^{35}S-labelled arylsulfate esters, *Biochem. Pharmacol.,* 18, 205, 1969.

19. **Brooks, S. C., Leithauser, G., de Loecker, W. C., and de Wever, F.,** In vitro stimulation of protein synthesis in uterine microsomal supernatant by estrone sulfate, *Endocrinology,* 84, 901, 1969.

20. **Harper, M. J. K.,** Estragenic effects of dehydroepiandrosterone and its sulfate in rats, *Endocrinology,* 84, 229, 1969.

21. **Puche, R. C. and Romano, M. C.,** The effect of dehydroepiandrosterone sulfate and testosterone on the development of chick embryo frontal bones *in vitro, Calcif. Tissue Res.,* 2, 133, 1968.

22. **Dessypris, A. G.,** Testosterone sulfate, its biosynthesis, metabolism, measurement, functions and properties, *J. Steroid Biochem.,* 6, 1287, 1975.

23. **Hidaka, H., Nagatsu, T., Takeya, K., Matsumoto, S., and Yagi, K.,** Inactivation of serotonin by sulfotransferase system, *J. Pharmacol. Exp. Ther.,* 166, 272, 1969.

24. **Sahashi, Y., Suzuki, T., Higaki, M., and Asano, T.,** Metabolism of vitamin D in animals. V. Isolation of vitamin D sulfate from mammalian milk, *J. Vitamindol.,* 13, 33, 1967.

25. **Mumma, R. O., McKee, E. E., Verlangieri, A. J., and Barron, G. P.,** Anti-scorbutic effect of ascorbic acid 2-sulfate in the guinea pig, *Nutr. Rep. Int.,* 6, 133, 1972.

26. **Campeau, J. D., March, S. C., and Tolbert, B. M.,** Urinary excretion of ascorbate sulfate in rats: rate and chemical form, *Fed. Proc. Abstr.,* 32, 931, 1973.

27. **Verlangieri, A. J. and Mumma, R. O.,** *In vivo* sulfation of cholesterol by ascorbic acid 2-sulfate, *Atherosclerosis,* 17, 37, 1973.

28. **Hornig, D.,** Recent advances in vitamin C metabolism, in *Vitamin C: Recent Aspects of its Physiological and Technological Importance,* Birch, G. G. and Parker, K., Eds., Applied Science Publishers, Barking, Essex, U. K., 1974, 91.

29. **Shapiro, S. S. and Poon, J. P.,** Apparent sulfation of glycosaminoglycans by ascorbic acid 2-[^{35}S]sulfate: an explanation, *Biochim. Biophys. Acta,* 385, 221, 1975.

30. **Himmelsbach, C. K. and Andrews, H. L.,** Studies on modification of the morphine abstinence syndrome by drugs, *J. Pharmacol. Exp. Ther.,* 77, 17, 1943.

31. **Knowlton, G. C. and Gross, E. G.,** A method for studying the analgesic effect of drugs in animals, *J. Pharmacol. Exp. Ther.,* 78, 93, 1943.

32. **Oberst, F. W. and Gross, E. G.,** Studies on the fate of morphine sulfuric ether, *J. Pharmacol. Exp. Ther.,* 80, 188, 1944.

33. **Bishop, P. M. F., Richards, N. A., and Perry, W. L. M.,** Stilboestrol sulfate, oestrone, and equalin; further observations in the potency and clinical assessment of oestrogens, *Lancet,* 260, 818, 1951.

34. **Barford, P. A., Olavesen, A. H., Curtis, C. G., and Powell, G. M.,** Metabolic fates of diethylstilboestrol sulfates in the rat, *Biochem. J.,* 164, 423, 1977.

35. **Barford, P. A., Olavesen, A. H., Curtis, C. G., and Powell, G. M.,** Biliary excretion of some anionic derivatives of diethylstilboestrol and phenolphthalein in the guinea pig, *Biochem. J.,* 168, 373, 1977.

36. **Stiehl, A., Raedsch, R., and Kommerell, B.,** Increased sulfation of lithocholate in patients with cholesterol gallstones during chenodeoxycholate treatment, *Digestion,* 12, 105, 1975.

37. **John, R. A. and Fasella, P.,** The reaction of L-serine *O*-sulfate with aspartate aminotransferase, *Biochemistry,* 8, 4477, 1969.

38. **Fowler, L. J. and John, R. A.,** Active-site-directed irreversible inhibition of rat brain 4-aminobutyrate aminotransferase by ethanolamine *O*-sulfate *in vitro* and *in vivo, Biochem. J.,* 130, 569, 1972.

39. **Ohl, V. S. and Litwack, G.,** Selective inhibition of glutathione S-transferase by 17β-estradiol disulfate, *Arch. Biochem. Biophys.,* 180, 186, 1977.

40. **Mulder, G. J.,** Detoxification or toxification? Modification of the toxicity of foreign compounds by conjugation in the liver, *Trends Biochem. Sci.,* 4, 86, 1979.
41. **DeBaun, J. R., Miller, E. C., and Miller, J. A.,** N-hydroxy-2-acetylaminofluorene sulfotransferase: its probable role in carcinogenesis and in protein-(methion-S-yl) binding in rat liver, *Cancer Res.,* 30, 577, 1970.
42. **Weisburger, J. H., Yamamoto, R. S., Williams, G. M., Grantham, P. M., Matsushima, T., and Weisburger, E. K.,** On the sulfate ester of N-hydroxy-N-2-fluorenyl-acetamide as a key ultimate hepatocarcinogen in the rat, *Cancer Res.,* 32, 491, 1972.
43. **Austin, J. H., Balasubramanian, A. S., Pattabiramanan, T. N., Saraswathi, S., Basu, D. J., and Bachhawat, B. K.,** A controlled study of enzyme activities in thee human diseases of glycolipid metabolism, *J. Neurochem.,* 10, 305, 1963.
44. **Neufeld, E. F.,** The enzymology of inherited mucopolysaccharide storage disorders, *Trends Biochem. Sci.,* 2, 25, 1977.
45. **Roy, A. B.,** Sulfatases, lysosomes and disease, *Aust. J. Exp. Biol Med. Sci.,* 54, 111, 1976.
46. **Austin, J., Armstrong, D., and Shearer, L.,** Metachromatic form of diffuse cerebral sclerosis. V. The nature and significance of sulfatase activity: a controlled study of brain, liver and kidney in four patients with metachromatic lecuodystrophy, *Arch. Neurol. (Chicago),* 13, 593, 1965.
47. **France, J. T., Seddon, R. J., and Liggins, G. C.,** A study of a pregnancy with low oestrogen production due to placental sulfatase deficiency, *J. Clin. Endocrinol. Metab.,* 36, 1, 1973.
48. **Dodgson, K. S. and Spencer, B.,** Sulfatases, *Rep. Prog. Chem.,* 53, 318, 1957.
49. **Roy, A. B.,** The hydrolysis of sulfate esters, in *The Enzymes,* Academic Press, New York, 1971, chap. 1.
50. **Dodgson, K. S. and Rose, F. A.,** Sulfoconjugation and sulfohydrolysis, in *Metabolic Conjugation and Metabolic Hydrolysis,* Vol. 1, Fishman, W. H., Ed., Academic Press, New York, 1970, 239.
51. **Nicholls, R. G. and Roy, A. B.,** Arylsulfatases, in *The Enzymes,* Vol. 5, 3rd ed., Boyer, P. D., Ed., Academic Press, New York, 1971, 21.
52. **Roy, A. B.,** The purification and properties of sulfatase A, *Biochem. J.,* 55, 653, 1953.
53. **Dodgson, K. S. and Spencer, B.,** The impure nature of nitrocatechol sulfate, *Biochim. Biophys. Acta,* 21, 175, 1956.
54. **Dodgson, K. S. and Spencer, B.,** Assay of sulfatases, *Methods Biochem. Anal.,* 4, 211, 1957.
55. **Dodgson, K. S. and Rose, F. A.,** Sulfohydrolases, in *Metabolic Pathways,* Vol. 9, 3rd ed., Fishman, W. H., Ed., Academic Press, New York, 1975, chap. 9.
56. **Dodgson, K. S. and Rose, F. A.,** Observations on the biological roles of sulfatases, in Ciba Foundation Symposium Number 72, *Sulphur in Biology,* Excerpta Medica, Amsterdam, 1980.
57. **Roy, A. B.,** Steroid sulfatase, *Biochem. J.,* 66, 700, 1957.
58. **Mehl, E. and Jatzkewitz, H.,** Cerebroside 3-sulfate as a physiological substrate for arylsulfatase A, *Biochim. Biophys. Acta,* 151, 619, 1968.
59. **Gorham, S. D. and Cantz, M.,** Arylsulphatase B, an exo-sulphatase for chondroitin 4-sulphate tetrasaccharide, *Hoppe-Seylers Z. Physiol. Chem.,* 359, 1811, 1978.
60. **Rogers, K. M., White, G. F., and Dodgson, K. S.,** Purification and properties of bovine liver lysosomal adenosine 5'-phosphosulfate sulfohydrolase, *Biochim. Biophys. Acta,* 527, 70, 1978.
61. **Dollefeld, E. and Breuer, H.,** Vorkommen, biogenese und ståffwechsel von Steroid sulfaten, *Z. Vitam. Horm. Fermentforsch.,* 14,193, 1966.
62. **Janne, O.,** Identification and quantitation of C_{19} and C_{21} steroid triol sulfates in adult human urine, *J. Steroid Biochem.,* 2, 33, 1971.
63. **Adlercreutz, H.,** Estimation of oestrogen sulfates in pregnancy urine, *Scand. J. Clin. Lab. Invest.,* 17, 121, 1965.
64. **Lefèbvre, Y., Chapdelaine, A., and Bolté, E.,** Effects of labor on plasma dehydroepiandrosterone sulfate and cortisol, *Gynecol. Invest.,* 1, 57, 1970.
65. **Feher, T. and Halmy, L.,** Dehydroepiandrosterone and dehydroepiandrosterone sulfate dynamics in obesity, *Can. J. Biochem.,* 53, 215, 1975.
66. **Cardiff, C., Uden, V., and Killinger, D. W.,** Steroid biosynthesis in gonadal tissue from patients with testicular feminization, *Can. J. Biochem.,* 50, 849, 1972.
67. **Shao, A., Nowaczynski, W., Kuchel, O. and Genest, J.,** Secretion rate of dehydroepiandrosterone and dehydroepiandrosterone sulfate in benign essential hypertension as compared to normal subjects, *Can. J. Biochem.,* 48, 1308, 1970.
68. **Adams, J. B. and Salasoo, S.,** A major pathway of adrenal C_{19}-Δ^5-steroid metabolism under conditions of stress: formation of 16α-hydroxyandrost-5-enes, *Acta Endocrinol.,* 72, 319, 1976.
69. **Yamaji, T. and Ibayashi, H.,** Plasma dehydroepiandrosterone sulfate in normal and pathological conditions, *J. Clin. Endocrinol. Metab.,* 29, 273, 1969.

70. **Rose, D. P. and Liskowski, L.,** Corticosteroid sulfate excretion and estrogen receptors in breast cancer, *Clin. Chim. Acta,* 67, 183, 1976.

71. **Fahl, W. E. and Rose, D. P.,** Effect of estrogen-containing oral contraceptives on urinary corticosteroid sulfate excretion, *Clin. Chim. Acta,* 63, 189, 1975.

72. **Boström, H., Gustafsson, B. E., and Wengle, B.,** Studies on ester sulfates. 18. Ester sulfate formation in the germfree rat, *Proc. Soc. Exp. Biol. Med.,* 114, 742, 1963.

73. **Curzon, G. and Pratt, R. T. C.,** Origin of urinary resorcinol sulfate, *Nature* (London), 204, 383, 1964.

74. **Boström, H.,** Sulfate conjugation and conjugated sulfates, *Scand. J. Clin. Lab. Invest.,* 17, 33, 1965.

75. **Tallan, H. H., Bella, S. T., Stein, W. H., and Moore, S.,** Tyrosine-*O*-sulfate as a constituent of normal human urine, *J. Biol. Chem.,* 217, 703, 1955.

76. **John, R. A., Rose, F. A., Wusteman, F. S., and Dodgson, K. S.,** The detection and determination of L-tyrosine *O*-sulfate in rabbit and other mammalian urine, *Biochem. J.,* 100, 278, 1966.

77. **Hext, P. M., Thomas, S., Rose, F. A., and Dodgson, K. S.,** Determination and significance of L-tyrosine *O*-sulfate and its deaminated metabolites in normal human and mouse urine, *Biochem. J.,* 134, 629, 1973.

78. **Schachter, B. and Marrian, G. F.,** The isolation of estrone sulfate from the urine of pregnant mares, *J. Biol. Chem.,* 126, 663, 1938.

79. **McKenna, J., Menini, E., and Norymberski, J. K.,** Oestrone sulfate in human pregnancy, *Biochem. J.,* 79, 11P, 1961.

80. **Davis, V. E., Huff, J. A., and Brown, H.,** Isolation of serotonin-*O*-sulfate from human urine, *Clin. Chim. Acta,* 13, 380, 1966.

81. **Dalgliesh, C. E.,** Excretion of conjugated 2-amino-3-hydroxyacetophenone by man, and its significance in tryptophan metabolism, *Biochem. J.,* 61, 334, 1955.

82. **Chadwick, B. T. and Wilkinson, J. H.,** Some aspects of the metabolism of 5-hydroxytryptamine, *Biochem. J.,* 76, 102, 1960.

83. **Merits, I.,** Formation and metabolism of [^{14}C] dopamine 3-*O*-sulfate in dog, rat and guinea pig, *Biochem. Pharmacol.,* 25, 829, 1976.

84. **Baker, E. M., Hammer, D. C., March, S. C., Tolbert, B. M., and Canham, J. E.,** Ascorbate sulfate-urinary metabolite of ascorbic acid in man, *Science,* 173, 826, 1971.

85. **Garton, G. A. and Williams, R. T.,** Studies in detoxication. 26. The fates of phenol, phenylsulfuric acid and phenylglucuronide in the rabbit, in relation to the metabolism of benzene, *Biochem. J.,* 45, 158, 1949.

86. **Hawkins, J. B. and Young, L.,** Biochemical studies of toxic agents. 5. Observations on the fate of ^{35}S-labelled arylsulfuric acids following their administration to the rat, *Biochem. J.,* 56, 166, 1954.

87. **Lloyd, A. G., Large, P. J., James, A. M., and Dodgson, K. S.,** The metabolic fate of hexose-6-*O*-[S^{35}]-sulfates and related compounds, *J. Biochem. (Tokyo),* 55, 669, 1964.

88. **Lloyd, A. G.,** The metabolism of exogenous *N*-acetyl-D-glucosamine 6-*O*[^{35}S]-sulfate in the normal rat, *Biochem. J.,* 80, 572, 1961.

89. **Lloyd, A. G.,** The metabolism of *N*-acetyl-D-galactosamine 6-*O*[^{35}S]-sulfate in rat, *Biochim. Biophys. Acta,* 58, 1, 1962.

90. **Rose, F. A. and Bleszynski, W.** The metabolism of 5-hydroxytryptamine *O*[^{35}S]-sulfate in the rat, *Biochem. J.,* 122, 601, 1971.

91. **Powell, G. M. and Olavesen, A. H.,** unpublished results.

92. **Powell, G. M., Parry, T. J., and Curtis, C. G.,** An enterogastric circulation, *Biochem. Soc. Trans.,* 6, 141, 1978.

93. **Hirom, P. C., Millburn, P., Smith, R. L. and Williams, R. T.,** Species variations in the threshold molecular-weight factor for the biliary excretion of organic anions, *Biochem. J.,* 129, 1071, 1972.

94. **Powell, G. M., Gregory, P. A., Olavesen, A. H., and Jones, J. G.,** Studies on the mechanism of biliary excretion of aryl sulfates in the rat, *Biochem. Soc. Trans.,* 1, 1165, 1973.

95. **Levy, G. and Matsuzawa, T.,** Role of sulfate formation in biotransformation of salicylamide in man, *J. Pharm. Sci.,* 55, 222, 1966.

96. **Morgan, C. D., Ruthven, C. R. J., and Sandler, M.,** The quantitative assessment of isoprenaline metabolism in man, *Clin. Chim. Acta,* 26, 381, 1969.

97. **Ishiguro, I., Naito, J., Ishikura, A., and Shiotani, T.,** Isolation and identification of 3-OH-anthranilamide-*O*-sulfate and 5-OH-anthranilamide-*O*-sulfate as urinary metabolites of anthranilamide in rat, *J. Pharm. Soc. Jpn.,* 94, 1224, 1974.

98. **Ikeda, G. J.,** Metabolism of 5-(para-hydroxyanilino)-1,2,3,4-thiatriazole in rats, *J. Med. Chem.,* 16, 1157, 1973.

99. **Nilsson, H. T., Persson, K., and Tegner, K.,** Metabolism of terbutaline in man, *Xenobiotica,* 2, 363, 1972.

100. **Arndts, D. and Pollmann, W.,** Pharmacokinetics and metabolism of K0592 in man, dog and rat, *Arch. Pharmacol.,* 277, 349, 1973.

101. **Shane, B. and Snell, E. E.**, Metabolism of 5'-deoxypyridoxine in rats: 5'-deoxypyridoxine 4'-sulfate as a major urinary metabolite, *Biochem. Biophys. Res. Commun.*, 66, 1295, 1975.
102. **Daniel, J. W., Green, T., and Phillips, P. J.**, Metabolism of phenolic antioxidant 3,5-di-tert-butyl-4-hydroxyanisole (Topanol-354). 2. Biotransformation in man, rat and dog, *Food Cosmet. Toxicol.*, 11, 781, 1973.
103. **Dalezois, J. I. and Wogan, G. N.**, Metabolism of aflatoxin-B-1 in rhesus monkeys, *Cancer Res.*, 32, 2297, 1972.
104. **Roche, J., Michel, R., Closon, J., and Michel, O.**, Sur la sulfoconjugaison hépatique de la 3,5,3'-triiodo-L-thyronine et la présence d'un ester sulfurique de cette hormone dans la bile et la plasma, *Biochim. Biophys. Acta,* 33, 461, 1959.
105. **Hearse, D. J., Powell, G. M., Olavesen, A. H., and Dodgson, K. S.**, The influence of some physicochemical factors on the biliary excretion of a series of structurally related aryl sulfate esters, *Biochem. Pharmacol.*, 18, 181, 1969.
106. **Hanahan, D. J., Everett, N. B., and Davis, C. D.**, Fate of S^{35}-Na estrone sulfate in pregnant and non-pregnant rats, *Arch. Biochem.*, 23, 501, 1949.
107. **Dolly, J. O., Curtis, C. G., Dodgson, K. S., and Rose, F. A.**, Metabolism of sodium oestrone [^{35}S]-sulfate in the rat, *Biochem. J.*, 123, 261, 1971.
108. **Twombly, G. H. and Levitz, M.**, Metabolism of oestrone-C^{14}-16-sulfate in women, *Am. J. Obstet. Gynecol.*, 80, 889, 1960.
109. **Dolly, J. O., Curtis, C. G., Dodgson, K. S., and Rose, F. A.**, Metabolism of sodium oestrone [^{35}S]-sulfate in the guinea pig, *Biochem. J.*, 128, 347, 1972.
110. **Dolly, J. O., Dodgson, K. S., and Rose, F. A.**, Studies on the oestrogen sulfatase and arylsulfatase C activities of rat liver, *Biochem. J.*, 128, 337, 1972.
111. **Flynn, T. G., Dodgson, K. S., Powell, G. M., and Rose, F. A.**, The metabolism of dipotassium 2-hydroxy-5-nitrophenyl [^{35}S]-sulfate, a substrate for lysosomal arylsulfatases A and B, *Biochem. J.*, 105, 1003, 1967.
112. **Wang, D. Y. and Bulbrook, R. D.**, Binding of sulfate esters of dehydroepiandrosterone, testosterone, 17-acetoxypregnenolone and pregnenolone in plasma, *J. Endocrinol.*, 39, 405, 1967.
113. **Curtis, C. G., Hearse, D. J., and Powell, G. M.**, Renal excretion of some aryl sulfate esters in the rat, *Xenobiotica*, 4, 595, 1974.
114. **Curtis, C. G.**, The Transport and Metabolism of Sulfuric Acid Esters in Mammalian Organisms, Ph.D. thesis, University of Wales, Cardiff, 1966.
115. **Sperber, I.**, Secretion of organic anions in the formation of urine and bile, *Pharmacol. Rev.*, 11, 109, 1959.
116. **Puche, R. C.**, The Renal Handling of Dehydroepiandrosterone sulfate in the rat, *Eur. J. Steroids,* 2, 261, 1967.
117. **May, D. G., Fujimoto, J. M., and Inturris, C. E.**, Tubular transport and metabolism of morphine-*N*-methyl-C^{14} by chicken kidney, *J. Pharmacol. Exp. Ther.*, 157, 626, 1967.
118. **Rennick, B. R. and Quebbemann, A. J.**, Site of excretion of catechol and catecholamines—renal metabolism of catechol, *Am. J. Physiol.*, 218, 1307, 1970.
119. **Quebbemann, A. J. and Anders, M. W.**, Renal tubular conjugation and excretion of phenol and para-nitrophenol in chicken—differing mechanisms of renal transfer, *J. Pharmacol. Exp. Ther.*, 184, 695, 1973.
120. **Menini, E. and Diczfalusy, E.**, Isolation and identification of sodium oestriol-3-sulfate in human meconium, *Endocrinology*, 68, 492, 1961.
121. **Laatikainen, T., Peltokallio, P., and Vihko, R.**, Steroid sulfates in human bile, *Steroids,* 12, 407, 1968.
122. **Laatikainen, T.**, Quantitative studies on the excretion of glucuronide and mono- and disulfate conjugates of neutral steroids in human bile, *Ann. Clin. Res.*, 2, 338, 1970.
123. **Cronholm, T., Eriksson, H., and Gustafsson, J.-Å.**, Excretion of endogenous steroids and metabolites of [4-^{14}C] pregnenolone in bile of female rats, *Eur. J. Biochem.*, 19, 424, 1971.
124. **Cronholm, T., Eriksson, H., and Gustafsson, J.-Å.**, Excretion of steroid-hormone metabolites in bile of male rats, *Steroids,* 19, 455, 1972.
125. **Baulieu, E. E. and Corpéchot, C.**, Métabolisme "direct" du sulfate de déhydroépiandrostérone, *Bull. Soc. Chim. Biol.*, 47, 443, 1965.
126. **Laatikainen, T.**, Disulfate fractions of human bile, *Steroids,* 15, 139, 1970.
127. **Noir, B. A. and Nanet, H.**, A study of the ethyl anthranilate a20 derivatives of bilirubin sulfate; confirmation of the existence of the bilirubin sulfate conjugates in bile, *Biochim. Biophys. Acta*, 372, 230, 1974.
128. **Palmer, R. H. and Bolt, M. G.**, Bile acid sulfates. 1. Synthesis of lithocholic acid sulfates and their identification in human bile, *J. Lipid Res.*, 12, 671, 1971.
129. **Eyssen, H. J., Parmentier, G. G., and Markens, J. A.**, Sulfated bile acids in germ-free and conventional mice, *Eur. J. Biochem.*, 66, 507, 1976.

130. **Peterson, R. E. and Fujimoto, J. M.,** Biliary excretion of morphine-3-glucuronide and morphine-3-ethereal sulfate by different pathways in the rat, *J. Pharmacol. Exp. Ther.*, 184, 409, 1973.

131. **Smith, D. S., Peterson, R. E., and Fujimoti, J. M.,** Species differences in the biliary excretion of morphine, morphine-3-glucuronide and morphine-3-ethereal sulfate in the cat and rat, *Biochem. Pharmacol.*, 22, 485, 1973.

132. **Smith, D. S. and Fujimoto, J. M.,** Alterations produced by movobiocin during biliary excretion of morphine, morphine-3-glucuronie and other compounds, *J. Pharmacol. Exp. Ther.*, 188, 504, 1974.

133. **Nikai, K., Shirakawa, Y., Tamayama, S., Fujita, T., Suzuoki, Z., Kato, S., and Hayashi, N.,** Metabolism of a thyroxine analogue, 3,-diiodo-4-(4'-acetoxy-3'-iodo phenoxy) benzoic acid in rats, *Xenobiotica*, 2, 277, 1972.

134. **Terayama, H., Naruke, T., Kasai, S., Numata, M., Nakayama, H., Saito, T., and Irikura, T.,** Studies on analgesic agents. 13. Metabolic fate of 1-butyryl-4-cinnamylpiperazine hydrochloride (BCP-CCl) in rats, *Chem. Pharm. Bull. (Tokyo)*, 21, 12, 1973.

135. **Iveson, P., Lundrup, W. E., Parke, D. V., and Williams, R. T.,** The metabolism of carbenoxolone in the rat, *Xenobiotica*, 1, 79, 1971.

136. **Smith, R. L. and Williams, R. T.,** Implication of the conjugation of drugs and other exogenous compounds, in *Glucuronic Acid, Free and Combined,* Dutton, G. J. Ed., Academic Press, New York, 1966, chap. 7.

137. **Millburn, P., Smith, R. L., and Williams, R. T.,** Biliary excretion of foreign compounds; biphenyl, stilboestrol and phenophthalein in the rat: molecular weight, polarity and metabolism as factors in biliary excretion, *Biochem. J.*, 105, 1275, 1967.

138. **Gatehouse, P. W., Roy, A. B., Dodgson, K. S. Powell, G. M., Lloyd, A. G., and Olavesen, A. H.,** The metabolism of sodium cortisone 21-[^{35}S]-sulfate in the rat, *Biochem. J.*, 127, 661, 1972.

139. **Millburn, P.,** Factors in the biliary excretion of organic compounds, in *Metabolic Conjugation and Metabolic Hydrolysis,* Vol. 2, Fishman, W. H. Ed., Academic Press, New York, 1970, 1.

140. **Powell, G. M., Olavesen, A. H., and Curtis, C. G.,** Biliary excretion of cyclohexylphenyl 4-[^{35}S]-sulfate in the guinea pig, *Biochem. J.*, 176, 443, 1978.

141. **Powell, G. M., Jones, J. G., Olavesen, A. H., and Curtis, C. G.,** A model system for investigating the biliary excretion of an anion in the rat, *Biochem. J.*, 148, 303, 1975.

142. **Hirom, P. C., Millburn, P., and Smith, R. L.,** Bile and urine as complementary pathways for the excretion of foreign organic compounds, *Xenobiotica*, 6, 55, 1976.

143. **Jorritsma, J., Meerman, J. H. N., Vonk, R. J., and Mulder, G. J.,** Biliary and urinary excretion of drug conjugates: effect of diuresis and choleresis on excretion of harmol sulfate and harmol glucuronide in the rat, *Xenobiotica*, 9, 247, 1979.

144. **Tudball, N.,** The metabolism of potassium L-serine O-[^{35}S]-sulfate in the rat, *Biochem. J.*, 85, 456, 1962.

145. **Thomas, J. H. and Tudball, N.,** Studies on the enzymic degradation of L-serine O-sulfate by a rat liver preparation, *Biochem. J.*, 105, 467, 1967.

146. **Tudball, N., Noda, Y., and Dodgson, K. S.,** The metabolism of glycyl-L-serine O-[^{35}S]-sulfate in the rat, *Biochem. J.*, 90, 439, 1964.

147. **Tudball, N., Noda, Y., and Dodgson, K. S.,** The metabolism of L-serylglycine O-[^{35}S]-sulfate in the rat, *Biochem. J.*, 95, 678, 1965.

148. **Tudball, N.,** Studies on the metabolism *in vivo* of L-threonine O-[^{35}S]-sulfate in the rat, *Biochem. Biophys. Acta*, 97, 345, 1965.

149. **Denner, W. H. B., Olavesen, A. H., Powell, G. M., and Dodgson, K. S.,** The metabolism of potassium dodecyl [^{35}S]-sulfate in the rat, *Biochem. J.*, 111, 43, 1969.

150. **Burke, B., Olavesen, A. H., Curtis, C. G., and Powell, G. M.,** The biodegradation of some anionic detergents in the rat: a common metabolic pathway, *Xenobiotica*, 5, 573, 1975.

151. **Burke, B., Olavesen, A. H., Curtis, C. G., and Powell, G. M.,** The biodegradation of the surfactant undecyl sulfate, *Xenobiotica*, 6, 667, 1976.

152. **Merits, I.,** The metabolism of labelled hexadecyl sulfate salts in the rat, dog and human, *Biochem. J.*, 148, 219, 1975.

153. **Ottery, J., Olavesen, A. H., and Dodgson, K. S.,** Metabolism of dodecyl sulfate in the rat: non-enzymic liberation of sulfate and γ-butyrolactone from the major metabolite, butyric acid 4-sulfate, *Life Sci.*, 9, 1335, 1970.

154. **Knaak, J. B., Kozbelt, S. J., and Sullivan, L. J.,** Metabolism of 2-ethylhexyl sulfate by the rat and rabbit, *Toxicol. Appl. Pharmacol.*, 8, 369, 1966.

155. **Maggs, J. L.,** unpublished results.

156. **Buu, N. T. and Kuchel, O.,** The direct conversion of dopamine 3-O-sulfate to norepinephrine by dopamine-β-hydroxylase, *Life Sci.*, 24, 783, 1979.

157. **Hatinaka, H., Egami, F., Kato, T., and Nagatsu, T.,** Ascorbate 2-sulfate inhibits dopamine β-hydroxylase reaction, but not ascorbate oxidase reaction, *J. Biochem. (Tokyo)*, 78, 821, 1975.

158. **Jenner, W. N. and Rose, F. A.**, Dopamine 3-*O*-sulfate, an end product of L-dopa metabolism in Parkinson patients, *Nature (London)*, 252, 237, 1974.

159. **Jenner, W. N. and Rose, F. A.**, Dopamine 3- and 4-*O*-[35S] sulfates as substrates for arylsulfatases *in vitro* and their metabolism by the rat *in vivo*, in *Conjugation Reactions in Drug Biotransformation*, Aitio, A. Ed., Elsevier/North Holland, Amsterdam, 1978, 501.

160. **Hyde, C. W. and Young, L.**, Biochemical studies of toxic agents; the metabolic formation of 1- and 2-menaphthylmercapturic acid, *Biochem. J.*, 107, 519, 1968.

161. **Clapp, J. J. and Young, L.**, Formation of mercapturic acids in rats after the administration of aralkyl esters, *Biochem. J.*, 118, 765, 1970.

162. **Gillham, B.**, The reaction of aralkyl sulfate esters with glutathione catalysed by rat liver preparations, *Biochem. J.*, 121, 667, 1971.

163. **Woodman, J. and Young, L.**, Mercapturic acid formation from sodium alkyl sulfates in the rat, *Biochem. J.*, 125, 78P, 1971.

164. **Kaye, C. M.**, The synthesis of mercapturic acids from diethyl sulfate and di-*n*-propyl sulfate in the rat, *Xenobiotica*, 4, 329, 1974.

165. **Dodgson, K. S., Powell, G. M., Rose, F. A., and Tudball, N.**, Observations on the metabolism of tyrosine *O*-[35S]-sulfate in the rat, *Biochem. J.*, 79, 209, 1961.

166. **Powell, G. M., Rose, F. A., and Dodgson, K. S.**, Studies on L-tyrosine *O*-sulfate. 2. Identification of *p*-hydroxyphenylpyruvic acid [35S]-sulfate as a metabolite of L-tyrosine *O*-[35S]-sulfate in the rat, *Biochem. J.*, 87, 545, 1963.

167. **Roberts, K. D., Bandi, L., Calvin, H. I., Drucker, W. D., and Lieberman, S.** Evidence that cholesterol sulfate is a precursor of steroid hormones, *J. Am. Chem. Soc.*, 86, 958, 1964.

168. **Pasqualini, J. R.**, Metabolic conjugation and hydrolysis of steroid hormones in the fetoplacental unit, in *Metabolic Conjugation and Metabolic Hydrolysis*, Vol. 2, Fishman, W. H. Ed., Academic Press, New York, 1970, 153.

169. **Dominguez, O. V., Valencia, S. A., and Loza, A. C.**, On the role of steroid sulfates in hormone biosynthesis, *J. Steroid Biochem.*, 6, 301, 1975.

170. **Schwenk, M., Delpino, V. L., and Bolt, H. M.**, The kinetics of hepatocellular transport and metabolism of estrogens (comparison between estrone sulfate, estrone, and ethinylestradiol), *J. Steroid Biochem.*, 10, 37, 1979.

171. **Wortmann, W., Johnston, D. E., Wortmann, B., and Touchstone, J. C.**, Metabolism of 3H-estrone sulfate perfused *in vivo* through a rhesus monkey liver, *J. Steroid Biochem.*, 4, 271, 1973.

172. **Holler, M., Napp, M., and Breuer, H.**, Comparative studies on the metabolism of radioactive estrone and estrone sulfate in the isolated perfused rat liver, *Biochem. Soc. Trans.*, 3, 890, 1975.

173. **Kishimoto, Y. and Hoshi, M.**, Dehydroepiandrosterone sulfate in rat brain—incorporation from blood and metabolism *in vivo*, *J. Neurochem.*, 19, 2207, 1972.

174. **Kishimoto, Y.**, Estrone sulfate in rat brain—uptake from blood and metabolism *in vivo*, *J. Neurochem.*, 20, 1489, 1973.

175. **Levitz, M. and Katz, J.**, Enterohepatic metabolism of estriol-3-sulfate-16-glucosiduronate in women, *J. Clin. Endocrinol. Metab.*, 28, 862, 1968.

176. **Taylor, A. J., Powell, G. M., Howes, D., Black, J. G., and Olavesen, A. H.**, Metabolism of the surfactants sodium undecyltriethoxy sulfate and sodium dodecyltriethoxy sulfate in the rat, *Biochem. J.*, 174, 405, 1978.

177. **Powell, G. M., Curtis, C. G., and Dodgson, K. S.**, The distribution of 35S-labelled sulfuric acid esters administered to mice and rats, *Biochem. Pharmacol.*, 16, 1997, 1967.

178. **Powell, G. M., Lloyd, A. G., Large, P. J., and Dodgson, K. S.**, Radioautographic studies on the metabolism of D-glucose 6-*O*-[35S]-sulfate in the mouse, *J. Biochem. Tokyo*, 55, 677, 1964.

179. **Wood, K. M., Wusteman, F. S., and Curtis, C. G.**, The Degradation of intravenously injected chondroitin 4-sulfate in the rat, *Biochem. J.*, 134, 1009, 1973.

180. **Perry, M. A., Powell, G. M., Wusteman, F. S., and Curtis, C. G.**, The catabolism of intravenously injected heparan *N*-[35S]-sulfate in the rat, *Biochem. J.*, 166, 373, 1977.

181. **Powell, G. M. and Curtis, C. G.**, Comparative Studies on the Fate of L-Tyrosine *O*-[35S]-sulfate in Mice and Rats, Abstr. 3rd Meeting Fed. Eur. Biochem. Soc., Warsaw, 1966.

182. **Powell, G. M., Rose, F. A., and Dodgson, K. S.**, The fate of L-tyrosine *O*-[35S]-sulfate in the mouse, *Biochem. J.*, 91, 6P, 1964.

183. **Curtis, C. G., Powell, G. M., and Dodgson, K. S.**, The site of metabolism of potassium L-tyrosine *O*-[35S]-sulfate in the rat, *Biochem. Pharmacol.*, 18, 2551, 1969.

184. **Jones, J. G., Powell, G. M., Curtis, C. G., and Basford, J. M.**, The fate and distribution of L-tyrosylglycine *O*-[35S]-sulfate in mice and rats, *Biochem. J.*, 99, 35P, 1966.

185. **Powell, G. M., Miller, J. J., Olavesen, A. H., and Curtis, C. G.**, Liver as major organ of phenol detoxication?, *Nature (London)*, 252, 234, 1974.

186. **Conway, W. D., Minatoya, H., Lands, A. M., and Shekosky, J. M.,** Absorption and elimination profile of isoproterenol. III. The metabolic fate of de-isoproterenol-7-^{3}H in the dog, *J. Pharmacol. Sci.,* 57, 1135, 1968.

187. **Connolly, M. E., Davies, D. S., Dollery, C. T., Morgan, C. D., Patterson, J. W., and Sandler, M.,** Metabolism of isoprenaline in dog and man, *Br. J. Pharmacol.,* 46, 458, 1972.

188. **George, C. F., Blackwell, E. W., and Davies, D. S.,** Metabolism of isoprenaline in intestine, *J. Pharmacol.,* 26, 265, 1974.

189. **Cohen, G. M., Haws, S. M., Moore, B. P., and Bridges, J. W.,** Benzo (*a*) pyren-3-yl hydrogen sulfate, a major ethyl acetate — extractable metabolite of benzo(*a*)pyrene in human, hamster and rat lung cultures, *Biochem. Pharmacol.,* 25, 2561, 1976.

190. **Powell, G. M.,** unpublished data.

191. **Briant, R. H., Blackwell, E. W., Williams, F. N., Davies, D. S., and Dollery, C. T.,** The metabolism of sympathomimetic bronchodilator drugs by the isolated perfused dog lung, *Xenobiotica,* 3, 787, 1973.

192. **Davies, D. S.,** Drug metabolism in man, in *Drug Metabolism: From Microbe to Man,* Parke, D. V. and Smith, R. L., Eds., Taylor & Francis, London, 1977, 357.

193. **Holler, M., Grochtmann, W., Napp, M., and Breuer, H.,** Studies on the metabolism of estrone sulfate. Comparative perfusions of estrone and estrone sulfate through isolated rat livers, *Biochem. J.,* 166, 363, 1977.

194. **Mulder, G. J., Hayen-Keulemans, K., and Sluiter, N. E.,** UDP-glucuronyltransferase and phenol sulfotransferase from rat liver *in vivo* and *in vitro* — characterization of conjugation and biliary excretion of harmol *in vivo* and in perfused liver, *Biochem. Pharmacol.,* 24, 103, 1975.

195. **Upshall, D. G.** unpublished data.

196. **Stiehl, A., Ast, E., Czygan, P., and Liersch, M.,** Formation, metabolism, and excretion of bile salt sulfates in man, in *The Hepatobiliary System,* Vol. 7, 2nd ed., Taylor, W., Ed., Plenum Press, New York, 1976, 453.

197. **Admirand, W. H., Stiehl, A., and Thaler, M. M.,** Sulfation of bile salts. An important metabolic pathway in cholestasis, *Gastroenterology,* 62, 190, 1972.

198. **Makino, I., Shinozaki, K., Nakagawa, S., and Mashimo, K.,** Measurement of sulfate and non-sulfated bile acids in human serum and urine, *J. Lipid Res.,* 15, 132, 1974.

199. **Summerfield, J. A., Gollan, J. L., and Billing, B. H.,** Synthesis of bile acid monosulfates by the isolated perfused rat kidney, *Biochem. J.,* 156, 339, 1976.

200. **Martensen, T. M. and Mansur, T. E.,** Fructose 1-phosphate-6-sulfate as an alternative substrate for aldolase and fructose-1,6-diphosphatase, *Biochem. Biophys. Res. Commun.,* 69, 844, 1976.

201. **Grazi, E., Barbieri, G., and Gagliona, R.,** Dihydroxyacetone sulfate as substrate analogue for α-glycerol phosphate dehydrogenase, *Biochim. Biophys. Acta,* 341, 248, 1974.

202. **Martensen, T. M. and Mansur, T. E.,** Studies on heart phosphofructokinase. Use of fructose 6-sulfate as an alternative substrate to study the mechanism of action and active site specificity, *J. Biol. Chem.,* 251, 3664, 1976.

Chapter 8

GENERATION OF REACTIVE INTERMEDIATES FROM XENOBIOTICS BY SULFATE CONJUGATION—THEIR POTENTIAL ROLE IN CHEMICAL CARCINOGENESIS

G. J. Mulder

TABLE OF CONTENTS

I. INTRODUCTION

Sulfate conjugates are usually less stable than glucuronide conjugates of the same substrate because sulfate (in an ester-type linkage) is a better leaving group than glucuronate (in a β-glycosidic bond). Some of the sulfate conjugates are so labile under physiological conditions that their formation in vivo, if it occurs, cannot be detected. For instance, the *N-O*-sulfate conjugate of *N*-hydroxy-*N*-acetyl-2-aminofluorene (*N*-hydroxy-2AAF) has a halflife of less than 1 min in aqueous media at pH 7;[1] therefore, the formation of this sulfate conjugate cannot be measured directly in vivo. Its *N-O*-glucuronide counterpart can be measured since it is much more stable at that pH.[2] The formation of labile conjugates was not given much consideration before the finding in 1968 that a labile *N-O*-sulfate ester might be involved in the carcinogenic action of *N*-hydroxy-2AAF (and its precursor *N*-acetyl-2-aminofluorene, 2AAF). This type of compound is now receiving much more attention, especially the sulfate conjugates of *N*-hydroxyarylamines.

The possible involvement of the *N-O*-sulfate conjugate of *N*-hydroxy-2AAF as an ultimate carcinogen of 2AAF was first suggested by King and Phillips.[3] They showed that sulfation of *N*-hydroxy-2AAF by a rat liver cytosolic preparation formed an intermediate, presumably the *N-O*-sulfate conjugate, that bound to RNA and protein. Using radioactive labels in different positions of the molecule, they showed that both the fluorene ring and the *N*-acetyl group were covalently bound to these macromolecules. Independently, De Baun et al.[4] reported similar findings: the cosubstrate of sulfation, PAPS, increased covalent binding of *N*-hydroxy-2AAF to DNA, RNA, and protein. They measured sulfation of this substrate by the PAPS-dependent formation of 1- and 3-methylmercapto-2AAF (Figure 1).[5] These products result from the initial formation of the *N-O*-sulfate conjugate, which breaks down to generate a reactive electrophilic intermediate following loss of the sulfate group. A correlation was suggested between carcinogenic response to *N*-hydroxy-2AAF and sulfotransferase activity towards this substrate in various species. These findings proved that sulfation of the *N*-hydroxy group of *N*-hydroxy-2AAF led to a labile sulfate conjugate that generates a reactive breakdown (rearrangement) product, reacting with available nucleophilic groups.

Later, sulfate conjugates of several other *N*-hydroxy compounds were shown to be reactive and to bind covalently to nucleophilic groups in DNA, RNA, protein, or low-molecular weight compounds. More extensively characterized were *N*-hydroxy-*N*-acetyl-2-aminophenanthrene,[6] *N*-hydroxy-*N*-methyl-4-aminoazobenzene[7] *N*-hydroxyphenacetin,[8] and *N*-hydroxyxanthine.[9] Also a C−O−sulfate ester has been shown to be reactive, namely that of 1′-hydroxysafrole[10] (Figure 2).

The chemical mechanism for the generation of reactive intermediates from sulfate conjugates seems to be the loss of the sulfate group, resulting in nitrenium ion or carbonium ion resonance forms.

Since these sulfate conjugates are very labile, their formation in vivo or in vitro has to be detected by an indirect method. This is usually achieved by the addition of nucleophilic compounds such as glutathione, methionine, or a macromolecule such as RNA, which can trap the nitrenium or carbonium ions formed by the breakdown of the sulfate conjugate. The trapping efficiency in most cases will not be 100%, and may vary considerably from one compound to the other. Thus, 100 mM methionine trapped only 5 to 15% of the total amount of reactive intermediate formed from sulfation of *N*-hydroxy-*N*-methyl-4-aminoazobenzene, whereas 20 mM methionine trapped 65 to 85% of the reactive sulfate ester of *N*-hydroxy-2AAF.[7] Furthermore, some methylmercapto derivatives may not be stable, like those of 2-naphthylamine that are

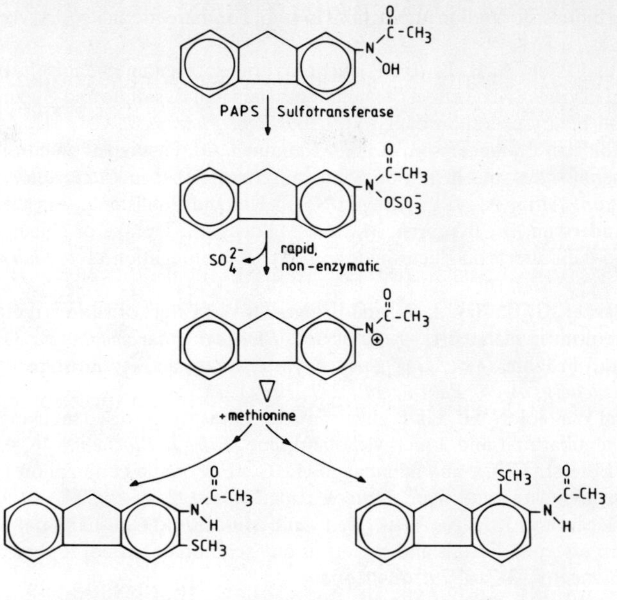

FIGURE 1. Formation of 1- and 3-methylmercapto-2 AAF from
N-hydroxy-2AAF by sulfation in the presence of methionine.

oxidized by air.[7] Glutathione trapped the reactive intermediate generated from
sulfation of N-hydroxyphenacetin much more effectively than methionine.[11] Therefore,
PAPS-dependent substrate disappearance may be a more reliable assay for the
determination of the rate of sulfation of a particular substrate that forms a reactive
sulfate ester. Alternatively, 4-nitrophenyl sulfate may be used as the donor of the
sulfate group for sulfation, in which case the

$$\text{4-nitrophenyl sulfate} + \text{PAP} \rightleftharpoons \text{4-nitrophenol} + \text{PAPS} \tag{1}$$

$$R_1R_2\text{-}N\text{-OH} + \text{PAPS} \rightleftharpoons R_1R_2\text{-}NO\text{-sulfate} + \text{PAP} \tag{2}$$

$$R_1R_2\text{-}NO\text{-sulfate} \rightarrow R_1R_2\text{-}N\text{-X} + \text{sulfate} \tag{3}$$

rate of generation of free 4-nitrophenol (yellow at alkaline pH) indicates the rate of
sulfation.[8] However, this method has its drawbacks (see Chapter 5, Section IID). If the
amount of substrate trapped by some nucleophilic agent is used to assay the formation
of reactive sulfate esters, it is important to compare the amount of the sulfate conjugate
that is trapped, with the rate of PAPS-dependent substrate disappearance. It is
important to realize that any increase or decrease of this covalent binding may be due to
an effect on trapping efficiency rather than on sulfotransferase activity as illustrated by
the following examples. Low-molecular weight compounds like methionine may
compete effectively with RNA or protein for trapping reactive intermediates.[7,8,11] The
presence of varying concentrations of strongly nucleophilic compounds in enzyme
preparations from various species or organs might affect the trapping efficiency in an
unpredictable fashion. Furthermore, reducing compounds like ascorbate may decrease
covalent binding to RNA and protein.[11,12] Because the reactive N-methylaminoazo-
benzene nitrenium ion, which (presumably) is the reactive species generated from
N-hydroxy-N-methyl-4-aminobenzene by sulfation, is reduced to N-methylaminoazo-
benzene by unreacted N-hydroxy-N-methyl-4-aminoazobenzene, its covalent binding

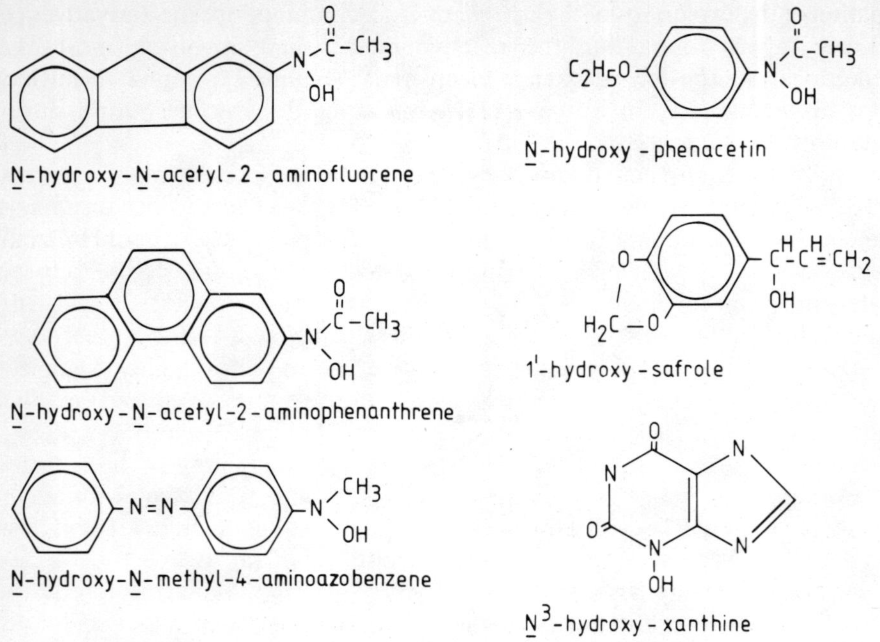

N-hydroxy-N-acetyl-2-aminofluorene

N-hydroxy-phenacetin

N-hydroxy-N-acetyl-2-aminophenanthrene

1'-hydroxy-safrole

N-hydroxy-N-methyl-4-aminoazobenzene

N^3-hydroxy-xanthine

FIGURE 2. Some substrates that generate reactive sulfate esters.

to methionine is prevented.[7] Any effect on this reduction may affect trapping efficiency, and thus produce errors in the determination of sulfation rate. Usually, very impure sulfotransferase preparations such as a 100,000 × g (60 min) postmicrosomal supernatant are used for estimation of the sulfation capacity of a tissue. Obviously, many factors in such a complex mixture of many enzymes and other compounds may interfere with the sulfation assay. Therefore, PAPS-dependent disappearance of substrate seems to be the best estimation of the sulfation capacity of a tissue, provided the PAPS concentration is optimum, and the PAPS–independent disappearance rate is small compared to the PAPS-dependent rate. One has to be aware, however, of the instability of many *N*-hydroxy compounds.[13,14]

II.   *N*-HYDROXY-2-ACETYLAMINOFLUORENE

As mentioned above, the first reactive *N-O*-sulfate ester reported was that of *N*-hydroxy-2AAF, in 1968. Some years before, this hydroxamic acid had been shown to be a necessary intermediary in the generation of ultimate carcinogens from 2AAF. However, it was not an ultimate carcinogen itself (see Reference 15 for a review), whereas its *N-O*-sulfate seemed a promising candidate.

The *N-O*-sulfate conjugate of *N*-hydroxy-2AAF has been synthesized chemically. It is very unstable in aqueous media with a halflife of less than 1 min at pH 7.[1] Moreover, this conjugate bound spontaneously (i.e., not enzyme-catalyzed) to DNA and caused mutations in a bacterial transformation test.[1] The formation of this reactive conjugate by sulfotransferase preparations from rat liver was detected by PAPS-dependent covalent binding of the radiolabeled substrate to RNA and methionine.[3,4] Because of this dependence on sulfation, the conclusion was that the *N-O*-sulfate (which was the only possible product, since no other acceptor groups for sulfate were present in the substrate molecule) generated a reactive species that bound to groups in DNA, RNA, or methionine. The binding to methionine occurred at its sulfur atom, resulting in the formation of the two *ortho*-methylmercapto-2-acetylaminofluorene derivatives (Figure 1). Later it was found that the reactive intermediate involved, most likely, a nitrenium-carbonium ion resonance electrophile (Figure 1), bound to nucleophilic groups in general.[15] Even a dimer of 2-acetylaminofluorene may form during the sulfation of *N*-hydroxy-2AAF in vitro.[16]

The sulfotransferase activity for *N*-hydroxy-2AAF is especially high in the male rat liver, is rather high in male rabbit liver, but much lower in livers from hamsters, guinea pig and mouse. A pronounced sex difference was observed in the liver of Holtzman and Sprague-Dawley rats, male rats having a much higher sulfotransferase activity than females; in Wistar or Fischer rats the difference was much smaller.[4,17-21] Only the liver contains a high sulfotransferase activity towards *N*-hydroxy-2AAF.[22] Notably devoid of this sulfotransferase activity are two tissues that are most highly susceptible to carcinogenesis by 2AAF and *N*-hydroxy-2AAF, the mammary gland and the sebaceous glands associated with the external auditory meatus (Zymbal's gland).[18] Kidney, lung, spleen, muscle, blood, and small intestinal mucosa similarly had almost no sulfotransferase activity for *N*-hydroxy-2AAF.[7,22] Some activity was found in fetal human liver, adrenals, pancreas, and ovary, and in fetal guinea-pig kidney; however, these activities were very low when compared to adult rat liver.[23]

After initial characterization of some properties of this sulfotransferase in rat liver postmicrosomal supernatant by De Baun et al.,[22] it was purified about 2000-fold from male rat-liver cytosol.[24] The activities towards *N*-hydroxy-2AAF and 4-nitrophenol copurified as a homogeneous protein, whereas the steroid sulfotransferase activity was lost. Much less enzyme could be isolated from female rat liver, confirming that the sex difference mentioned above was due to a difference in amount of sulfotransferase enzyme properly. Further details on properties of this enzyme can be found in Chapter 5, Section IX.

The major adducts formed from the reaction of the *N-O*-sulfate ester with DNA, RNA, and protein have been characterized. King and Philips[25] showed that 2′-(3′)-GMP effectively competed with RNA in trapping the reactive intermediate generated from the *N-O*-sulfate conjugate. They analyzed the GMP-adduct and found that the AAF moiety was bound to C_8 of guanosine. The adduct had retained the *N*-acetyl group. When RNA was reacted with the sulfate conjugate of *N*-hydroxy-2AAF (generated *in situ* by the sulfotransferase), an AAF adduct at the C_8 of guanosine was identified after hydrolysis of the RNA. AMP, CMP, and UMP did not compete with RNA for the reactive intermediate, confirming that binding to guanosine was the main adduct-forming reaction.

The adduct to protein was identified by De Baun et al.[22] In alkaline digests of solvent-extracted liver protein from rats given 2AAF or *N*-hydroxy-2AAF, 1- and 3-methylmercapto-2AAF (Figure 1) were found. When the *N-O*-sulfate conjugate was reacted in vitro with methionine, the same products resulted, with about 30% as the 1-isomer and 70% as the 3-isomer. This shows that the main point of attack of the reactive intermediate in proteins is the sulfur atom of methionine.

These data show that the *N-O*-sulfate conjugate has sufficient reactivity to bind covalently to DNA, RNA, and protein in vivo. Indeed, when *N*-hydroxy-2AAF or its precursor 2AAF is injected in vivo, it does become covalently bound to tissue macromolecules. The percentage of the dose that becomes bound will depend on the dose and route of administration. The question then is: what is the role of sulfation in this covalent binding? Several other biotransformation reactions also lead to reactive metabolites of *N*-hydroxy-2AAF that may bind covalently to macromolecules (for a review see Reference 15 and 26). When 2AAF or *N*-hydroxy-2AAF is injected in vivo, the major part of the adducts to DNA are deacetylated, 2AF, adducts, showing that at least two different reactive metabolites react with DNA.[27] It is generally assumed that the formation of certain of these adducts is the cause of the carcinogenicity of *N*-hydroxy-2AAF. The question, therefore, is to what extent each of these metabolites of *N*-hydroxy-2AAF contributes to the covalent binding in vivo and, by implication, is responsible for its carcinogenic effects.

One approach to the evaluation of the role of *N*-*O*-sulfation in the metabolism and carcinogenicity of *N*-hydroxy-2AAF has been an attempt to change sulfate availability in vivo by depleting and supplementing inorganic sulfate. De Baun et al.[28] have tried to deplete the sulfate pool in rats with paracetamol (acetaminophen or 4-hydroxyacetanilide). The high dose they used may indeed have caused a decrease in serum sulfate, but this was not determined. In these presumably sulfate-depleted rats a high intraperitoneal dose of inorganic sulfate (about 5 mmol/kg) caused a consistent increase in radioactively labeled *N*-hydroxy-2AAF covalently bound to protein, RNA or DNA, as compared to controls that received sodium chloride instead of sodium sulfate. Even normally nontoxic doses of *N*-hydroxy-2AAF became very toxic upon sodium sulfate injection, suggesting that the toxicity of *N*-hydroxy-2AAF is increased at high serum sulfate levels, presumably by increased sulfation. These findings were confirmed in another experiment which demonstrated that the LD_{50} of *N*-hydroxy-2AAF was much higher in female than in male Sprague Dawley rats,[21] which correlated with the fact that the sulfotransferase activity towards *N*-hydroxy-2AAF is much higher in males than in females. In Wistar or Fischer rats the sex difference was much smaller, both in LD_{50} and sulfotransferase activity for *N*-hydroxy-2AAF.

De Baun et al.[22] have accumulated much suggestive evidence for a possible correlation between carcinogenicity of *N*-hydroxy-2AAF and its sulfation. They observed some relationship between high sulfotransferase activity and hepato-carcinogenicity of this compound, confirming earlier findings in different species.[4] Various changes in the hormonal status of rats, by castration, injection of steroid sex hormones, hypophysectomy, or thyroidectomy changed sulfotransferase activity towards *N*-hydroxy-2AAF and protein-bound radioactive 2AAF in the liver in parallel, which suggested that covalent binding to protein was a result of sulfation of *N*-hydroxy-2AAF. Moreover, all those ablations that caused a decrease in hepatic tumor induction, also were found to decrease *N*-hydroxy-2AAF sulfotransferase in the liver. Further, sex differences in rats for hepatocarcinogenesis seemed to correlate with sulfotransferase activity.[19] These data, therefore, suggested that sulfation might be the (a?) causative factor in protein-binding of 2AAF and carcinogenicity of this compound in the liver in vivo. However, the kidney had no detectable sulfotransferase activity of *N*-hydroxy-2AAF and yet contained protein-bound 2AAF at about 15 to 25% of the level found in the liver, when *N*-hydroxy-2AAF was administered to rats. Two other organs without measurable sulfotransferase activity, the mammary gland and Zymbal's gland, are main targets for the carcinogenic action of *N*-hydroxy-2AAF.[18] In addition, several other potentially carcinogenic metabolites of *N*-hydroxy-2AAF had been discovered.[2,15,26] Therefore, this correlation of sulfotransferase activity with carcinogenicity does not give an answer to the problem.

The Weisburger group has attempted to get more information about the role of sulfation in carcinogenicity of *N*-hydroxy-2AAF by altering the availability of inorganic sulfate for sulfation.[29-31] The significant finding was that acetanilide inhibited liver tumor formation by *N*-hydroxy-2AAF, and that the addition of inorganic sulfate to the diet restored the hepatocarcinogenic action of *N*-hydroxy-2AAF.[29] Acetanilide is mainly converted in vivo to 4-hydroxyacetanilide (paracetamol) which is subsequently glucuronidated and sulfated. The Weisburgers explained their finding by a decrease of sulfation of *N*-hydroxy-2AAF as the result of either depletion of inorganic sulfate by acetanilide (for sulfation of the product 4-hydroxyacetanilide) or competition of this product with N-hydroxy-2AAF for sulfation. Addition of inorganic sulfate in the diet would either replenish the sulfate pool, or relieve the inhibition by increasing the sulfate concentration, and presumably that of PAPS in the liver.

A problem in the interpretation of this and a later study by the same group[30] is that the rats were not pair-fed; Mohan et al.[31] (from the same group) showed later that there were clear-cut differences in food consumption, and therefore in carcinogen dose, between the variously treated groups. Moreover, a relatively mild decrease of 2AAF-tumor generation in the liver by the product of acetanilide, 4-hydroxyacetanilide, could not be overcome by sulfate in the diet.[30] Therefore, the authors concluded that liver tumor induction was mediated only in part by the sulfate ester, and that other activated esters might also be instrumental in the carcinogenic process. Indeed, Mohan et al.[31] could not find clear indications for inhibition of sulfation in the 4-hydroxyacetanilide-fed rats; however, 4-hydroxyacetanilide induced UDP-glucuronosyltransferase, thus increasing the formation of the presumably much less carcinogenic N-O-glucuronide conjugate of N-hydroxy-2AAF. Further, competition for binding to macromolecules between reactive intermediates from N-hydroxy-2AAF and 4-hydroxyacetanilide might occur[31] which might affect toxicity of N-hydroxy-2AAF. Taken together, these results of the Weisburger group give no clear-cut assessment of the role of sulfation in hepatocarcinogenesis. Moreover, the problem with this type of experiment is that combination of two or more drugs, especially when given orally, provides many levels of interaction and makes analysis of the results very difficult. In addition to the various explanations given by the above authors for their findings, the possibility that feeding inorganic sulfate affects the metabolism of N-hydroxyacetanilide rather than that of N-hydroxy-2AAF should be considered. In that case the inhibitor of the carcinogenic action would be more rapidly eliminated at the higher sulfate levels. Indeed, Galinsky et al.[32] found that at increased serum sulfate levels the elimination rate of 4-hydroxyacetanilide was enhanced. Moreover, the difference in effectivity between acetanilide and 4-hydroxyacetanilide may be related to different pharmacokinetics and elimination rates. All these factors have to be considered in the analysis of the data, and they make it hard to draw any definite conclusion. Finally, the increase in serum sulfate concentration in rats fed a diet containing 0.8% (w/w) sodium sulfate was probably very limited, although it has not been measured in any of the studies so far. Recent work by Tullis et al. showed that the serum sulfate concentration in rats increased only by about 30% under these conditions.[33]

A completely unrelated hypothesis about the effect of sulfate on chemical carcinogenesis has been forwarded by Hadler et al.,[34,35] who showed that 1.5 mM sulfate influences mitochondrial oxidative phosphorylation. They suggest that there is a confluence between oxidative phosphorylation and chemical carcinogenesis; sulfate disturbs oxidative phosphorylation and thereby may, somehow, enhance chemical carcinogenesis.

Since in recent years several other 2AAF metabolites have been implicated in the carcinogenesis by N-hydroxy-2AAF,[15,26] it remains as yet undecided whether sulfation of N-hydroxy-2AAF plays a major or only a minor role in the carcinogenesis by this compound in various organs and species.

Although, as pointed out above, it is difficult to assess the role of sulfation in vivo, isolated hepatocytes offer an alternative preparation in which sulfate levels can be controlled much easier than in vivo. King et al.[36] have measured binding of N-hydroxy-2AAF to RNA and protein in rat hepatocytes as a function of sulfate concentration in the incubation medium. They found that both binding to RNA (five- to tenfold) and protein (threefold) were increased when the sulfate in the incubation medium was increased from 0.00 mM to the normal 0.8 mM. DNA binding was not determined in that study. This shows that a drastic reduction of sulfate certainly will lead to a reduction in covalent binding to RNA and protein. For unknown reasons, other authors[37] were not able to reproduce these findings.

Even though it is very likely that sulfation of N-hydroxy-2AAF takes place in vivo, it is not known what percentage of the dose is being converted to the sulfate conjugate. Most likely, of course, this percentage will vary with the dose and the route of administration. Meerman et al.[38,39] have tried to estimate the quantitative role of sulfation in two ways. First, they have studied the metabolism of N-hydroxy-2AAF after selective inhibition of sulfation by pentachlorophenol or 2,6-dichloro-4-nitro-phenol in vivo. In the second place they have compared the metabolism of N-hydroxy-2AAF in the perfused rat liver with and without sulfate in the perfusion medium. Both the pretreatment with the sulfation inhibitors and the perfusion without sulfate showed a great increase in the N-O-glucuronide conjugate of N-hydroxy-2AAF as compared with controls. Some as yet unidentified water-soluble metabolite of N-hydroxy-2AAF was decreased to the same extent as the glucuronide was increased. These results tentatively suggested that in the rat about 40 to 50% of an i.v. dose of 60 μmol/kg was converted to the N-O-sulfate conjugate. Further, these authors found that the covalent binding of N-hydroxy-2AAF to macromolecules was decreased under conditions where sulfation was decreased. Clearly, however, more work is needed in this area.

Recently the Ames *Salmonella* mutagenesis test system has received much attention because it has some predictive value for the in vivo carcinogenicity of the tested compounds.[40] When N-hydroxy-2AAF is tested in this system, without further additions, it is only very weakly mutagenic. If, however, a postmicrosomal supernatant from rat liver is added, the mutagenic effect increases very greatly, most likely due to deacetylaction and transacetylation reactions. When cofactors for sulfation were subsequently added to this system, they did not cause the expected increase in mutagenicity, but resulted in a marked decrease.[41] One explanation for this is that the N-O-sulfate conjugate of N-hydroxy-2AAF is so extremely reactive that it breaks down too rapidly to allow the reactive nitrenium ion to reach the nucleus and cause a mutation. It may react immediately with nucleophiles outside the microorganisms, in which case the reactive intermediate is detoxified. This mechanism implies that sulfation competes efficiently with the other, activating enzyme systems in the postmicrosomal supernatant. These findings have been extended and studied in greater depth.[12,42-45] There is, of course, no straightforward relationship between chemical carcinogensis and mutagenesis, but these results very forcefully pose the question: is the N-O-sulfate of N-hydroxy-2AAF stable enough to reach the DNA inside the nucleus of the hepatocyte? Weisburger et al.[29] could not find any sulfotransferase activity towards N-hydroxy-2AAF in rat liver nuclei, and therefore the sulfate conjugate of N-hydroxy-2AAF would have to be synthesized in the cytosol and to diffuse into the nucleus before it could bind to DNA. However, recently a relatively low sulfotransferase activity towards N-hydroxy-2AAF in rat liver nuclei was reported;[46] this report requires further confirmation.

In conclusion, the combined results show that N-hydroxy-2AAF may be converted to a reactive N-O-sulfate conjugate in vivo. Several pieces of (circumstantial) evidence implicate this sulfate conjugate in the carcinogenic action of (N-hydroxy)-2AAF. Possibly this is limited to hepatocarcinogenicity: N-hydroxy-3-acetylaminofluorene is not a hepatocarcinogen and is not converted into a reactive intermediate by sulfation,[47] but yet this compound causes cancer in the mammary gland.[47] Thus, the role of sulfation needs to be further clarified since the evidence for its involvement until now seems to be more of a negative quality: if nothing else can be the ultimate carcinogen, it has to be the N-O-sulfate conjugate. An illustration of the problem is that the N-O-sulfate causes no tumors at its site of injection;[48,49] this procedure is often used to detect ultimate carcinogens. A further complication is that prolonged administration of N-hydroxy-2AAF decreases the sulfotransferase activity in the liver considerably.[50]

III. OTHER REACTIVE SULFATE ESTERS

Several other sulfate esters, especially N-O-sulfate esters, are very reactive, and some of them have been implicated in chemical carcinogenesis. An example of the latter group is N-hydroxy-N-methyl-4-aminoazobenzene (N-hydroxy-MAB). This compound is not a hydroxamic acid like N-hydroxy-2AAF, but a substituted hydroxylamine; the latter are in general much less stable in aqueous solution than the hydroxamic acids. Kadlubar et al.[7] provided evidence that sulfation of the very labile N-hydroxy-MAB generated a reactive intermediate that bound covalently to methionine and guanosine. They studied some properties of the sulfation reaction, such as species differences and tissue distribution. Only 5 to 20% of the PAPS-dependent loss of substrate was trapped by methionine as methylmercapto-derivatives, which illustrates the poor efficiency of methionine as trapping agent for the sulfate ester of this compound. Male rat liver had the highest sulfating activity, but several other species also had relatively high activity in the liver. In kidney and intestinal mucosa of the male rat about 20% of the activity in the liver was found. Since no other metabolic reaction seemed to convert N-hydroxy-MAB to a reactive intermediate that bound covalently to DNA (under conditions in which the N-hydroxy-MAB was stabilized by working in an argon atmosphere), the authors suggest that the N-O-sulfate conjugate of this compound is an ultimate carcinogen. This was supported by the findings of Blunck and Crowther[51] that sulfate in the diet of rats fed a MAB-analog (3′-methyl-4-N,N-dimethylaminoazobenzene) strongly enhanced carcinogenicity of this compound. Therefore, the N-O-sulfate of N-hydroxy-MAB was postulated to be an ultimate carcinogen of MAB. Later work with 3′-methyl-4-N,N-dimethylaminoazobenzene in vitro suggested that sulfation was required for binding to RNA, whereas covalent binding to protein did not require prior sulfation.[52] Glutathione and cysteine inhibited this binding to RNA in vitro.

Safrole (Figure 2) is a naturally occurring plant constituent that is hepatotoxic to animals and has a weak hepatocarcinogenic action in rats and mice. Wislocki et al.[10] discovered that a reactive conjugate which bound covalently to RNA resulted from sulfation of the 1′-hydroxy group. Several other metabolites of this compound also yield reactive metabolites, so that it is not known to what extent each of them may contribute to the carcinogenic effect of safrole.[53]

Sulfation of the carcinogen 3-hydroxyxanthine in the presence of methionine leads to the formation of 8-methylmercaptoxanthine (Figure 3);[54] 3-hydroxyguanine showed an analogous reaction. Since 8-methylmercaptoxanthine is one of the metabolites of 3-hydroxyxanthine found in urine,[55] sulfation might play a role in the generation of this compound in vivo and probably of a carcinogenic species from 3-hydroxyxanthine as well. The chemistry of this type of compounds has been extensively studied by the group of Brown (see, e.g., Reference 56), who also synthesized the N-O-sulfate conjugate of 3-hydroxyxanthine.[57] The susceptibility of a series of purine-N-oxide derivatives to a rat liver sulfotransferase preparation has been correlated with the carcinogenic potency of these compounds.[9] The sulfation rate was determined by substrate-induced release of inorganic $^{35}SO_4^{2-}$ from PAPS. There appeared to be no proportionality between both parameters, so that the authors concluded that sulfation might not be involved in

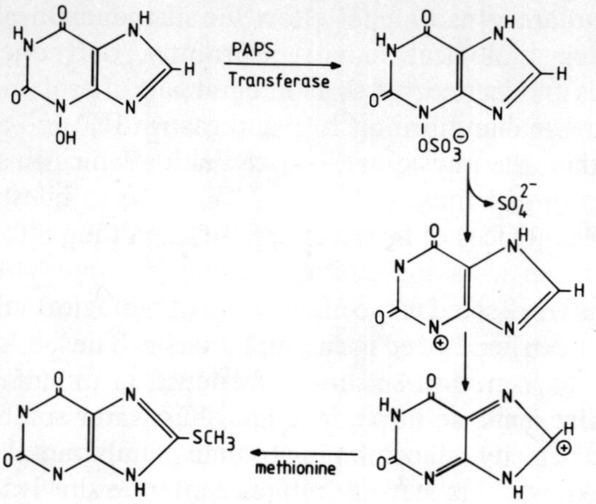

FIGURE 3. Generation of 8-methylmercaptoxanthine by sulfation of N^3-hydroxyxanthine in the presence of methionine.

carcinogensis by all of these compounds, even though many of the sulfate conjugates were reactive (a prerequisite in this assay, of course, because stable sulfate conjugates would not be measured).

N-hydroxy-*N,N'*-diacetylbenzidine has been shown to be an in vitro metabolite of benzidine in several rodent species. It is converted into a reactive metabolite by sulfation in a rat-liver supernatant, but not in hamster liver. With methionine methylmercapto derivatives were formed during sulfation.[58]

Reactive sulfate conjugates of several other *N*-hydroxy compounds were detected by incubating the radiolabeled substrates with a sulfotransferase preparation, and measuring the radioactivity covalently bound to protein, RNA, DNA, or methionine. Thus, Mulder et al.[8,11] found that sulfation of *N*-hydroxyphenacetin led to a sequence of reactions as shown in Figure 4. The proposed reactive imidoquinone bound to protein or glutathione.

N-hydroxy-4-acetylaminobiphenyl forms a reactive conjugate when it is sulfated.[22,36] However, the sulfation reaction seemed to be less important than the deacetylation reaction in covalent binding of *N*-hydroxy-4-acetylaminobiphenyl to protein or RNA in isolated hepatocytes.[36]

The *N-O*-sulfate ester of *N*-hydroxy-2-acetylaminophenanthrene reacted with methionine, adenosine, and guanosine.[6,22] These reactions, and their products, have been identified by Scribner and Naimy.[6] *N*-hydroxy-4-acetylaminostilbene was also mildly reactive, whereas *N*-hydroxy-2-acetylaminonaphthalene was marginally active,[8,22] and *N*-hydroxyacetanilide or *N*-hydroxy-*p*-chloroacetanilide were not at all reactive after sulfation.[8] *N*-hydroxy-4-aminobiphenyl, *N*–hydroxy-2-naphthylamine, *N*-hydroxy-4-aminoazobenzene, and *N*-hydroxy-*N*-ethyl-4-aminoazobenzene bound to methionine in varying amounts after sulfate conjugation.[7,17]

A final example is the generation of an aziridine from a β-amine alcohol, catalyzed by sulfation of the alcoholic-OH group (Figure 5).[59] This might be important because several biogenic amines have a similar structure.

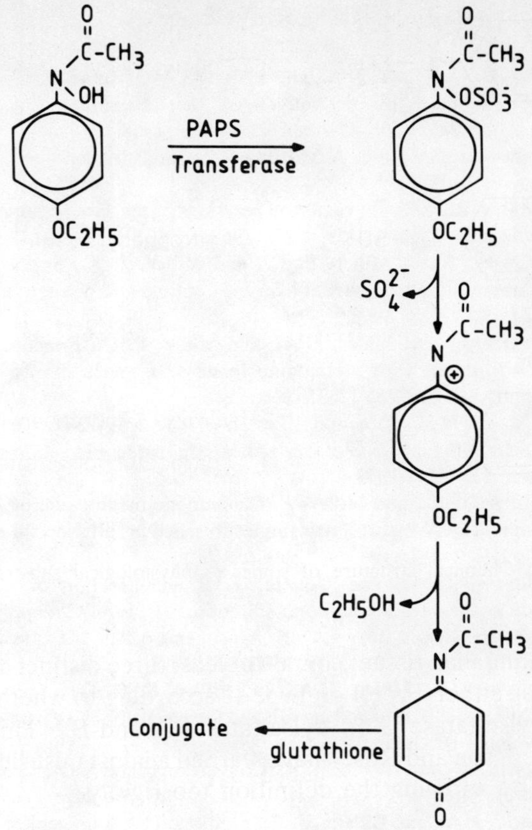

FIGURE 4. Generation of a glutathione conjugate from *N*-hydroxyphenacetin by sulfation in the presence of glutathione.

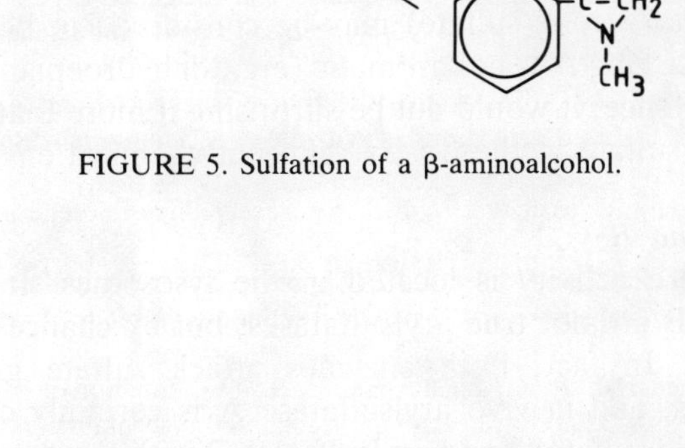

FIGURE 5. Sulfation of a β-aminoalcohol.

REFERENCES

1. **Maher, V. M., Miller, E. C., Miller, J. A., and Szybalski, W.,** Mutations and decreases in density of transforming DNA produced by derivatives of the carcinogen 2-acetylaminofluorene and N-methyl-4-aminoazobenzene, *Mol. Pharmacol.*, 4, 411, 1968.
2. **Irving, C. C.,** Metabolic activation of N-hydroxy compounds by conjugation, *Xenobiotica*, 1, 387, 1971.
3. **King, C. M. and Phillips, B.,** Enzyme-catalyzed reactions of the carcinogen N-hydroxy-2-fluorenylacetamide with nucleic acid, *Science*, 159, 1351, 1968.
4. **De Baun, J. R., Rowley, J. Y., Miller, E. C., and Miller, J. A.,** Sulfotransferase activation of N-hydroxy-2-acetylaminofluorene in rodent livers susceptible and resistent to this carcinogen, *Proc. Soc. Exp. Biol. Med.*, 129, 268, 1968.
5. **Lotlikar, P. D., Scribner, J. D., Miller, J. A., and Miller, E. C.,** Reactions of esters of aromatic N-hydroxyamines and amides with methionine *in vitro:* a model for *in vivo* binding of amine carcinogens to protein, *Life Sci.*, 5, 1263, 1966.
6. **Scribner, J. D. and Naimy, N. K.,** Reactions of esters of N-hydroxy-2-acetylaminophenanthrene with cellular nucleophiles and the formation of free radicals upon decomposition of N-acetoxy-N-arylacetamides, *Cancer Res.*, 33, 1159, 1973.
7. **Kadlubar, F. F., Miller, J. A., and Miller, E. C.,** Hepatic metabolism of N-hydroxy-N-methyl-4-aminoazobenzene and other N-hydroxy arylamines to reactive sulfuric acid esters, *Cancer Res.*, 36, 2350, 1976.
8. **Mulder, G. J., Hinson, J. A., and Gillette, J. R.,** Generation of reactive metabolites of N-hydroxyphenacetin by glucuronidation and sulfation, *Biochem. Pharmacol.*, 26, 189, 1977.
9. **McDonald, J. J., Stöhrer, G., and Brown, G. B.,** Oncogenic purine N-oxide derivatives as substrates for sulfotransferase, *Cancer Res.*, 33, 3319, 1973.
10. **Wislocki, P. G., Borchert, P., Miller, J. A., and Miller, E. C.,** The metabolic activation of the carcinogen 1'-hydroxy safrole *in vivo* and *in vitro* and the electrophilic reactivities of possible ultimate carcinogens, *Cancer Res.*, 36, 1686, 1976.
11. **Mulder, G. J., Hinson, J. A., and Gillette, J. R.,** Conversion of the N-O-glucuronide and N-O-sulfate conjugated of N-hydroxy phenacetin to reactive intermediates, *Biochem. Pharmacol.*, 27, 1641, 1978.
12. **Andrews, L. S., Hinson, J. A., and Gillette, J. R.,** Studies on the mutagenicity of N-hydroxy-2-acetylaminofluorene in the Ames–*Salmonella* mutagenesis test system, *Biochem. Pharmacol.*, 27, 2399, 1978.
13. **Beckett, A. H., Navas, G. E., Hutt, A. J., and Farag, M.,** Disappearing N-hydroxy compounds, *J. Pharm. Pharmacol.*, 31, 476, 1979.
14. **Gorrod, J. W.,** Ed., *The Biological Oxidation of Nitrogen*, Elsevier, Amsterdam, 1978.
15. **Miller, E. C.,** Some current perspectives on chemical carcinogenesis in humans and experimental animals, *Cancer Res.*, 38, 1469, 1978.
16. **Andrews, L. S., Pohl, L. R., Hinson, J. A., Fisk, C. L., and Gillette, J. R.,** Production of a dimer of 2-acetylaminofluorene during the sulfation of N-hydroxy-2-acetylaminofluorene *in vitro*, *Drug Metab. Dispos.*, 7, 296, 1979.
17. **Lotlikar, P. D.,** Effect of sex hormones on enzymatic esterification of 2-(N-hydroxyacetamido) fluorene by rat liver cytosol, *Biochem. J.*, 120, 409, 1970.
18. **Irving, C. C., Janss, D. H., and Russell, L. T.,** Lack of N-hydroxy-2-acetylaminofluorene sulfotransferase activity in the mammary gland and Zymbal's gland of the rat, *Cancer Res.*, 31, 387, 1971.
19. **Gutmann, H. R., Malejka-Giganti, D., Barry, E. J., and Rydell, R. E.,** On the correlation between hepatocarcinogenicity of the carcinogen N-2-fluorenylacetamide and its metabolic activation by the rat, *Cancer Res.*, 32, 1554, 1972.
20. **King, C. M. and Olive, C. W.,** Comparative effects of strain, species and sex on the acyltransferase- and sulfotransferase-catalyzed activations of N-hydroxy-N-2-fluorenylacetamide, *Cancer Res.*, 35, 906, 1975.
21. **Irving, C. C.,** Comparative toxicity of N-hydroxy-2-acetylaminofluorene in several strains of rats, *Cancer Res.*, 35, 2959, 1975.
22. **De Baun, J. R., Miller, E. C., and Miller, J. A.,** N-hydroxy-2-acetylaminofluorene sulfotransferase: its probable role in the carcinogenesis and in protein-(methion-S-yl) binding in rat liver, *Cancer Res.*, 30, 577, 1970.
23. **Namkung, M. J., Zachariah, P. K., and Juchau, M. R.,** O-sulfonation of N-hydroxy-2-fluorenylacetamide and 7-hydroxy-N-2-fluorenylacetamide in fetal and placental tissues of humans and guinea pigs, *Drug Metab. Dispos.*, 5, 288, 1977.

24. **Wu, S. G. and Straub, K. D.**, Purification and characterization of N-hydroxy-2-acetylaminofluorene sulfotransferase from rat liver, *J. Biol. Chem.*, 251, 6529, 1976.
25. **King, C. M. and Phillips, B.**, N-hydroxy-2-fluorenylacetamide. Reaction of the carcinogen with guanosin, ribonucleic acid, deoxyribonucleic acid and protein, following enzymatic deacetylation or esterification, *J. Biol. Chem.*, 244, 6209, 1969.
26. **Clayson, D. B. and Garner, R. C.**, Carcinogenic aromatic amines and related compounds, in *Chemical Carcinogens,* Searle, C. E., Ed., American Chemical Society, Washington D.C., 1976, 366.
27. **Kriek, E.**, Carcinogenesis by aromatic amines, *Biochim. Biophys. Acta,* 355, 177, 1974.
28. **De Baun, J. R., Smith, J. Y. R., Miller, E. C., and Miller, J. A.**, Reactivity *in vivo* of the carcinogen N-hydroxy-2-acetylaminofluorene: increase by sulfate ion, *Science,* 167, 184, 1970.
29. **Weisburger, J. H., Yamamoto, C. S., Williams, G. M., Grantham, P. H., Matsushima, T., and Weisburger, E. K.**, On the sulfate ester of N-hydroxy-N-2-fluorenylacetamide as a key ultimate hepatocarcinogen in the rat, *Cancer Res.,* 32, 491, 1972.
30. **Yamamoto, R. S., Williams, G. M., Richardson, H. L., Weisburger, E. K., and Weisburger, J. H.**, Effect of p-hydroxyacetanilide on liver cancer induction by N-hydroxy-N-2-fluorenylacetamide, *Cancer Res.,* 33, 454, 1973.
31. **Mohan, L. C., Grantham, P. H., Weisburger, E. K., Weisburger, J. H., and Idoine, J. B.**, Mechanisms of the inhibitory action of p-hydroxy-acetanilide on carcinogenesis by N-2-fluorenylacetamide or N-hydroxy-N-2-fluorenyl-acetamide, *J. Nat. Cancer Inst.,* 56, 763, 1976.
32. **Galinsky, R. E., Slattery, J. T., and Levy, G.**, Effect of sodium sulfate on acetaminophen elimination by rats, *J. Pharm. Sci.,* 68, 803, 1979.
33. **Tullis, L.**, Ph.D. thesis, University of Arkansas, Little Rock, 1981.
34. **Hadler, H. I. and Cook, G. L.**, The mitochondrial activation of sulfate and arsenate and their role in carcinogenesis, *J. Environ. Pathol. Toxicol.,* 2, 601, 1979.
35. **Hadler, H. I., Daniel, B. G., and Pratt, R. D.**, The induction of ATP energized mitochondrial volume changes by carcinogenic N-hydroxy-N-acetylaminofluorenes when combined with showdomycin. A unitary hypothesis for carcinogenesis, *J. Antibiot.,* 24, 405, 1971.
36. **King, C. M., Traub, N. R., Cardona, R. A., and Howard, R. B.**, Comparative adduct formation of 4-aminobiphenyl and 2-aminofluorene derivatives with macromolecules of isolated liver parenchymal cells, *Cancer Res.,* 36, 2374, 1976.
37. **Dybing, E., Søderlund, E., Haug, L. T., and Thorgeirsson, S. S.**, Metabolism and activation of 2-acetylaminofluorene in isolated rat hepatocytes, *Cancer Res.,* 39, 3268, 1979.
38. **Meerman, J. H. N., Van Doorn, A. B. D., and Mulder, G. J.**, Effect of pentachlorophenol and 2,6-dichloro-4-nitrophenol on the metabolism of the carcinogen N-hydroxy-2-acetylaminofluorene in the rat, *Proc. 20th Dutch Fed. Meet.,* (Abstr.), Dutch Foundation Fed. Medical Sci. Soc., Nÿmegan, The Netherlands, 1979, 278.
39. **Meerman, J. H. N., Van Doorn, A. B. D., and Mulder, G. J.**, Inhibition of sulfate conjugation of N-hydroxy-2-acetylaminofluorene in the isolated perfused rat liver and in the rat *in vivo* by pentachlorophenol and low-sulfate, *Cancer Res.,* 40, 3772, 1980.
40. **Ames, B. N., Mccann, J., and Yamasahi, E.**, Methods for detecting carcinogens and mutagens with the *Salmonella*/mammalian-microsome mutagenicity test, *Mutat. Res.,* 31, 347, 1975.
41. **Mulder, G. J., Hinson, J. A., Nelson, W. L., and Thorgeirsson, S. S.**, Role of sulfotransferase from rat liver in the mutagenicity of N-hydroxy-2-acetylaminofluorene in *Salmonella typhimurium, Biochem. Pharmacol.,* 26, 1356, 1977.
42. **Sakai, S., Reinhold, C. E., Wirth, P. J., and Thorgeirsson, S. S.**, Mechanism of *in vitro* mutagenic activation and covalent binding of N-hydroxy-2-acetylaminofluorene in isolated cell nuclei from rat and mouse, *Cancer Res.,* 38, 2058, 1978.
43. **Schut, H. A. J. and Thorgeirsson, S. S.**, *In vitro* metabolism and mutagenic activation of 2-acetylaminofluorene by subcellular liver fractions from Cotton Rats, *Cancer Res.,* 38, 2501, 1978.
44. **Andrews, L. S., Fysh, J. M., Hinson, J. A., and Gillette, J. R.**, Ascorbic acid inhibits covalent binding of enzymatically generated 2-acetylaminofluorene-N-sulfate to DNA under conditions in which it increases mutagenesis in *Salmonella* TA-1538, *Life Sci.,* 24, 59, 1979.
45. **Hinson, J. A., Andrews, L. S., Mulder, G. J., and Gillette, J. R.**, Decomposition mechanisms of N-O-glucuronide and N-O-sulfate conjugates of phenacetin and other arylamides, in *Conjugation Reactions in Drug Metabolism,* Aitio, A., Ed., Elsevier, Amsterdam, 1978, 455.
46. **Stöhrer, G., Harmonay, L. A., and Brown, G. B.**, Sulfotransferase in rat liver nuclei, *Proc. 17th Ann. Meet. Am. Soc. Cancer Res.,* 20, (Abstr. 1157), 285, 1979.
47. **Zieve, F. J. and Gutman, H. R.**, Reactivities of the carcinogens N-hydroxy-2-fluorenylacetamide and N-hydroxy-3-fluorenylacetamide with tissue nucleophiles, *Cancer Res.,* 31, 471, 1971.
48. **Miller, J. A. and Miller, E. C.**, The metabolic activation of carcinogenic aromatic amines and amides, *Prog. Exp. Tumor Res.,* 11, 273, 1969.

49. **Bartsch, H., Malaveille, C., Stich, H. F., Miller, E. C., and Miller, J. A.,** Comparative electrophilicity, mutagenicity, DNA repair induction activity, and carcinogenicity of some *N*- and *O*-acyl derivatives of *N*-hydroxy-2-aminofluorene, *Cancer Res.,* 37, 1461, 1977.

50. **Jackson, C. D. and Irving, C. C.,** Sex differences in cell proliferation and *N*-hydroxy-2-acetylamino-fluorene sulfotransferase levels in rat liver during 2-acetylaminofluorene administration, *Cancer Res.,* 32, 1590, 1972.

51. **Blunck, J. M. and Crowther, C. E.,** Enhancement of azo dye carcinogenesis by dietary sodium sulphate, *Eur. J. Cancer,* 11, 23, 1975.

52. **Labuc, G. E. and Blunck, J. M.,** Metabolic activation of the hepatocarcinogen 3′-methyl-4-dimethyl-aminoazobenzene by a rat liver cellfree system, *Biochem. Pharmacol.,* 28, 2367, 1979.

53. **Wislocki, P. G., Miller, E. C., Miller, J. A., McCoy, E. C., and Rosenkranz, H. S.,** Carcinogenic and mutagenic activities of safrole, 1′-hydroxysafrole, and some known or possible metabolites, *Cancer Res.,* 37, 1883, 1977.

54. **Stöhrer, G., Corbin, E., and Brown, G. B.,** Enzymatic activation of the oncogen 3-hydroxyxanthine, *Cancer Res.,* 32, 637, 1972.

55. **Stöhrer, G. and Brown, G. B.,** Oncogenic purine derivatives: evidence for a possible proximate oncogen, *Science,* 167, 1622, 1970.

56. **Lee, T. C., Salemnick, G., and Brown, G. B.,** Reactions of an *N*-hydroxy-quinazoline structurally analogous to oncogenic *N*-hydroxypurines, *J. Org. Chem.,* 38, 3102, 1973.

57. **Stöhrer, G. and Salemnick, G.,** Oxidizing action of purine *N*-oxide esters, *Cancer Res.,* 35, 122, 1975.

58. **Morton, K. C., Beland, F. E., Evans, F. E., Hulse, N. F., and Kadlubar, F. F.,** Metabolic activation of *N*-hydroxy-*N,N*′-diacetylbenzidine by hepatic sulfotransferase, *Cancer Res.,* 40, 751, 1980.

59. **Bicker, U. and Fischer, W.,** Enzymatic aziridine synthesis from β-aminoalcohols—a new example of endogenous carcinogen formation, *Nature,* 249, 344, 1974.

LIST OF ABBREVIATIONS

In addition to the conventional abbreviations (see e.g., *Biochem. J.*, 169, 1, 1978), the following have been used:

APS	adenosine 5′-sulfatophosphate
APSe	adenosine 5′-selenophosphate
GPS	guanosine 5′-sulfatophosphate
IPS	inosine 5′-sulfatophosphate
N-hydroxy AAF	*N*-hydroxy-*N*-acetyl-2-aminofluorene
PAP	adenosine 3′-phosphate 5′-phosphate (adenosine 3′, 5′-bisphosphate)
PAPS	adenosine 3′-phosphate 5′-sulfatophosphate
PCMB	*p*-chloromercuribenzoate
PIPS	inosine 3′-phosphate 5′-sulfatophosphate

INDEX

A

B

Q

R

S